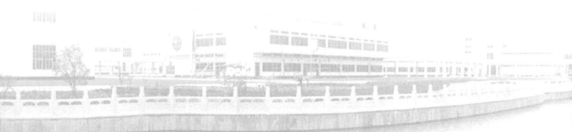

Full View of Yangtze River Pharmaceuticals Group（Taizhou, Jiangsu, China）

扬子江药业集团全景（中国·江苏·泰州）

A Newly Compiled
Practical English-Chinese Library
of Traditional Chinese Medicine
（英汉对照）新编实用中医文库

General Compiler-in-Chief Zuo Yanfu
总主编　左言富

Translators-in-Chief
Zhu Zhongbao Huang Yuezhong Tao Jinwen Li Zhaoguo
总编译　朱忠宝　黄月中　陶锦文　李照国（执行）

Compiled by Nanjing University of
Traditional Chinese Medicine
Translated by Shanghai University
of Traditional Chinese Medicine
南 京 中 医 药 大 学　主 编
上 海 中 医 药 大 学　主 译

SCIENCE OF PRESCRIPTIONS

方 剂 学

Examiner-in-Chief	Li Fei
Compiler-in-Chief	Fan Qiaoling
Translator-in-Chief	Zhu Zhongbao
Vice-Translator-in-Chief	Zhao Junqing
Translator	Zhu Wenxiao

主　审	李　飞
主　编	樊巧玲
主　译	朱忠宝
副 主 译	赵俊卿
译　者	朱文晓

PUBLISHING HOUSE OF SHANGHAI UNIVERSITY
OF TRADITIONAL CHINESE MEDICINE
上海中医药大学出版社

Publishing House of Shanghai University of Traditional Chinese Medicine

530 Lingling Road，Shanghai，200032，China

Science of Prescriptions

Compiler-in-Chief　Fan Qiaoling　Translators-in-Chief　Zhu Zhongbao

(A Newly Compiled Practical English-Chinese Library of Traditional Chinese Medicine

General Compiler-in-Chief　Zuo Yanfu)

ISBN 7 - 81010 - 650 - 3/R • 616　paperback

ISBN 7 - 81010 - 682 - 1/R • 647　hardback

Printed in Shanghai Xinhua printing works

图书在版编目(CIP)数据

方剂学/樊巧玲主编；朱忠宝主译 . —上海：上海中医药大学出版社，2002

(英汉对照新编实用中医文库/左言富总主编)

ISBN 7 - 81010 - 650 - 3

Ⅰ.方...　Ⅱ.①樊...②朱...　Ⅲ.方剂学－英、汉　Ⅳ.R289

中国版本图书馆 CIP 数据核字(2002)第 064850 号

方剂学　　　　　　　　　　主编 樊巧玲　主译 朱忠宝

上海中医药大学出版社出版发行　　　　（零陵路 530 号　邮政编码 200032）
新华书店上海发行所经销　　　　　　　　　上海新华印刷厂印刷
开本　787mm×1092mm　1/18　印张 23.666　字数　千字　印数 1—3 600 册
版次 2002 年 11 月第 1 版　　　　　印次 2002 年 11 月第 1 次印刷

ISBN 7 - 81010 - 650 - 3/R • 616　　　　　定价 48.40 元

Compilation Board of the Library

《(英汉对照)新编实用中医文库》编纂委员会

《（英汉对照）新编实用中医文库》编译委员会

顾　　　问　邵循道　欧　明

总　编　译　朱忠宝　黄月中　陶锦文

执行总编译　李照国

副总编译　（按姓氏笔画为序）

寻建英　李永安　张庆荣　张登峰　杨洪英　黄国琪　谢金华

编　译　者　（按姓氏笔画为序）

于　新　王瑞辉　田开宇　申　光　兰凤利　成培莉　朱文晓
朱玉琴　朱金江　朱桂香　乐毅敏　刘升鹏　李经蕴　杨　莹
杨明山　何迎春　张　杰　张海峡　张　维　陈仁英　周永明
周素贞　屈榆生　赵俊卿　荆　蓁　胡克武　徐启龙　徐　瑶
郭小民　黄熙璇　曹丽娟　康　勤　董　晶　覃百长　曾海苹
楼建华　赖月珍　鲍　白　裴慧华　薛俊梅　戴文军　魏　敏

编译委员会办公室

主　任　杨明山

秘　书　徐林娣　陈　力

Approval Committee of the Library

Director   Li Zhenji

Vice-Directors   Shen Zhixiang   Chen Xiaogu   Zhou Zhongying   Wang Canhui   Gan Zuwang   Jiang Yuren

Members (Listed in the order of the number of strokes in the Chinese names)

Ding Renqiang	Ding Xiaohong	Wang Xinhua	You Benlin
Shi Yanhua	Qiao Wenlei	Yi Sumei	Li Fei
Li Guoding	Yang Zhaomin	Lu Mianmian	Chen Songyu
Shao Mingxi	Shi Bingbing	Yao Xin	Xia Guicheng
Gu Yuehua	Xu Fusong	Gao Yuanhang	Zhu Fangshou
Tao Jinwen	Huang Yage	Fu Zhiwen	Cai Li

General Compiler-in-Chief   Zuo Yanfu

Executive Vice-General-Compilers-in-Chief   Ma Jian   Du Wendong

Vice-General-Compilers-in-Chief   (Listed in the order of the number of strokes in the Chinese names)

Ding Shuhua	Wang Xudong	Wang Lufen	Yan Daonan
Wu Changguo	Wang Shouchuan	Wang Yue	Chen Yonghui
Jin Hongzhu	Zhao Jingsheng	Tang Decai	Tan Yong
Huang Guicheng	Zhai Yachun	Fan Qiaoling	

Office of the Compilation Board Committee

Directors   Ma Jian   Du Wendong

Vice-Directors   Wu Jianlong   Zhu Changren

Publisher   Zhu Bangxian

Chinese Editors   (Listed in the order of the number of strokes in the Chinese names)

Ma Shengying	Wang Lingli	Wang Deliang	He Qianqian
Shen Chunhui	Zhang Xingjie	Zhou Dunhua	Shan Baozhi
Jiang Shuiyin	Qin Baoping	Qian Jingzhuang	Fan Yuqi
Pan Zhaoxi			

English Editors   Shan Baozhi   Jiang Shuiyin   Xiao Yuanchun

Cover Designer   Wang Lei

Layout Designer   Xu Guomin

Foreword Ⅰ

As we are walking into the 21st century, "health for all" is still an important task for the World Health Organization (WHO) to accomplish in the new century. The realization of "health for all" requires mutual cooperation and concerted efforts of various medical sciences, including traditional medicine. WHO has increasingly emphasized the development of traditional medicine and has made fruitful efforts to promote its development. Currently the spectrum of diseases is changing and an increasing number of diseases are difficult to cure. The side effects of chemical drugs have become more and more evident. Furthermore, both the governments and peoples in all countries are faced with the problem of high cost of medical treatment. Traditional Chinese medicine (TCM), the complete system of traditional medicine in the world with unique theory and excellent clinical curative effects, basically meets the need to solve such problems. Therefore, bringing TCM into full play in medical treatment and healthcare will certainly become one of the hot points in the world medical business in the 21st century.

Various aspects of work need to be done to promote the course of the internationalization of TCM, especially the compilation of works and textbooks suitable for international readers. The impending new century has witnessed the compilation of such a

序　一

人类即将迈入 21 世纪,"人人享有卫生保健"仍然是新世纪世界卫生工作面临的重要任务。实现"人人享有卫生保健"的宏伟目标,需要包括传统医药学在内的多种医学学科的相互协作与共同努力。世界卫生组织越来越重视传统医药学的发展,并为推动其发展做出了卓有成效的工作。目前,疾病谱正在发生变化,难治疾病不断增多,化学药品的毒副作用日益显现,日趋沉重的医疗费用困扰着各国政府和民众。中医药学是世界传统医学体系中最完整的传统医学,其独到的学科理论和突出的临床疗效,较符合当代社会和人们解决上述难题的需要。因此,科学有效地发挥中医药学的医疗保健作用,必将成为 21 世纪世界卫生工作的特点之一。

加快中医药走向世界的步伐,还有很多的工作要做,特别是适合国外读者学习的中医药著作、教材的编写是极其重要的方面。在新千年来临之际,由南京中医药大学

series of books known as *A Newly Compiled Practical English-Chinese Library of Traditional Chinese Medicine* published by the Publishing House of Shanghai University of TCM, compiled by Nanjing University of TCM and translated by Shanghai University of TCM. Professor Zuo Yanfu, the general compiler-in-chief of this Library, is a person who sets his mind on the international dissemination of TCM. He has compiled *General Survey on TCM Abroad*, a monograph on the development and state of TCM abroad. This Library is another important works written by the experts organized by him with the support of Nanjing University of TCM and Shanghai University of TCM. The compilation of this Library is done with consummate ingenuity and according to the development of TCM abroad. The compilers, based on the premise of preserving the genuineness and gist of TCM, have tried to make the contents concise, practical and easy to understand, making great efforts to introduce the abstruse ideas of TCM in a scientific and simple way as well as expounding the prevention and treatment of diseases which are commonly encountered abroad and can be effectively treated by TCM.

This Library encompasses a systematic summarization of the teaching experience accumulated in Nanjing University of TCM and Shanghai University of TCM that run the collaborating centers of traditional medicine and the international training centers on acupuncture and moxibustion set by WHO. I am sure that the publication of this Library will further promote the development of traditional Chinese med-

主编、上海中医药大学主译、上海中医药大学出版社出版的《(英汉对照)新编实用中医文库》的即将问世,正是新世纪中医药国际传播更快发展的预示。本套文库总主编左言富教授是中医药学国际传播事业的有心人,曾主编研究国外中医药发展状况的专著《国外中医药概览》。本套文库的编撰,是他在南京中医药大学和上海中医药大学支持下,组织许多著名专家共同完成的又一重要专著。本套文库的作者们深谙国外的中医药发展现状,编写颇具匠心,在注重真实,不失精华的前提下,突出内容的简明、实用,易于掌握,力求科学而又通俗地介绍中医药学的深奥内容,重点阐述国外常见而中医药颇具疗效的疾病的防治。

本套文库蕴含了南京中医药大学和上海中医药大学作为 WHO 传统医学合作中心、国际针灸培训中心多年留学生教学的实践经验和系统总结,更为全面、系统、准确地向世界传播中医药学。相信本书的出版将对中医更好地走向世界,让世界更好地了解中医产生更

icine abroad and enable the whole world to have a better understanding of traditional Chinese medicine.

为积极的影响。

Professor Zhu Qingsheng

Vice-Minister of Health Ministry of the People's Republic of China

Director of the State Administrative Bureau of TCM

December 14, 2000 Beijing

朱庆生教授

中华人民共和国卫生部副部长

国家中医药管理局局长

2000 年 12 月 14 日于北京

Foreword II

Before the existence of the modern medicine, human beings depended solely on herbal medicines and other therapeutic methods to treat diseases and preserve health. Such a practice gave rise to the establishment of various kinds of traditional medicine with unique theory and practice, such as traditional Chinese medicine, Indian medicine and Arabian medicine, etc. Among these traditional systems of medicine, traditional Chinese medicine is a most extraordinary one based on which traditional Korean medicine and Japanese medicine have evolved.

Even in the 21st century, traditional medicine is still of great vitality. In spite of the fast development of modern medicine, traditional medicine is still disseminated far and wide. In many developing countries, most of the people in the rural areas still depend on traditional medicine and traditional medical practitioners to meet the need for primary healthcare. Even in the countries with advanced modern medicine, more and more people have begun to accept traditional medicine and other therapeutic methods, such as homeopathy, osteopathy and naturopathy, etc.

With the change of the economy, culture and living style in various regions as well as the aging in the world population, the disease spectrum has changed. And such a change has paved the way for the new application of traditional medicine. Besides,

序 二

在现代医学形成之前,人类一直依赖草药和其他一些疗法治病强身,从而发展出许多有理论、有实践的传统医学,例如中医学、印度医学、阿拉伯医学等。中医学是世界林林总总的传统医学中的一支奇葩,在它的基础上还衍生出朝鲜传统医学和日本汉方医学。在跨入 21 世纪的今天,古老的传统医学依然焕发着活力,非但没有因现代医学的发展而式微,其影响还有增无减,人们对传统医学的价值也有了更深刻的体会和认识。在许多贫穷国家,大多数农村人口仍然依赖传统医学疗法和传统医务工作者来满足他们对初级卫生保健的需求。在现代医学占主导地位的许多国家,传统医学及其他一些"另类疗法",诸如顺势疗法、整骨疗法、自然疗法等,也越来越被人们所接受。

伴随着世界各地经济、文化和生活的变革以及世界人口的老龄化,世界疾病谱也发生了变化。传统医学有了新的应用,而新疾病所引起的新需求以及现代医学的成

the new requirements initiated by the new diseases and the achievements and limitations of modern medicine have also created challenges for traditional medicine.

WHO sensed the importance of traditional medicine to human health early in the 1970s and have made great efforts to develop traditional medicine. At the 29th world health congress held in 1976, the item of traditional medicine was adopted in the working plan of WHO. In the following world health congresses, a series of resolutions were passed to demand the member countries to develop, utilize and study traditional medicine according to their specific conditions so as to reduce medical expenses for the realization of "health for all".

WHO has laid great stress on the scientific content, safe and effective application of traditional medicine. It has published and distributed a series of booklets on the scientific, safe and effective use of herbs and acupuncture and moxibustion. It has also made great contributions to the international standardization of traditional medical terms. The safe and effective application of traditional medicine has much to do with the skills of traditional medical practitioners. That is why WHO has made great efforts to train them. WHO has run 27 collaborating centers in the world which have made great contributions to the training of acupuncturists and traditional medical practitioners. Nanjing University of TCM and Shanghai University of TCM run the collaborating centers with WHO. In recent years it has, with the cooperation of WHO and other countries, trained about ten thousand international students from over

就与局限又向传统医学提出了挑战，推动它进一步发展。世界卫生组织早在 20 世纪 70 年代就意识到传统医学对人类健康的重要性，并为推动传统医学的发展做了努力。1976 年举行的第二十九届世界卫生大会将传统医学项目纳入世界卫生组织的工作计划。其后的各届世界卫生大会又通过了一系列决议，要求各成员国根据本国的条件发展、使用和研究传统医学，以降低医疗费用，促进"人人享有初级卫生保健"这一目标的实现。

世界卫生组织历来重视传统医学的科学、安全和有效使用。它出版和发行了一系列有关科学、安全、有效使用草药和针灸的技术指南，并在专用术语的标准化方面做了许多工作。传统医学的使用是否做到安全和有效，是与使用传统疗法的医务工作者的水平密不可分的。因此，世界卫生组织也十分重视传统医学培训工作。它在全世界有 27 个传统医学合作中心，这些中心对培训合格的针灸师及使用传统疗法的其他医务工作者做出了积极的贡献。南京中医药大学、上海中医药大学是世界卫生组织传统医学合作中心之一，近年来与世界卫生组织和其他国家合作，培训了近万名来自 90 多个国

90 countries.

In order to further promote the dissemination of traditional Chinese medicine in the world, *A Newly Compiled Practical English-Chinese Library of Traditional Chinese Medicine*, compiled by Nanjing University of TCM with Professor Zuo Yanfu as the general compiler-in-chief and published by the Publishing House of Shanghai University of TCM, aims at systematic, accurate and concise expounding of traditional Chinese medical theory and introducing clinical therapeutic methods of traditional medicine according to modern medical nomenclature of diseases. Undoubtedly, this series of books will be the practical textbooks for the beginners with certain English level and the international enthusiasts with certain level of Chinese to study traditional Chinese medicine. Besides, this series of books can also serve as reference books for WHO to internationally standardize the nomenclature of acupuncture and moxibustion.

The scientific, safe and effective use of traditional medicine will certainly further promote the development of traditional medicine and traditional medicine will undoubtedly make more and more contributions to human health in the 21st century.

Zhang Xiaorui

WHO Coordination Officer

December, 2000

家和地区的留学生。

在南京中医药大学左言富教授主持下编纂的、由上海中医药大学出版社出版的《(英汉对照)新编实用中医文库》,旨在全面、系统、准确、简要地阐述中医基础理论,并结合西医病名介绍中医临床治疗方法。因此,这套文库可望成为具有一定英语水平的初学中医者和具有一定中文水平的外国中医爱好者学习基础中医学的系列教材。这套文库也可供世界卫生组织在编写国际针灸标准术语时参考。

传统医学的科学、安全、有效使用必将进一步推动传统医学的发展。传统医学一定会在 21 世纪为人类健康做出更大的贡献。

张小瑞

世界卫生组织传统医学协调官员

2000 年 12 月

Preface

The Publishing House of Shanghai University of TCM published *A Practical English-Chinese Library of Traditional Chinese Medicine* in 1990. The Library has been well-known in the world ever since and has made great contributions to the dissemination of traditional Chinese medicine in the world. In view of the fact that 10 years has passed since its publication and that there are certain errors in the explanation of traditional Chinese medicine in the Library, the Publishing House has invited Nanjing University of TCM and Shanghai University of TCM to organize experts to recompile and translate the Library.

Nanjing University of TCM and Shanghai University of TCM are well-known for their advantages in higher education of traditional Chinese medicine and compilation of traditional Chinese medical textbooks. The compilation of *A Newly Compiled Practical English-Chinese Library of Traditional Chinese Medicine* has absorbed the rich experience accumulated by Nanjing University of Traditional Chinese Medicine in training international students of traditional Chinese medicine. Compared with the previous Library, the Newly Compiled Library has made great improvements in many aspects, fully demonstrating the academic system of traditional Chinese medicine. The whole series of books has systematically introduced the basic theory and thera-

前　言

上海中医药大学出版社于1990年出版了一套《（英汉对照）实用中医文库》，发行10年来，在海内外产生了较大影响，对推动中医学走向世界起了积极作用。考虑到该套丛书发行已久，对中医学术体系的介绍还有一些欠妥之处，因此，上海中医药大学出版社特邀南京中医药大学主编、上海中医药大学主译，组织全国有关专家编译出版《（英汉对照）新编实用中医文库》。

《（英汉对照）新编实用中医文库》的编纂，充分发挥了南京中医药大学和上海中医药大学在高等中医药教育教学和教材编写方面的优势，吸收了作为WHO传统医学合作中心之一的两校，多年来从事中医药学国际培训和留学生学历教育的经验，对原《（英汉对照）实用中医文库》整体结构作了大幅度调整，以突出中医学术主体内容。全套丛书系统介绍了中医基础理论和中医辨证论治方法，讲解了中药学和方剂学的基本理论，详细介绍了236味中药、152首常用方剂和100种常用中成药；详述

peutic methods based on syndrome differentiation, expounding traditional Chinese pharmacy and prescriptions; explaining 236 herbs, 152 prescriptions and 100 commonly-used patent drugs; elucidating 264 methods for differentiating syndromes and treating commonly-encountered and frequently-encountered diseases in internal medicine, surgery, gynecology, pediatrics, traumatology and orthopedics, ophthalmology and otorhinolaryngology; introducing the basic methods and theory of acupuncture and moxibustion, massage (tuina), life cultivation and rehabilitation, including 70 kinds of diseases suitable for acupuncture and moxibustion, 38 kinds of diseases for massage, examples of life cultivation and over 20 kinds of commonly encountered diseases treated by rehabilitation therapies in traditional Chinese medicine. For better understanding of traditional Chinese medicine, the books are neatly illustrated. There are 296 line graphs and 30 colored pictures in the Library with necessary indexes, making it more comprehensive, accurate and systematic in disseminating traditional Chinese medicine in the countries and regions where English is the official language.

This Library is characterized by following features:

1. Scientific　Based on the development of TCM in education and research in the past 10 years, efforts have been made in the compilation to highlight the gist of TCM through accurate theoretical exposition and clinical practice, aiming at introducing authentic theory and practice to the world.

2. Systematic　This Library contains 14 sepa-

264 种临床内、外、妇、儿、骨伤、眼、耳鼻喉各科常见病与多发病的中医辨证论治方法；系统论述针灸、推拿、中医养生康复的基本理论和基本技能，介绍针灸治疗病种 70 种、推拿治疗病种 38 种、各类养生实例及 20 余种常见病证的中医康复实例。为了更加直观地介绍中医药学术，全书选用线图 296 幅、彩图 30 幅，并附有必要的索引，从而更加全面、系统、准确地向使用英语的国家和地区传播中医学术，推进中医学走向世界，造福全人类。

　　本丛书主要具有以下特色：(1) 科学性：在充分吸收近 10 余年来中医教学和科学研究最新进展的基础上，坚持突出中医学术精华，理论阐述准确，临床切合实用，向世界各国介绍“原汁原味”的中医药学术；(2) 系统性：本套丛书包括《中医基础理论》、《中医诊断学》、《中药学》、《方剂学》、《中医内

rate fascicles, i. e. *Basic Theory of Traditional Chinese Medicine*, *Diagnostics of Traditional Chinese Medicine*, *Science of Chinese Materia Medica*, *Science of Prescriptions*, *Internal Medicine of Traditional Chinese Medicine*, *Surgery of Traditional Chinese Medicine*, *Gynecology of Traditional Chinese Medicine*, *Pediatrics of Traditional Chinese Medicine*, *Traumatology and Orthopedics of Traditional Chinese Medicine*, *Ophthalmology of Traditional Chinese Medicine*, *Otorhinolaryngology of Traditional Chinese Medicine*, *Chinese Acupuncture and Moxibustion*, *Chinese Tuina (Massage)*, *and Life Cultivation and Rehabilitation of Traditional Chinese Medicine*.

3. Practical Compared with the previous Library, the Newly Compiled Library has made great improvements and supplements, systematically introducing therapeutic methods for treating over 200 kinds of commonly and frequently encountered diseases, focusing on training basic clinical skills in acupuncture and moxibustion, tuina therapy, life cultivation and rehabilitation with clinical case reports.

4. Standard This Library is reasonable in structure, distinct in categorization, standard in terminology and accurate in translation with full consideration of habitual expressions used in countries and regions with English language as the mother tongue.

This series of books is not only practical for the beginners with certain competence of English to study TCM, but also can serve as authentic textbooks for international students in universities and colleges of TCM in China to study and practice TCM. For those from TCM field who are going to go

科学》、《中医外科学》、《中医妇科学》、《中医儿科学》、《中医骨伤科学》、《中医眼科学》、《中医耳鼻喉科学》、《中国针灸》、《中国推拿》、《中医养生康复学》14 个分册,系统反映了中医各学科建设与发展的最新成果;(3) 实用性:临床各科由原来的上下两册,根据学科的发展进行大幅度的调整和增补,比较详细地介绍了 200 多种各科常见病、多发病的中医治疗方法,重点突出了针灸、推拿、养生康复等临床基本技能训练,并附有部分临证实例;(4) 规范性:全书结构合理,层次清晰,对中医各学科名词术语表述规范,对中医英语翻译执行了更为严格的标准化方案,同时又充分考虑到使用英语国家和地区人们的语言习惯和表达方式。

本丛书不仅能满足具有一定英语水平的初学中医者系统学习中医之用,而且也为中医院校外国留学生教育及国内外开展中医双语教学提供了目前最具权威的系列教材,同时也是中医出国人员进

abroad to do academic exchange, this series of books will provide them with unexpected convenience.

Professor Xiang Ping, President of Nanjing University of TCM, is the director of the Compilation Board. Professor Zuo Yanfu from Nanjing University of TCM, General Compiler-in-Chief, is in charge of the compilation. Zhang Wenkang, Minister of Health Ministry, is invited to be the honorary director of the Editorial Board. Li Zhenji, Vice-Director of the State Administrative Bureau of TCM, is invited to be the director of the Approval Committee. Chen Keji, academician of China Academy, is invited to be the General Advisor. International advisors invited are Mr. M. S. Khan, Chairman of Ireland Acupuncture and Moxibustion Fund; Miss Alessandra Gulí, Chairman of "Nanjing Association" in Rome, Italy; Doctor Secondo Scarsella, Chief Editor of YI DAO ZA ZHI; President Raymond K. Carroll from Australian Oriental Touching Therapy College; Ms. Shulan Tang, Academic Executive of ATCM in Britain; Mr. Glovanni Maciocia from Britain; Mr. David, Chairman of American Association of TCM; Mr. Tzu Kuo Shih, director of Chinese Medical Technique Center in Connecticut, America; Mr. Helmut Ziegler, director of TCM Center in Germany; and Mr. Isigami Hiroshi from Japan. Chen Ken, official of WHO responsible for the Western Pacific Region, has greatly encouraged the compilers in compiling this series of books. After the accomplishment of the compilation, Professor Zhu Qingsheng, Vice-Minister of Health Ministry and Director of the State Administrative Bureau of TCM, has set a high value on the books in his fore-

行中医药国际交流的重要工具书。

全书由南京中医药大学校长项平教授担任编委会主任、左言富教授任总主编，主持全书的编写。中华人民共和国卫生部张文康部长担任本丛书编委会名誉主任，国家中医药管理局李振吉副局长担任审定委员会主任，陈可冀院士欣然担任本丛书总顾问指导全书的编纂。爱尔兰针灸基金会主席萨利姆先生、意大利罗马"南京协会"主席亚历山大·古丽女士、意大利《医道》杂志主编卡塞拉·塞肯多博士、澳大利亚东方触觉疗法学院雷蒙特·凯·卡罗院长、英国中医药学会学术部长汤淑兰女士、英国马万里先生、美国中医师公会主席大卫先生、美国康州中华医疗技术中心主任施祖谷先生、德国中医中心主任赫尔木特先生、日本石上博先生担任本丛书特邀外籍顾问。世界卫生组织西太平洋地区官员陈恳先生对本丛书的编写给予了热情鼓励。全书完成后，卫生部副部长兼国家中医药管理局局长朱庆生教授给予了高度评价，并欣然为本书作序；WHO 传统医学协调官员张小瑞对于本丛书的编写给予高度关注，百忙中也专为本书作序。我国驻外教育机构，特别是中国驻英国曼彻斯特领事张益群先生、中国驻美国休斯敦领事严美华

word for the Library. Zhang Xiaorui，an official from WHO's Traditional Medicine Program，has paid great attention to the compilation and written a foreword for the Library. The officials from the educational organizations of China in other countries have provided us with some useful materials in our compilation. They are Mr. Zhang Yiqun, China Consul to Manchester in Britain；Miss Yan Meihua, Consul to Houston in America；Mr. Wang Jiping, First Secretary in the Educational Department in the Embassy of China to France；and Mr. Gu Shengying，the Second Secretary in the Educational Department in the Embassy of China to Germany. We are grateful to them all.

The Compilers
December，2000

女士、中国驻法国使馆教育处一秘王季平先生、中国驻德国使馆教育处二秘郭胜英先生在与我们工作联系中，间接提供了不少有益资料。在此一并致以衷心感谢！

编　者
2000 年 12 月

Note for Compilation

This book aims to introduce systematically the basic knowledge of Science of prescriptions so that those who are studying Traditional Chinese Medicine home and abroad can have a general idea of the essential formulating principles and specific application of the prescriptions as well as the typical prescriptions commonly used in clinic. It is meant to lay a foundation for further using syndrome differentiation and treatment in accordance with the TCM theories.

It is divided into General Introduction, Specific Discussions and Appendix. Basic theories of science of prescriptions are presented in the General Introduction, while Specific discussions mainly focuses on the source, ingredients, directions, actions, clinical application, elucidation, cautions of 152 typical prescriptions commonly used in clinical practice under 16 categories. Listed under the item of Source is the name of works wherein a certain recipe was earliest recorded. Ingredients and Directions are based primarily on the original works, with dosages converted into the metric system accordingly, and including only the preparation of drugs commonly used in clinic. Since there is only a brief account of the preparation of some pill and powder prescriptions, readers who want to know the details about it may refer to the *Pharmacopoeia of the People's Republic of China*. The powder can be prepared into decoction, which is not indicated again. In the Clinical Application, syndromes and the chief symptoms are listed first,

编写说明

本书旨在系统介绍中医方剂学基本知识，使众多海内外学习中医的人士借此了解方剂组成的基本原理、使用方法和临床常用代表方，为进一步运用中医药理论进行辨证论治奠定基础。

全书分为总论、各论与附录三部分。总论介绍了方剂学的基本理论。各论根据功用将 152 首临床常用代表方剂分为 16 类，重点介绍其方源、组成、用法、功用、临床应用、方解、注意事项等内容。每首正方的"方源"注明最早记载该方的著作。"组成"及"用法"基本参照原书，用药剂量按照原书折算为公制，药物的炮制只收录目前临床常用者；部分丸、散剂的制法书中叙述较简，欲知其详者，可参阅《中华人民共和国药典》；散剂可作汤剂服用，文中不再注明。"临床应用"首列适应证候及其主要症状，次叙目前临床常用该方治疗的疾病，如为汤剂再简述其常用加减方法，以便学者进一步理解方剂的应用变化。"方解"先扼要概括主治证候的病机要点，再重点阐述药

followed with names of diseases treated clinically. In the case of decoction, its modification is briefed so as to enable the learners to have a further understanding of the application and variation of the recipe. After summarizing the main points of pathogenesis the meaning and feature of the compatibility among drugs are dwelt on in Elucidation. The item of Cautions is omitted when it is consistent with what is related in the summary of each chapter or if no special problems should be noted. Thus readers may make cross-references sometimes. One hundred kinds of Chinese patent medicines commonly-used are introduced in the Appendix in the form of chart including their ingredients, actions, indications, directions and dosages, and specifications. The dosages listed in the book are for the adult use, if not specially noted. Therefore, they should be reduced appropriately in the case of children. For the convenience of retrieval, a Chinese stroke index is attached at the end of the book, which covers all the prescriptions mentioned in this book.

This book is distinct in its focal points and terse in its writing, elucidating the profound in simple language. Thus, it can be adopted as a rudimentary course for the beginners and provide references for the physicians as well in their selection of prescriptions and drugs in practice.

Compilers
December, 2000

物的配伍意义与配伍特点。"注意事项"与每章概述所论相同者不复赘述,读者应前后互参,如无特殊需要注意的问题则此项略之。附录中以列表的形式介绍了 100 种临床常用中成药的组成、功用、主治、用法用量及其规格。书中方剂剂量如未特别注明者均为成人用量,小儿用时酌减。最后附有本书涉及到的所有方剂的中文笔画索引,以便检索。

全书重点突出,文字精炼,深入浅出,既可作为初学者入门学习之用,又可为临床中医师选方用药提供参考。

编　者
2000 年 12 月

CONTENTS

目 录

1 General Introduction 总　论

1.1 Introduction 第一章　导言

Science of Prescriptions is a subject dealing with treatment and the theories of compatibility of prescriptions as well as the clinical application. In TCM, it is one of the important basic courses and has a close relationship with all other clinical branches, linking up the basic theories with clinical practices.

A prescription is composed of selected drugs and suitable doses based on syndrome differentiation for etiology and the composition of therapies in accordance with the principle of formulating a prescription. It serves as a chief means of treating diseases clinically.

The formation of prescriptions has undergone a considerably long history. As early as in the Chinese primitive society, our ancestors discovered, while going in search of food, drugs and used them for curative purposes. Initially they only used a single drug in a dose. But through long clinical practice, they recognized that a recipe composed of two or more drugs proved more advantageous for treatment of diseases, and various prescriptions were gradually formed. *Wushi'er Bingfang* (*The Prescriptions for Fifty-two Kinds of Diseases*) is the oldest extant medical formulary with a collection of over 280 prescriptions, most of which consist of less ingredients, rough dosages, simple forms of preparations and unnamed prescriptions, all reflecting the simplicity of early prescriptions. *Huangdi Neijing* (*Huangdi's Classic on Medicine*) written in the Spring and Autumn Period and the Warring

方剂学是研究治法与方剂配伍理论及其临床运用的一门学科,在中医专业中,既是一门重要的基础课,又与临床各科紧密相连,起着沟通基础与临床的桥梁作用。

方剂是由药物组成的,是在辨证审因、确定治法之后,选择适宜的药物,酌定用量,按照组方原则配伍而成,是中医临床治疗疾病的主要工具。

方剂的起源历史悠久。早在中国的原始社会时期,先人们在寻找食物的过程中就发现了药物的作用,并用以治疗疾病。最初只是使用单味药,经过长期实践,认识到运用数味中药组成复方治病具有更多的优越性,于是逐渐形成了方剂。在现存医学典籍中,《五十二病方》是最古老的一部方书。该书收录医方280余首,多数方剂组成药物较少,用量粗略,剂型简单,且没有方名,反映了早期方剂的古朴特征。成书于春秋战国时代的《黄帝内经》虽然仅载方

States Period, though recording only 13 prescriptions with simple ingredients, includes such dosage forms as decoction, pill, powder, ointment, pellet and medicinal liquor. Besides it summed up the theories of therapeutic principles based on syndrome differentiation, therapeutic methods, principles of formulating prescriptions as well as the incompatibility of drugs, laying a preliminary theoretical foundation for the formation and development of the science of prescriptions. The book *Shanghan Zabing Lun* (*Treatise on Febrile and Miscellaneous Diseases*), complied by Zhang Zhongjing in the Eastern Han Dynasty, creatively merged the theories, methods, prescriptions and drugs into a single whole and is thus honored as "the forerunner of prescription books" by the later generations. The book recorded 314 prescriptions with a rigorous compatibility, precise selection of drugs and remarkable therapeutic effect. It has a far-reaching influence upon the development of this science and it is known as a "classic on prescriptions".

　　Along with the increasing accumulation of the clinical experiences in using prescriptions, the number of prescriptions also appeared one after another, and prescription books were published in almost each dynasty, in which all previous prescriptions were synthesized and brought to their highest development. For example, *Beiji Qianjin Yaofang* (*Valuable Prescriptions for Emergencies*) and *Qianjin Yifang* (*Supplement to Valuable Prescriptions*) complied by Sun Simiao and *Waitai Miyao* (*The Medical Secrets of An Official*) by Wang Tao in the Tang Dynasty, *Taiping Shenghui Fang* (*the Peaceful Holy Benevolent Prescriptions*) by Wang Huaiyin and *Shengji Zonglu* (*General Collection for Holy Relief*) by Zhao Jie in the Song Dynasty and *Puji Fang* (*The Prescriptions for Universal Relief*) by Zhu Su in the Ming

13 首,组成药物亦较简单,但其剂型已有汤、丸、散、膏、丹、药酒之分,并总结出有关辨证治则、治疗方法、方剂组成原则、配伍宜忌等理论,为方剂学的形成与发展奠定了初步的理论基础。东汉张仲景所著的《伤寒杂病论》创造性地融理、法、方、药于一体,被后世誉为"方书之祖",书中共载方 314 首,配伍严谨,选药精当,疗效卓著,人们称之为"经方",对方剂学的发展产生了深远的影响。

　　随着临床运用方剂经验的积累,方剂的数量日益增多,几乎每个朝代均有集前人方剂之大成的总结性方书问世。如唐代有孙思邈编著的《备急千金要方》、《千金翼方》,王焘编著的《外台秘要》;宋代有王怀隐等编著的《太平圣惠方》,赵佶等编著的《圣济总录》;明代有朱橚等编著的《普济方》,计收载 61 739 首方剂,是我国古代收录方剂数量最多的一部方书。近年来出版的由南京中医药大学主编的《中医方剂大辞典》,对历代

Dynasty. The last one is the most voluminous prescription book with 61,739 prescriptions in ancient China. Recently, *Zhongyi Fangji Daci Dian* (*A Dictionary of Traditional Chinese Prescriptions*) compiled by the Nanjing University of Traditional Chinese Medicine summarizes all the prescriptions appearing in the previous medical works in history. The dictionary collects, systematizes and studies all the entitled prescriptions from the Qin and Han dynasties up to the present (1986) with a record of nearly 100 thousand prescriptions, filling in the gaps in prescription works between the Ming Dynasty and today.

　　Prescription books before the Song Dynasty usually embody only the ingredients, dosages, administration and indications, but give little interpretation to the compatibility of drugs in a prescription and the therapeutic principles. Therefore, physicians of later generations often have divergent understandings in the application of some of the prescriptions, or lay them aside due to the failure in understanding certain prescriptions. It was Cheng Wuji of Jin Dynasty who first applied the compatible principle of monarch, minister, adjuvant and guiding drugs mentioned in *Neijing* (*Huangdi's Classic on Medicine*) to analyzing and studying the principle of formulating a prescription, aiming at relating syndrome differentiation and establishment of prescriptions and the compatible law. In addition, he compiled, on the basis of what he had learned from his study of 20 prescriptions in *Shanghan Lun* (*Treatise on Exogenous Febrile Diseases*), a book entitled *Concise Exposition of Febrile Diseases*. This is the first monograph dealing with the compatible theory of prescriptions in the history of traditional Chinese medicine (also known as "*Treatise on Prescriptions*"), thereby carrying the theory to a new phase. Hereafter, came out a lot of monographs about prescriptions, in which all the previous

医著中收录的中医方剂进行了又一次大的总结,该书对我国上自秦、汉,下迄现代(1986年)的所有有方名的方剂加以系统的整理研究,收载方剂近10万首,填补了明代以来中医方剂文献荟萃集结的空白。

　　宋代以前的方书大多只收录方剂的组成药物、用量用法及其适应病证,对这些方剂中药物的配伍作用、治病原理阐述较少,使后人在运用其中某些方剂时常常产生一些认识上的分歧,甚至因不明其制方之义而束之高阁。金代成无己首次将《内经》君臣佐使的组方原则用于分析研究方剂的组方原理,以阐明前人的辨证立方原则和遣药配伍法度,并将其中 20 首《伤寒论》方剂的研究心得编著成卷,即《伤寒明理论·药方论》,这是中医学史上第一部研究方剂配伍理论的专著(又称"方论"),将方剂学理论推进到一个新的阶段。此后陆续有多部方论著作问世,从各个不同侧面对历代著名方剂进行了证治机理与组方原理的阐发,为后人正确理解和运用这些

famous prescriptions were expounded from different aspects in terms of their therapeutic mechanism of syndromes and principle of formulation. These books provided valuable reference materials for the later physicians to understand and apply these prescriptions correctly. Meanwhile they greatly enriched and developed the theories of prescriptions, thus making the science of prescriptions gradually become a subject with an integrated theoretical system.

Likewise, the application of prescriptions also went through the process from experience to theory. At first people chose prescriptions and drugs in the light of syndrome only. But with the increasing number of prescriptions and long-term clinical practices, they gradually summarized some regularity of functions of the prescriptions, thus the therapeutic theory came into being. By the therapeutic method is meant a guiding principle of treatment for different syndromes. It is established on the basis of differentiating syndromes for etiology and selecting treatment. For instance, heat-clearing therapy is used for treating interior-heat syndrome, the interior-warming therapy for treating interior-cold syndrome, and the activating blood to resolve stasis therapy is used for the syndrome of blood stasis. Once the therapeutic theory is developed, it will be looked upon as an important principle and theoretical basis to guide people in the application of extant prescriptions or creation of new ones. If a disease is marked by aversion to cold, fever, headache and aching body, anhidrosis and asthma, thin and whitish tongue fur, superficial and tense pulse, it may be determined as exterior-cold syndrome caused by exogenous wind-cold through comprehensive analysis of the four diagnostic methods. It should be treated by pungent and warm prescriptions for relieving exterior syndrome in accordance with the principles

方剂提供了宝贵的参考资料，同时也极大地充实和发展了方剂学理论，使方剂学逐步成为一门具有完整理论体系的学科。

方剂的应用也经历了一个由经验上升到理论的过程。最初人们只是针对病证来选药用方，随着方剂数量的增加以及大量的临床实践，逐渐总结出了方剂功用的一些规律性的认识，在此基础上产生了治法理论。治法就是针对不同的病证，通过辨证求因、审因论治而确定的治疗指导原则。例如针对里热证候要采用清热法，针对里寒证候要采用温里法，针对血瘀证候要采用活血化瘀法等等。治法理论一经形成之后，便成为指导人们运用成方或创制新方的重要理论依据。例如：一位患者，临床表现为恶寒发热，头痛身疼，无汗而喘，舌苔薄白，脉浮而紧，医师经过四诊合参，确定其为外感风寒引起的表寒证。根据表证宜用汗法，治寒当用温药的原则，确定使用辛温解表法治疗，这时候就可以拟定治疗处方了；或者是

of diaphoretic therapy for exterior syndromes and drugs of warm nature for cold syndromes. In this case, the physician may either adopt a set prescription (Mahuang Tang) with modification, or draw up, by himself, a pungent and warm prescription for relieving exterior syndrome with proper drugs in the light of the principle of formulating a prescription. And the patient will get recovered after taking the drugs that are decocted as required. Thus it can be seen that the therapeutic method is the theoretical basis for formulating a prescription and the prescription is the concrete embodiment of the former, namely "prescriptions come from and are guided by therapeutic methods". The two aspects interrelate closely with each other, constituting the two important links in the process of treatment based on syndrome differentiation.

按照治法的要求选用相应的辛温解表成方加减（如麻黄汤），或者是自行选择合适的药物，根据方剂的组成原则组成辛温解表剂，患者如法煎服，便能汗出病解，邪去人安。由此可见，治法是组方的理论依据，方剂是治法的具体体现，即"方从法出，以法统方"，二者密切相连，构成了中医辨证论治过程中的两个重要环节。

How do you differentiate syndromes, establish the therapeutic methods and formulate a prescription? How do you conduct reasonable compatibility of drugs? How do you apply prescriptions to treating various diseases? If you want completely to answer the above questions, you must learn Science of Prescriptions of TCM after finishing with Basic Theory of TCM, Diagnostics of TCM and Science of Chinese Materia Medica. Through the study of the book, you will learn the basic theory of formulating a prescription, the rudimentary knowledge of dosage forms, and basic requirements for administration. What's more, many illustrations of famous prescriptions will help you have a deeper understanding of the composition and clinical application of the prescriptions, thus laying a solid foundation for your studies of clinical courses.

那么，如何辨证立法组方呢？如何对中药进行合理配伍呢？如何运用方剂去治疗各种疾病呢？如果您想了解上述问题，如果您已经学完了中医基础理论、中医诊断学和中药学三门课程，那么就开始学习方剂学吧！本书将告诉您方剂组成的基本理论，方剂剂型的基本知识，方剂服用的基本要求，并通过大量历代名方的介绍与分析，帮助您深入了解中医方剂的组成及其临床应用，为您进入临床课程的学习奠定坚实的基础。

1.2 Composition and Modification of the Prescriptions

Apart from very few single drugs of all the prescriptions used clinically, the great majority of them are compound drugs consisting of two or more drugs. The reasons are that the action of a single drug is usually limited, and some of them may produce certain side effects or even toxicity. But when several drugs are applied together, ensuring a full play of their advantages and inhibiting the disadvantages, they will display their superiority over a single drug in the treatment of diseases. This can be illustrated in the following three aspects. Firstly, drugs of similar action, if used simultaneously, can strengthen the therapeutic effect for serious diseases. For example, the synergism of Mangxiao (*Natrii Sulphas*) and Dahuang (*Radix et Rhizoma Rhei*) can enhance the therapeutic effects of eliminating pathogenic factors by purgation in the treatment of serious heat accumulation syndrome, e.g. Da Chengqi Tang. Secondly, drugs of different actions in combination can broaden the therapeutic scope in the treatment of complex conditions. For example, Renshen (*Radix Ginseng*) capable of reinforcing qi and Maimendong (*Radix Ophiopogonis*) of nourishing yin in combination has the action of reinforcing both qi and yin for deficiency of both qi and yin, e. g. Shengmai San. Thirdly, drastic or noxious drugs may be applied with some drugs capable of reducing or removing their side effect or toxicity so that they are not likely to generate or

第二章 方剂的组成与变化

目前临床使用的方剂中，除了极少数单味药方（俗称"单方"）之外，大多是由两味或两味以上的中药所组成的复方。这是因为单味中药的作用是有限的，有些对人体还会产生一些副作用甚至毒性，如果将若干味中药配合起来应用，相互之间扬长抑短，显然较之仅用一味药物治疗疾病有着更多的优越性。这种优越性具体表现在以下三个方面：其一，将功效相近的药物配伍同用，可以增强疗效，以适应较为严重的病证，例如大黄与芒硝合用，可以加强泻下逐邪的作用，治疗热结重证，方如大承气汤；其二，将功效不同的药物配伍同用，可以扩大治疗范围，适应较为复杂的病变，例如人参补气，麦门冬滋阴，两者合用，则有气阴双补作用，治疗气阴两虚证候，方如生脉散；其三，在使用药性峻烈或有毒性的药物时，配伍一些能够减轻或消除其

at least produce less damage to the body resistance or toxic reaction. For instance, Gansui (*Euphorbia*) has the function of eliminating retained fluid, but is drastic and toxic in property. If Dazao (*Fructus Ziziphi Jujubae*) are added to it, they can alleviate its side effect, e. g. Shizao Tang. Hence, it's obvious that a rational and appropriate compatibility of the drugs contributes to the full play of the drugs' efficacy and helps reduce to its maximum or get rid of the toxicity and side effect of drugs. That's why compound prescriptions are so widely used. To achieve the above requirement so that the made prescriptions can meet the clinical syndromes to the greatest extent, it is imperative that the drugs be chosen and prescriptions made with flexibility to suit the specific syndromes under the guidance of the formulation principle.

毒副作用的药物,则可以避免或减轻人体正气的损伤以及毒性反应,例如甘遂泻下逐水,但药性峻猛,且有毒性,使用时配伍大枣则能够缓和其对人体的不利影响,方如十枣汤。由此可见,方剂通过合理妥善的配伍,可以最大限度地发挥药物的治疗作用,最大限度地降低乃至消除药物的毒性和副作用,这就是复方被广泛使用的主要原因。要达到上述要求,使得所拟方剂尽可能地切合临床病证,就必须在方剂组成原则的指导下遣药制方,并且针对具体证候加以灵活的变化。

1.2.1 Composition of Prescriptions

第一节　方剂的组成

How to make prescriptions with different drugs based on their rational compatibility? Besides an accurate differentiation of syndromes, establishment of therapeutic method and appropriate choice of drugs and doses, it is necessary to follow the peculiar principle of monarch (jun), minister (chen), adjuvant (zuo) and guide (shi) drugs in a prescription.

Monarch drug: Being an essential ingredient in a prescription, it plays a leading curative role aiming at the cause or the main syndrome of a disease.

Minister drug: It helps strengthen the curative effect of the monarch drug.

如何将一些各不相同的中药合理配伍组成方剂呢?除了准确的辨证、立法以及合理选择药物,权衡用药剂量之外,还必须遵循方剂特有的组成原则,即"君臣佐使"。其具体涵义如下:

君药:即针对病因或主证起主要治疗作用的药物,是方剂组成中不可缺少的药物。

臣药:是协助君药以加强治疗作用的药物。

Adjuvant drug: It refers to: ① the ingredient to co-operate with the monarch and minister drugs to strengthen the therapeutic effects or treat the accompanying diseases or syndromes; ② the ingredient to inhibit the drastic effects or toxicity of the monarch and minister drugs; ③ the ingredient to possess the properties and flavor opposite to those of the monarch drug, but play supplementing effect in the treatment when serious diseases due to excessive pathogenic factors make patients refuse the drug.

Guiding drug: It refers to: ① the ingredient leading the other drugs in the prescription to the affected part; and ② the ingredient regulating the properties of other drugs in the prescription.

Take Mahuang Tang for example to explain the above principle of formulation. This recipe is composed of Mahuang (*Herba Ephedrae*) 9 g, Guizhi (*Ramulus Cinnamomi*) 6 g, Xingren (*Semen Armeniacae Amarum*) 6 g, and Gancao (*Radix Glycyrrhizae*) 3 g. It is used to treat exterior excess syndrome due to affection of exogenous pathogenic wind-cold, marked by aversion to cold, fever, headache, general aching, anhidrosis, asthma, thin and whitish fur, superficial and tense pulse. The syndrome herein is caused by exogenous wind-cold. Its chief syndrome is attack of wind-cold on the superficies, the accompanying one being the obstruction of the lung-qi. Thus the therapy for expelling cold to relieve exterior syndrome and facilitating the flow of lung-qi to relieve asthma should be employed. The first two ingredients of this recipe are both pungent in flavor and warm in property, capable of expelling cold to relieve the exterior syndrome. But Mahuang (*Herba Ephedrae*) bears a drastic efficacy with a large dosage, and is thus used as monarch drug to deal

佐药：有三种意义。① 佐助药，即配合君药、臣药以加强治疗作用，或治疗兼病与兼证的药物；② 佐制药，即起到制约君药、臣药的峻烈之性，或减轻与消除君药、臣药毒性反应的药物；③ 反佐药，即病重邪甚，可能拒药时，配用与君药性味相反而又能在治疗中起相成作用的药物。

使药：有两种意义。① 引经药，即能引导方中诸药达到病所的药物；② 调和药，即具有调和方中诸药性味的药物。

兹举麻黄汤为例对上述组成原则加以说明：麻黄汤由麻黄 9 g、桂枝 6 g、杏仁 6 g、甘草 3 g 组成，主治外感风寒表实证，症见恶寒发热，头痛身疼，无汗而喘，舌苔薄白，脉象浮紧。此证病因是外感风寒，主证为风寒束表，兼证为肺气失宣。治疗宜用散寒解表，宣肺平喘之法。方中麻黄与桂枝均味辛性温，可散寒解表，但麻黄发汗散邪力强，且药量较重，因而是在本方中针对病因和主证起主要治疗作用的药物，即君药；桂枝协助麻黄加强发汗散寒解表作用，故为臣药；杏仁降气止咳平喘，专门针对肺气失宣、咳嗽气喘的兼证而设，故为佐药（佐助

with the cause of the disease and the chief syndrome. Guizhi (*Ramulus Cinnamomi*) helps Mahuang (*Herba Epheadrae*) induce sweating to disperse cold and expel exterior pathogenic factors and functions as minister drug. Xingren (*Semen Armeniacae Amarum*) acts as adjuvant drug with the function of descending adversely rising qi, stopping cough and relieving asthma, and is specially supposed to treat accompanying symptoms. The last ingredient in this recipe can mediate drug properties on the one hand, belonging to a mediating drug of guiding drugs. On the other hand, it is sweet in flavor and mild in property, and can alleviate excessive diaphoretic effects induced by the first two ingredients that are pungent and warm in nature, so it is concurrently the adjuvant drug. Here is the outline of the formulation of the above recipe:

药);甘草可以调和药性,属于使药中的调和药,但其味甘性缓,又能缓和麻黄、桂枝辛温发散可能导致发汗太过之弊,兼作佐药。兹将上述麻黄汤的组方意义概括如下:

Mahuang Tang
- Monarch drug — Mahuang (*Herba Ephedrae*): Relieving exterior syndrome by means of diaphoresis, activating the flow of the lung-qi to relieve asthma
- Minister drug — Guizhi (*Ramulus Cinnamomi*): Assisting the monarch drug to induce diaphoresis, relieve exterior syndrome and expel cold
- Adjuvant drug — Xingren (*Semen Armeniacae Amarum*): Helping the monarch drug to promote the flow of lung-qi and stop asthma
- Guiding drug — Gancao (*Radix Glycyrrhizae*): Mediating the drug properties and preventing the impairment of vital qi due to excessive diaphoresis

麻黄汤
- 君药——麻黄:发汗解表,宣肺平喘。
- 臣药——桂枝:助麻黄发汗、解表、散寒。
- 佐药——杏仁:合麻黄宣降肺气,止咳平喘。
- 使药——甘草:调和药性,并防麻黄、桂枝过汗伤正(兼佐药)。

The above principle of forming a prescription shows that drugs in a prescription have their respective importance of effect in the order of the monarch, minister, adjuvant and guiding drugs. Besides, the drugs in a recipe are related to one another — the monarch and minister drugs cooperate with each other, the adjuvant drug coordinates or inhibits the monarch and minister drugs,

上述"君臣佐使"的组方原则告诉我们:① 方剂中药物的作用有主次之分,其中君药至为重要,臣药次之,佐、使药物又再次之。② 方剂中药物之间存在着多方面的联系,如君药与臣药之间的相互配

ensuring the optimum effect of the recipe by means of a
supplementary or opposite relationship. Moreover, not
every recipe comprises invariably the monarch, minister,
adjuvant and guiding drugs, nor does each of the four ingredients play a single role in a recipe. So the composition
of monarch, minister, adjuvant and guiding drugs depends
on therapeutic requirements. Although monarch drug is
indispensable to a recipe, it does not necessarily follow
that the rest three should be included in the recipe. If the
monarch drug has adequate potency, minister drug will
not be included in the recipe. If the first two ingredients
bear no toxic and drastic property, adjuvant drug is not
needed. If the drugs meant to treat the chief syndrome
can come to the affected part, no guiding drug will be in-
volved. Some minister drugs may have the function of the
adjuvant drug concurrently, so do some adjuvant drugs of
the guiding drug, e. g. , Gancao (*Radix Glycyrrhizae*) in
Mahuang Tang is a guiding drug in itself, but has a con-
current function with the adjuvant drug. Therefore, this
principle should never be applied mechanically.

　　The drugs in a prescription in accordance with the
compatible principle have their special effect and action.
They interact with and inhibit one another. In this way,
they form an organic whole with rigorous compatibility,
thereby producing significant therapeutic effect.

1.2.2　Modification of a Prescription

　　In the clinical application of a set prescription, it is
necessary to modify it flexibly under the guidance of the

合与协助,佐药与君药、臣药之间的协同或制约,通过相辅相成或相反相成的配伍关系,使方剂发挥最佳的治疗效应。③ 并非每首方剂均包含君、臣、佐、使各类药物,也不一定每味药只专任一职。这是因为"君臣佐使"是根据治疗的需要而设,除君药必不可缺外,其余类型药物并不一定必须具备,若君药药力足够,则不必以臣药辅之;若君、臣药无毒亦不峻烈时,亦无需以佐药制之;若主病药物能直达病所,则不必再加引经的使药;有的臣药兼有佐药之职,有的佐药兼有使药之能,如麻黄汤中的甘草既为使药又兼佐药之功,所以切不可机械地理解"君臣佐使"的组方原则。

　　遵循"君臣佐使"的组方原则配伍组方,能够使方中各药主从有序,既有明确的分工,又有密切的配合,相互之间协调制约,使方剂成为一个配伍法度严谨的有机整体,就能取得临床预期的疗效。

第二节　方剂的变化

　　临床在运用成方时,必须在君、臣、佐、使的组方原则指

compatible principle and in accordance with the condition of illness, constitution, age, sex of the patient and the occurring season, climate as well as patients' habits. Only when the principle is unified with flexibility can the prescription tally with the syndromes and the expected therapeutic goal be achieved. In other words, it is necessary to follow the principle but not adhere to the originally established prescription mechanically. The modification of a prescription includes the following three ways:

1.2.2.1 Modification of Drugs

This can be subdivided into two. One is the modification of the adjuvant drug, by which is meant subtracting some unsuitable drugs in the original prescription or adding some necessary drugs that are not in the original prescription to meet the need of treatment of present accompanying symptoms. But it should be carried out on the condition that the present chief syndrome is identical with that of the original prescription, but the accompanying symptoms are different. Since the adjuvant drug plays a minor role in a recipe, its modification is not likely to bring about a radical change of the original potency. This is also known as "the modification in the light of the symptoms". For instance, Si Junzi Tang is chiefly designed for qi-deficiency syndrome of the spleen and stomach, marked by pale complexion, faint voice, short breath, lack of strength, poor appetite, loose stool, pale tongue with whitish fur, thready and weak pulse. It is composed of Renshen (*Radix Ginseng*), Baizhu (*Rhizoma Atractylodis Macrocephalae*), Fuling (*Poria*) and Zhigancao (*Radix Glycyrrhizae Praeparatae*), and functions to replenish qi and invigorate the spleen. If the above symptoms are accompanied by oppressed sensation over the epigastrium and abdominal distention and obstruc-

导下,结合患者的病情、体质、年龄、性别与季节、气候以及生活习惯等,予以加减运用,灵活化裁,所谓"师其法而不泥其方",就是指原则性与灵活性的统一,才能使方药与病证相吻合,达到预期的治疗目的。方剂的组成变化,归纳起来主要有以下三种方式。

一、药味增减的变化

药味的增减变化有两种情况,一种是佐使药的加减,即在原方的主证与现证基本相同而兼证不同时,减去原方中某些不适宜的药物,或加上某些原方中没有但现证又需要的药物,以适应兼证的治疗要求;由于佐使药在方中的作用较为次要,其变化不致于引起原方功效的根本改变,故又称为"随证加减"。如四君子汤主治脾胃气虚证,症见面色萎白,语声低微,气短乏力,食少便溏,舌淡苔白,脉细弱,该方由人参、白术、茯苓、炙甘草组成,功在益气补脾,若在上述症状基础上又兼见脘闷腹胀,则为脾虚不运,又兼气滞之征,可在四君子汤中加入陈皮以行气消胀(此方亦名异功散),这就是根据兼证的变化,临床上予以随证加减的运用。

ted flow of qi, which results from dysfunction of spleen-qi, Chenpi (*Pericarpium Citri Reticulatae*) can be added to the above recipe to promote the flow of qi and relieve distention. This gives rise to another prescription entitled Yigong San.

The other refers to the modification of monarch and minister drugs or the change of the monarch drug and its compatibility by adding to or subtracting other drugs from the original prescription. Consequently radical changes will take place in terms of the potency. For example, when Guizhi (*Ramulus Cinnamomi*) in Mahuang Tang is substituted for Shigao (*Gypsum Fibrosum*), it is called Mahuang Xingren Gancao Shigao Tang. The former takes Mahuang (*Herba Ephedrae*) as the monarch drug, which is combined with Guizhi (*Ramulus Cinnamomi*) to treat exterior-excess syndrome caused by wind-cold through inducing diaphoresis and expelling cold. While the latter take Mahuang (*Herba Ephedrae*) and Shigao (*Gypsum Fibrosum*) together as the monarch drug to remove heat from the lung to relieve asthma. Thereby, it is effective for curing cough with asthma due to lung-heat. It can be seen that though the two are different only in one ingredient, because of the change of the relationship between monarch drug and its compatibility, the main action of the prescription changes accordingly. In that case, the prescription for relieving exterior syndrome with pungent and warm drugs is changed consequently into one for relieving exterior syndrome with pungent and cool drugs.

In the clinical application of set prescriptions, the above modifications can be conducted according to the actual requirements. Generally, "the modification in the light of the symptoms" is easy to master and conforms to the thought of the physicians, and is thus commonly used in clinical treatment.

另一种是君臣药的加减，或者君臣药虽然仍保留在方剂中，但由于其他药物的增减使方中的君药及其配伍关系发生了改变，从而使方剂的功效发生根本变化。例如将麻黄汤中的桂枝换成石膏，就成为麻黄杏仁甘草石膏汤。前者以麻黄为君药，与桂枝配伍以发汗散寒，治疗风寒表实证；后者以麻黄与石膏共为君药，两药配伍共同发挥清肺平喘作用，治疗肺热咳喘证。由此可见，虽然两方仅一药之差，但因为改变了君药及其配伍关系，结果使方剂的主要功用亦随之发生改变，由辛温解表之方一变而成为辛凉解表之剂。

在临床运用成方时，可以根据不同的需要选用相应的药味增减。一般来说，"随证加减"方法易于掌握，较为符合临床医师用方的思路，因而在临床实践中被广泛应用。

1. 2. 2. 2   Modification of Dosage

It refers to increasing or decreasing the dosage of a drug in an established prescription without any change in its ingredients so as to change its potency or even its compatibility as well as its action and indication. For instance, Sini Tang and Tongmai Sini Tang are both composed of Fuzi (*Radix Aconiti Lateralis*), Ganjiang (*Rhizoma Zingiberis*) and Zhigancao (*Radix Glycyrrhizae Praeparatae*), acting respectively as the monarch, minister and adjuvant drugs. Because the former contains less of the first two ingredients than the latter, and functions to recuperate depleted yang and rescue patients from collapse, it is used to treat the syndrome due to excessive yin and deficient yang marked by cold limbs, aversion to cold, lying in curl, dyspeptic diarrhea, deep faint and thready pulse. In the latter, however, both of the first two ingredients are increased. So it functions to warm the interior to recuperate depleted yang and promote blood circulation. It is mainly applied to treating the syndrome due to excessive yin repelling yang marked by cold limbs, no aversion to cold, flushed cheeks, dyspeptic diarrhea and extremely faint or even depleting pulse (see Table 1). Take Xiao chengqi Tang and Houpo Sanwu Tang for another example, both are composed of Dahuang (*Radix et Rhizoma Rhei*), Zhishi (*Fructus Aurantii Immaturus*) and Houpo (*Cortex Magnoliae Officinalis*). In the former prescription, Dahuang (*Radix et Rhizoma Rhei*) is in large dosage and used as the monarch drug, and Zhishi (*Fructus Aurantii Immaturus*) as the minister drug. Houpo (*Cortex Magnoliae Officinalis*) is in half the dosage of Dahuang (*Radix et Rhizoma Rhei*) and serves as the adjuvant drug. This recipe, with the function of purging away heat and relieving constipation, is indicated for

二、药量增减的变化

这种变化是指方剂的药物组成不变,仅通过增加或减少方中药物的剂量,以改变其药效的强弱乃至配伍关系,进而影响方剂的功用。如四逆汤和通脉四逆汤均由附子、干姜、炙甘草三药组成,且均以附子为君,干姜为臣,炙甘草为佐使。但前方附子、干姜用量相对较小,功能回阳救逆,主治阴盛阳微而致的四肢厥逆,恶寒蜷卧,下利清谷,脉沉微细的证候;后方附子、干姜用量较前方俱有增加,温里回阳之功增大,能够回阳通脉,主治阴盛格阳于外而致四肢厥逆,身反不恶寒,其人面色赤,下利清谷,脉微欲绝的证候(见表1)。又如小承气汤和厚朴三物汤,都由大黄、枳实、厚朴三味药物组成,但小承气汤中大黄用量较大,作为君药,枳实为臣药,厚朴用量较小,是大黄的二分之一,为佐使,功能泻热通便,主治阳明腑实轻证;厚朴三物汤中厚朴用量独重,为君药,枳实为臣药,用量亦较小承气汤中枳实为大,大黄为佐使,用量是厚朴的二分之一,全方功能行气通便,主治气滞便秘证(见表2)。

mild case with excess syndrome of the Yangming fu organs.
In the latter, however, Houpo (*Cortex Magnoliae Officinalis*) serves as the monarch drug with a larger dosage, Zhishi
(*Fructus Aurantii Immaturus*) as the minister with
the dose larger than that of the former prescription, and
Dahuang (*Radix et Rhizoma Rhei*) as the adjuvant drug
in half the dosage of Houpo (*Cortex Magnoliae Officinalis*). The latter prescription functions to promote the flow
of qi and relieve constipation and is mainly used to treat
constipation due to stagnation of qi (see Table 2).

Table 1　　　　　　**Comparison between Sini Tang and Tongmai Sini Tang**

Prescription	Ingredients			Actions	Indications
	Monarch drug	Minister drug	Adjuvant and Guiding drug		
	Radix Aconiti Lateralis	*Rhizoma Zingiberis*	*Radix Glycyrrhizae Praeparatae*		
Sini Tang	1 piece	1. 5 liang	2 liang	Recuperating the depleted yang and rescuing the patient from collapse	Cold limbs, aversion to cold with the body huddling up, dyspeptic diarrhea, deep and fine pulse due to excessive yin and deficient yang
Tongmai Sini Tang	1 piece (larger)	3 liang	2 liang	Recuperating the depleted yang and dredging pulse	Cold limbs, no aversion to cold, flushed complexion, dyspeptic diarrhea, faint and fading pulse due to excessive yin repelling yang

Notes: The above dosages are recorded from *Shanghan Lun* (*Treatise on Exogenous Febrile Diseases*) by Zhang
Zhongjing (same as below).

表1　　　　　　　　　　　　**四逆汤和通脉四逆汤比较**

方　名	组　成　药　物			功　用	主　治　病　证
	君	臣	佐　使		
	生附子	干　姜	炙甘草		
四逆汤	一　枚	一两五钱	二　两	回阳救逆	阴盛阳微所致四肢厥逆,恶寒蜷卧,下利清谷,脉沉微细。
通脉四逆汤	一枚(大者)	三　两	二　两	回阳通脉	阴盛格阳所致四肢厥逆,身反不恶寒,其人面色赤,下利清谷,脉微欲绝。

注：上述药物剂量,是汉代张仲景所著《伤寒论》中记载的用量(下同)。

Table 2　　　　　**Comparison between Xiao Chengqi Tang and Houpo Sanwu Tang**

Prescription	Ingredients			Actions	Indications
	Monarch Drug	Minister Drug	Adjuvant and Guiding Drug		
Xiao Chengqi Tang	*Radix et Rhizoma Rhei*, 4 liang	*Fructus Aurantii Immaturus*, 3 pieces	*Cortex Magnoliae Officinalis*, 2 liang	Purging away heat and relaxing the bowels	Excess syndrome of yangming fu organ (heat-accumulation): hectic fever, delirium, constipation, abdominal pain and tenderness
Houpo Sanwu Tang	*Cortex Magnoliae Officinalis*, 8 liang	*Fructus Aurantii Immaturus*, 5 pieces	*Radix et Rhizoma Rhei*, 4 liang	Promoting flow of qi and relaxing the bowels	Constipation due to qi stagnation: abdominal fullness and constipation

表 2　　　　　**小承气汤和厚朴三物汤比较**

方　名	组　成　药　物			功　用	主　治　病　证
	君	臣	佐　使		
小承气汤	大黄四两	枳实三枚	厚朴二两	泻热通便	阳明腑实证(热结)：潮热谵语，大便秘结，腹痛拒按。
厚朴三物汤	厚朴八两	枳实五枚	大黄四两	行气通便	气滞便秘证(气滞)：脘腹满痛不减，大便秘结。

It can be seen from the above that Sini Tang and Tongmai Sini Tang, though different in the doses of drugs, have the same compatibility. They differ only in their power of actions and pathologic conditions. However, in Table 2, because of modification of the quantity of the ingredients, the compatible relationships of the two prescriptions are changed, thus leading to the change of their actions and indications.

1. 2. 2. 3 Modification of Forms

The form of a prescription is closely related to its actions. With the same ingredients and doses, different forms of a prescription have different actions and indications. Generally speaking, decoction is of quick and

由上可见，四逆汤和通脉四逆汤的药量虽有轻重之异，但其剂量的改变并未影响原方君臣佐使的配伍关系，结果其作用仅有强弱的差别，主治证候亦是轻重之异；而小承气汤和厚朴三物汤则由于药量的增减导致了配伍关系改变，因而两方的功用和主治证发生了质的改变。

三、剂型更换的变化

方剂的剂型与功用密切相关，同一方剂的组成药物与剂量完全相同，但由于剂型不同，其作用和适应证亦有区

drastic effect and pill or bolus of slow action and lasting effect. They can be selected clinically as needed. For instance, Lizhong Wan and Renshen Tang are made up of the same ingredients with same doses. The former is fine particles made into honeyed bolus, used to treat deficiency-cold syndrome of the spleen and stomach marked by stomachache, epigastric and abdominal pain, poor appetite and loose stool in mild and chronic state. The latter is boiled with water to be taken orally, used for deficiency-cold syndrome of the upper and middle energizers marked by oppressed and stuffy sensation in the chest, upward adverse flow of qi from the hypochondria, suitable for an acute or a serious case (see Table 3).

别。一般来说,汤剂的作用快而力峻,而丸剂的作用慢而力缓,临床可根据需要随证选用。如理中丸和人参汤,两方组成、用量完全相同,前方共为细末,炼蜜为丸,治疗脾胃虚寒,脘腹疼痛,纳差便溏,虚寒较轻,病势较缓,取丸以缓治;后方水煎作汤内服,主治中上二焦虚寒之胸痹,症见心胸痞闷,自觉气从胁下上逆,虚寒较重,病势较急,取汤以速治(见表3)。

Table 3　　　　　　**Comparison between Lizhong Wan and Renshen Tang**

Prescription	Ingredients				Indications	Preparation & Application
	Radix Genseng	Rhizoma Zingiberis	Rhizoma Atractylodis Mactocphalae	Prepared Radix Glycyrrhizae		
Lizhong Wan	3 liang	3 liang	3 liang	3 liang	Deficient and cold midenergizer marked by abdominal pain, no thirst, spitting saliva after recovery from illness	Preparing them with honey into boluses as big as yolk; one bolus each time
Renshen Tang	3 liang	3 liang	3 liang	3 liang	Deficient and cold upper Energizer, and mid-energizer marked by oppressed and stuffysensation in the chest, upward adverse flow of qi from the hypochondria	Decocted for oral administration, 3 times daily

表3　　　　　　　　　　**理中丸与人参汤比较**

方　名	组　成　药　物				主　治　病　证	制　剂　用　法
	人　参	干　姜	白　术	炙甘草		
理中丸	三　两	三　两	三　两	三　两	中焦虚寒,脘腹疼痛,自利不渴,病后喜唾涎沫。	炼蜜为丸如鸡子黄大,每服1丸。
人参汤	三　两	三　两	三　两	三　两	中上二焦虚寒,心胸痞闷,气从胁下上逆。	水煎,分3次服。

To sum up, the modification of either the ingredients, or the dosage, or the forms will exert an effect to different extent on the action of the prescriptions. In particular, modification of the main ingredients and the dosage often changes the compatibility of the monarch and minister drugs in the original prescription so that radical changes take place in terms of the actions and indications. The above three modifications of an established prescription can be applied separately or simultaneously. Clinically it depends on the concrete conditions of the patients. What should be noted is to modify a prescription with a mastery of the compatible relationship between the monarch, minister, adjuvant and guiding drugs. Only in this way can the established principle be followed flexibly, modification is also made time and again.

综上所述,方剂的药味增减、药量增减或者剂型更换都会对其功用产生不同程度的影响,特别是主要药物的变更与药量的增减,常常改变原方君臣药物的配伍关系,以致其功效与主治证候发生较大的变化。上述变化形式既可以分别运用,也可以合并运用,临证可根据需要灵活选用。应当注意的是,在对成方进行加减化裁的同时,必须认真把握其君臣佐使的配伍关系,如此才能师古而不泥古,变化而不离宗。

1.3 Common Forms of Prescriptions

第三章 方剂的常用剂型

The forms of prescription refer to the definite patterns processed, after drugs are made up into a prescription in line with certain compatibility, according to the condition of the patient, the properties of the drugs and the route of administration as well. An appropriate form is indispensable to the action of a prescription and the efficacy of the drugs.

Here are the commonly used forms as follows:

将药物配伍成方之后,再根据病情的需要、药物的性质以及给药的途径,将原料药进行加工制成的型态,称为剂型。适宜的剂型是方剂治疗作用和药效发挥不可缺少的条件。

现将临床常用的方剂剂型简介如下:

1.3.1 Decoction

It refers to the medicinal solution obtained by removing the dregs after soaking and decocting the prepared herbal pieces in water for a period of time. It is chiefly for oral administration, e.g., Mahuang Tang, Guizhi Tang, etc. Besides it can be applied externally for washing, steaming and gargling. It bears the characteristics of being easily absorbed and producing quick curative effects. It is especially suitable for serious or unsteady cases. And it can be modified according to the changes of disease. It can meet the need of treatment based on syndrome differentiation, so it is one of the forms most widely used in clinical practice. Nevertheless it has its disadvantages. Firstly, it needs to be taken in large amount, and the effective compositions of some drugs are difficult to extract and easy to volatilize. Secondly, it takes a longer time to

一、汤剂

汤剂是将药物饮片混合加水浸泡,再煎煮一定时间,去渣取汁而成的液体剂型。汤剂主要供内服,如麻黄汤、桂枝汤等。外用的多作洗浴、薰蒸及含漱。汤剂的特点是吸收较快,能迅速发挥药效,特别是便于根据病情的变化而随证加减使用,适用于病证较重或病情不稳定的患者。汤剂有利于满足辨证论治的需要,是中医临床运用最广泛的一种剂型。汤剂的不足之处是服用量大,某些药物的有效成分不易煎出或易挥发散

boil the drugs and thus it is not beneficial to the rescue work of critical patients. Thirdly, it is inconvenient to carry and difficult for children to take for its bitter taste.

1.3.2 Powder

The drugs are ground into fine powder and well mixed for oral use and external use. Generally the powder for oral administration is usually ground into fine powder to be taken orally with warm boiled water or directly if in small dosage, such as Qili San, Xingjun San, and so on. Some drugs may be ground into coarse powder to be boiled with water and then the residue is removed to get the liquid for oral use. So they got the name of "boiled powder", e.g. Yinqiao San, Baidu San, etc. The powder for external use is generally applied to or sprinkled on a sore or affected part of the body. Jinhuang San and Shengji San are such examples. But some are for eye droppings or throat insufflation, e. g. Babao Yanyao, Bingpeng San, etc. Powder is prepared easily and absorbed quickly, stable in property, insusceptible of going bad, and convenient to use and carry with less drugs used.

1.3.3 Pill

It refers to the round solid preparation of drugs obtained by grinding drugs into fine powder or extracting medicinal materials and then mixing with excipient. Compared with decoction, pills have the advantages of slow absorption, lasting potency, small dosage, and are convenient to carry and take because of their small volumes. Therefore they are commonly adopted to treat chronic diseases or diseases with deficiency syndromes, e.g. Liuwei Dihuang Wan, Xiangsha Liujunzi Wan, etc. Sometimes they are also used for chronic treatment with drugs drastic

失,煎煮费时而不利于危重病人的抢救,口感较苦而小儿难以服用,亦不便于携带等。

二、散剂

散剂是将药物粉碎,混合均匀而制成的粉末状制剂。根据其用途,分内服和外用两类。内服散剂一般是研成细粉,以温开水冲服,量小者亦可直接吞服,如七厘散、行军散等。亦有制成粗末,临用时加水煎煮去渣取汁服的,称为煮散,如银翘散、败毒散等。外用散剂一般作为外敷、掺撒疮面或患病部位,如金黄散、生肌散等;亦有作点眼、吹喉等外用的,如八宝眼药、冰硼散等。散剂的特点是制备方法简便,吸收较快,节省药材,性质较稳定,不易变质,便于服用与携带。

三、丸剂

丸剂是将药物研成细粉或用药材提取物,加适宜的赋形剂制成的圆形固体剂型。丸剂与汤剂相比,吸收较慢,药效持久,节省药材,体积较小,便于携带与服用。适用于慢性、虚弱性疾病,如六味地黄丸、香砂六君子丸等;也有取峻药缓治而用丸剂的,如十枣丸、抵当丸等;还有因方剂

in properties, e. g. Shizao Wan, Didang Wan, etc. They may also contain drugs aromatic in flavor, and unsuitable to be boiled in water, e. g. Angong Niuhuang Wan, Suhexiang Wan, etc. The pills or boluses commonly used are listed as follows:

1.3.3.1   Honeyed Pills or Boluses

They are made by mixing fine powder of drugs with refined honey, inclusive of large and small ones. Since honeyed pills or boluses are soft and moist in property, moderate and lasting in action, they have the actions of rectifying taste, replenishing and nourishing. They are often applied in the treatment of chronic diseases or patients of weak constitution, such as Lizhong Wan, Liuwei Dihuang Wan and so on.

1.3.3.2   Water-paste Pills

This refers to the pills prepared by mixing the fine powder of drugs with such excipients as water (cold boiled or distilled water), wine, vinegar, or drug juice. Water-paste pills are easy to be decomposed, absorbed and swallowed, applicable to various diseases, Fangfeng Tongsheng Wan and Zuojin Wan are such examples.

1.3.3.3   Paste-pills

They are prepared by mixing up the drug powders and the excipients made of rice, flour, or yeast paste, characterized by strong adhesiveness, solid quality, slow decomposition and dissolution. They can prolong the therapeutic effect and reduce harmful reaction and irritation to the stomach generated from toxic and drastic drugs, e. g. Zhouche Wan, Heixi Dan, etc.

1.3.3.4   Condensed Pills

This refers to the pills prepared by decocting drugs until their decoction is concentrated to extract, then mixing the extract with the fine powder of other drugs, drying the mixed material and grinding it into powder,

中含较多芳香走窜药物,不宜入汤剂煎煮而制成丸剂的,如安宫牛黄丸、苏合香丸等。常用的丸剂有以下几类:

(一) 蜜丸

蜜丸是将药物细粉用炼制的蜂蜜为赋形剂制成的丸剂,分为大蜜丸和小蜜丸两种。蜜丸性质柔润,作用缓和持久,并有补益和矫味作用,常用于治疗慢性病和虚弱性疾病,如理中丸、六味地黄丸等。

(二) 水丸

水丸是将药物细粉用水(冷开水或蒸馏水)或酒、醋、药汁等为赋形剂制成的小丸。水丸较蜜丸易于崩解,吸收快,易于吞服,适用于多种疾病,如防风通圣丸、左金丸等。

(三) 糊丸

糊丸是将药物细粉用米糊、面糊、曲糊等为赋形剂制成的小丸。糊丸粘合力强,质地坚硬,崩解、溶散迟缓,内服可延长药效,减轻毒剧药的不良反应和对胃肠的刺激,如舟车丸、黑锡丹等。

(四) 浓缩丸

浓缩丸是将药物或方中部分药物煎汁浓缩成膏,再与其他药物细粉混合干燥、粉碎,用水或蜂蜜或药汁制成丸

which then is mixed with water or honey or drug juice. It is used to treat various diseases because it has a higher content of active constituents, small volume and dosage. It is also convenient to use.

There are other types of pills or boluses not mentioned here, such as wax-wrapped pill, water-honey pills, tiny pellet, and guttate pills, etc.

1.3.4　Extract, Ointment and Plaster

They are medicinal preparations made by decocting drugs in water or vegetable oil and discarding the dregs, for oral or external application. The former includes liquid extract, extract and decocted extract, and the latter ointment and plaster. Among them, liquid extract and extract mostly serve as a mediator for other preparations, such as mixture, syrup, granule and tablet. Here is a brief explanation of decocted extract, ointment and plaster.

1.3.4.1　Decocted Extract

It refers to the semi-liquid form of preparation made by decocting the drugs in water repeatedly, discarding the dregs, then concentrating and adding to it refined honey or sugar. Such paste is small in size, high in content, convenient to take and tasty with a nourishing action, applicable to patients with chronic disease and weak constitution, e.g. Lutai Gao, Bazhen Yimu Gao, etc.

1.3.4.2　Ointment

It refers to the semisolid form of preparation with certain viscosity made by mixing the drug powder with appropriate matrix, among which the one made with emulsion is also known as emulsive ointment, mostly applicable to the skin, mucous membrane or sores and scabs. Since

剂。因其有效成分含量高,体积小,剂量小,易于服用,可用于治疗多种疾病。

其他尚有蜡丸、水蜜丸、微丸、滴丸等,不一一列举。

四、膏剂

膏剂是将药物用水或植物油煎熬去渣而制成的剂型。有内服和外用两种,内服膏剂有流浸膏、浸膏、煎膏三种;外用膏剂分软膏、硬膏两种。其中流浸膏与浸膏多数用作调配其他制剂使用,如合剂、糖浆剂、冲剂、片剂等。现将煎膏与外用膏剂分述如下:

(一)煎膏

煎膏又称膏滋。是将药物加水反复煎煮,去渣浓缩后,加炼蜜或炼糖制成的半液体剂型。其特点是体积小,含量高,便于服用,口味甜美,有滋润补益作用,一般用于慢性虚弱性疾病的调理,有利于较长时间用药,如鹿胎膏、八珍益母膏等。

(二)软膏

软膏又称药膏。是将药物细粉与适宜的基质制成具有适当稠度的半固体外用制剂。其中用乳剂型基质的亦称乳膏剂。多用于皮肤、黏膜

ointment bears a certain viscosity, it will gradually soften or melt with drugs slowly absorbed and producing lasting therapeutic effect. It is applicable externally to sores and furuncles, ulcer and masses, and burns as well.

1.3.4.3　Plaster

It refers to the preparation obtained by boiling drugs in vegetable oil to certain extent, removing the residue, boiling again till it becomes so solid that the dripping water turns to beads, adding to it the yellow lead, mixing up and cooling it down. Before applied to the affected part or point, it should be heated and spreaded over a piece of cloth or paper till it softens. It is applicable to both local and general diseases, e. g. sores, ulcer and masses, injuries from falls, fractures, contusions and strains, rheumatic diseases, waist soreness and abdominal pain as well. The commonly used are Goupi Gao, Nuanqi Gao, etc.

1.3.5　Medicated Liquor

It is an alcoholic solution obtained by soaking drugs in liquor or rice / millet wine, or stewing them with a separation between water and drugs, then discarding the residue. The liquor is taken orally or applied externally. With the characteristics of promoting blood circulation to remove obstruction in the meridians, being apt to volatilize and helpful in bringing the potency into full play, it is often used for dispelling wind and dredging the collaterals, for example, Fengshi Yaojiu, Shenrong Yaojiu, and Wujiapi Jiu, etc. If applied externally, it may dispel wind to promote blood circulation, and to relieve pain and edema.

1.3.6　Dan (*a special form of pill*)

It is divided into two types, one for oral administra-

或创面。软膏具有一定的黏稠性,外涂后渐渐软化或溶化,使药物慢慢吸收,持久发挥疗效,适用于外科疮疡疖肿、烧烫伤等。

(三)硬膏

硬膏又称膏药。是以植物油将药物煎至一定程度,去渣,煎至滴水成珠,加黄丹等搅匀、冷却制成的硬膏。用时加温摊涂在布或纸上,软化后贴于患处或穴位上,可治疗局部疾病和全身性疾病,如疮疡肿毒、跌打损伤、风湿痹证以及腰痛、腹痛等。常用的有狗皮膏、暖脐膏等。

五、酒剂

酒剂又称药酒。是将药物用白酒或黄酒浸泡,或加温隔水炖煮,去渣取液供内服或外用。酒有活血通络,易于发散和助长药效的特性,故常于祛风通络和补益方剂中使用,如风湿药酒、参茸药酒、五加皮酒等。外用酒剂尚可祛风活血,止痛消肿。

六、丹剂

丹剂有内服与外用两种,

tion and the other external application. The former does not have a fixed form, inclusive of pellet and powder, and gets the name because it consists of rare drugs or bears remarkable effect, e. g. Zhibao Dan, Huoluo Dan, etc. The latter is also called Danyao, which refers to the crystal-like product of various shapes made by heating, under higher temperature, some medicinal minerals. It is often smashed into powder and sprinkled over the affected part in the treatment of sores and ulcer, carbuncle and gangrene. It can also be made into medicinal paper strip or thread for external application.

1.3.7   Medicated Tea

It refers to either the coarse granules processed by crushing the drugs, or the block preparation made by mixing the powder with appropriate adhesive, drunk as tea after infused with boiling water or boiled for juice. It is mostly applicable to cold, dyspepsia, and diarrhea. Recently, however, new products have come into being, some for building up the body and others for reducing weight, e. g. Wushi Cha, Ciwujia Cha, and Jianfei Cha, etc.

1.3.8   Medicinal Dew

It refers to the fragrant crystal-clear solution obtained by distilling fresh drugs containing volatile ingredients, to be used as drinks or for relieving summer heat, e. g. Jinyinhua Lu, Qinghao Lu, etc.

1.3.9   Pastille

It refers to the solid preparation with specific shapes obtained by crushing drugs into fine powder, or mixing up

内服丹剂没有固定剂型,有丸剂,也有散剂,每以药品贵重或药效显著而名之曰丹,如至宝丹、活络丹等。外用丹剂亦称丹药,是以某些矿物类药经高温烧炼制成的不同结晶形状的制品。常研粉涂撒疮面,治疗疮疡痈疽,亦可制成药条、药线和外用膏剂应用。

七、茶剂

茶剂是将药物经粉碎加工而制成的粗末状制品,或加入适宜赋形剂压制成块状制剂。应用时以沸水泡或煎取药汁,不定时饮用。一般多用于治疗感冒、食积、腹泻,近年来又有许多健身、减肥的新产品,如午时茶、刺五加茶、减肥茶等。

八、露剂

露剂亦称药露。是将新鲜含有挥发性成分的药物,用蒸馏法制成的芳香气味的澄明水溶液。一般作为饮料及清凉解暑剂,常用的有金银花露、青蒿露等。

九、锭剂

锭剂是将药物研成细粉,或加适当的赋形剂制成规定

the powder and certain adhesive, inclusive of spindle, cylinder and bar shapes. It is ground into fine powder or juice for oral administration or external application. The commonly seen are pastilles as Zijin Ding, Wanying Ding, and Chansu Ding, etc.

1.3.10　Lozenge

It is a form of preparation made by twisting medicated paper into a slender roll or by twisting paper into a slender roll and then medicating it. Clinically it is inserted into the opening of a sore or fistula to remove rotten tissue and pus and to promote tissue regeneration, such as Hongsheng Dan Yaotiao, etc.

1.3.11　Medicated Thread

It refers to a form of preparation for external application made by soaking and boiling silk or cotton thread in medicated liquid and then drying it. It is through the mild decomposing action of the contained drugs and mechanical fastening that medicated thread carries out its function of helping discharge or shrink pus or making it come off in the treatment of fistula, hemorrhoid and vegetation.

1.3.12　Liniment

It refers to a solution, lactescence, or suspension made up of drugs and appropriate menstruum, and specially designed for applying over the skin or on a dressing. It can protect skin, relieve pain and resist irritation, such as turpentine, camphor lotions, etc.

1.3.13　Suppository

It refers to a solid preparation of certain shape made

形状的固体剂型,有纺锤形、圆柱形、条形等。可供外用与内服,研末调服或磨汁服,外用则磨汁涂患处。常用的有紫金锭、万应锭、蟾酥锭等。

十、条剂

条剂亦称药捻,是将药物细粉用桑皮纸粘药后搓捻成细条,或将桑皮纸捻成细条再粘着药粉而成。使用时插入疮口或瘘管内,以化腐拔毒、生肌收口。常用的有红升丹药条等。

十一、线剂

线剂是将药丝线或棉线置药液中浸煮,经干燥制成的外用制剂。用于治疗瘘管、痔疮或赘生物,通过所含药物的轻度腐蚀作用和药线紧扎的剪切作用,使其引流通畅或萎缩、脱落。

十二、搽剂

搽剂是将药物与适宜溶媒制成的专供揉搽皮肤表面或涂于敷料贴用的溶液型、乳状液或混悬液制剂。有保护皮肤和镇痛及抗刺激作用。常用的有松节油搽剂、樟脑搽剂等。

十三、栓剂

栓剂古称坐药或塞药,是

by mixing drug powder with matrix, which is applied in the cavity and gets melted or dissolved to release drugs, capable of killing worms, relieving itching, moistening, and astringency. Since it is absorbed through rectal mucous (some through vagina), and 50%- 70% of the drugs get into blood circulation directly without passing through the liver, this actually lessens the metabolism of drugs within the liver. Simultaneously it reduces the toxic and side effect to the liver generated by the drugs, and can also prevent gastrointestinal juice from affecting the drugs and drugs from irritating the gastric mucosa. It is especially convenient for infants and babies, such as suppository to relieve fever of the babies, and that to remove hemorrhoid.

1.3.14　Granule

It refers to the dried particles or tiny blocks processed by mixing drug extracts with proper amount of excipients or fine powder of some drugs, to be taken after infused with boiled water. It has quick action and is tasty, small and convenient to use, therefore is very popular with patients, such as granule for cold and fever, and Fufang Yangjiao Chongji, etc.

1.3.15　Tablet

It refers to a flat preparation made by pressing the mixture of fine powder or extract of drugs with some excipients, small in size and accurate in dosage. Bitter drugs and drugs with an offensive odor can be made into sugar-coated tablets for convenient administration. If it is meant to act only in the intestinal tract, enteric fur can be used

将药物细粉与基质混合制成的一定形状的固体制剂。用于腔道并在其间融化或溶解而释放药物,有杀虫止痒、滑润、收敛等作用。栓剂的特点是通过直肠(也有用于阴道)黏膜吸收,有50%～70%的药物不经过肝脏而直接进入大循环,一方面减少药物在肝脏中的代谢作用,同时减少药物对肝脏的毒性和副作用,还可以避免胃肠液对药物的影响及药物对胃黏膜的刺激作用。婴幼儿直肠给药尤为方便。常用的有小儿解热栓、消痔栓等。

十四、冲剂

冲剂是将药材提取物加适量赋形剂或部分药物细粉制成的干燥颗粒状或块状制剂,用时以开水冲服。冲剂具有作用迅速,味道可口,体积较小,服用方便等特点,深受患者欢迎。常用的有感冒退热冲剂、复方羊角冲剂等。

十五、片剂

片剂是将药物细粉或药材提取物与辅料混合压制而成的片状制剂。片剂用量准确,体积小。味很苦或具恶臭的药物压片后可再包糖衣,使之易于服用。如需在肠道吸

so as to enable it to disintegrate wherein. Tablets also include buccal tablet, effervescent tablet, etc.

1.3.16　Syrup

It refers to the saturated solution of sugar, which is made by concentrating the boiled drug juice without residue and dissolving sugar in it. Syrup is sweet and convenient to use, in small dose and easily absorbed, and thus fits children best, e. g. Zhike Tangjiang, Guipi Tangjiang.

1.3.17　Oral Liquid

It is the refined liquid preparation obtained by extracting drugs by means of water or solvent, which pools up the features of decoction, syrup and injection and has its own merits of small dosage, quick absorption, convenient to use and agreeable taste. There has been an accelerative trend in its development, especially the steady rise in the amount of oral liquid for health care and tonics, e. g. Renshen Fengwangjiang Koufuye, Qiju Dihuang Koufuye, etc.

1.3.18　Injection

It refers to either the aseptic solution, or the aseptic suspension or the aseptic powder for preparing liquid, which has gone through the process of extracting, refining and preparing drugs. It is used for subcutaneous, muscular or intravenous injections, with the characteristics of being accurate in dosage, quick in action and not influenced by the digestive system. It is especially suitable to patients who suffer coma and have difficulty in taking

收的药物,则又可包肠溶衣,使之在肠道中崩解。此外,尚有口含片、泡腾片等。

十六、糖浆剂

糖浆剂是将药物煎煮去渣取汁浓缩后,加入适量蔗糖溶解制成的浓蔗糖水溶液。糖浆剂具有味甜量小,服用方便,吸收较快等特点,尤适用于儿童服用。如止咳糖浆、桂皮糖浆等。

十七、口服液

口服液是将药物用水或其他溶剂提取,经精制而成的内服液体制剂。该制剂集汤剂、糖浆剂、注射剂的特色于一体,具有剂量较小、吸收较快、服用方便、口感适宜等优点。近年来发展很快,尤其是保健与滋补性口服液日益增多,如人参蜂王浆口服液、杞菊地黄口服液等。

十八、注射剂

注射剂是将药物经过提取、精制、配制等步骤而制成的灭菌溶液、无菌混悬液或供配制成液体的无菌粉末,供皮下、肌肉、静脉注射的一种制剂。具有剂量准确,药效迅速,不受消化系统影响的特点,对于神志昏迷,难于口服

medicine，e. g. Qingkailing injection, Shengmai injection, etc.

All the forms mentioned above have their respective features and need to be applied clinically in the light of the pathological conditions and the drug properties in a recipe. In addition，such forms as capsule, moxa, press preparation, enema and spray are also widely used. At present the forms of Chinese Patent medicines have amounted to roughly 60 varieties. Moreover many traditional products have got new forms through renovation, which provide convenience for patients and improve clinical effect as well.

用药的病人尤为适宜。临床常用的有清开灵注射液、生脉注射液等。

以上剂型各有特点，临证应根据病情与方剂中药物特性酌情选用。此外，胶囊剂、灸剂、熨剂、灌肠剂、气雾剂等亦在临床广泛应用，目前中成药剂型已达 60 种左右，还有为数不少的中药传统产品，通过剂型改进研制成新剂型，进一步方便了广大患者，提高了临床药效。

1.4 Usage of Prescriptions

It mainly covers two aspects: the method of decocting drugs and the method of taking drugs, both can help bring about and even enhance the therapeutic effect if used properly. So special attention should be paid to.

1.4.1 Methods of Decocting Drugs

Of all the forms mentioned above, decoction is most commonly used. It should be prepared with suitable method in accordance with the drug properties and condition of illness. Otherwise, it will affect the therapeutic effect.

1.4.1.1 Utensil for Decocting Drugs

It is preferable to use an earthen jug or pot, and then comes the enamelware or aluminum product. But iron or copper wares are forbidden because some drugs, when heated together with iron or copper, may generate sediment, lower solubility or even lead to chemical reaction and side effect. It is also advisable to use a pot with large capacity so as to provide a favorable condition for boiling up drugs without boiling over, accelerating the extraction of active constituents. Besides a lid is necessary to prevent water from evaporating too fast, which is not good for the complete extraction of active constituents.

第四章 方剂的使用方法

方剂的使用方法主要包括煎药方法与服药方法,若用法得当,有助于发挥乃至增强治疗效果,故应加以重视。

第一节 煎药法

方剂在临床使用时最常用的是汤剂。制备汤剂时应根据药物的性质及病情的特点采取合适的煎煮方法,否则就有可能影响疗效。

一、煎药用具

煎药用具以瓦罐、沙锅为好,搪瓷器具或铝制品亦可,忌用铁器、铜器,因为有些药物与铜、铁一起加热之后,会产生沉淀,降低溶解度,甚至会引起化学变化,产生副作用。煎药器皿的容量稍大一些为宜,以利于药物沸腾时不断翻滚,促使有效成分加速浸出,并可避免外溢耗损药液。煎药器皿须加盖,以防水分蒸发过快,使药物的有效成分不能完全溶出。

1. 4. 1. 2　Water for Decocting Drugs

The water used must be pure and clean except some special need. Tap water, well water or distilled water can be used. Our forefathers used to take running water, spring water, wild cabbage-washing water and rice-washing water. Sometimes it is necessary to use liquor or watery wine according to the characteristic of drugs as well as the illness condition. The amount of water used depends on the amount and quality of drugs and time needed. As prepared herbal pieces are dry and able to absorb large amount of water once put in it, adequate amount of water must be put in the pot for boiling drugs. Usually a dose of drugs is decocted twice, some three times. For the first decocting, water is added until the drugs are 3 - 5 cm underwater, and less water may be used for the second and third decocting, each with 100 - 200 ml decoction.

1. 4. 1. 3　Fire for Decocting Drugs

It includes mild fire and strong fire, by the latter is meant quick decocting and by the former slow decocting. Usually strong fire is used until the water boils, followed by mild fire for certain duration. Besides the choice of fire should base on the drug property and time needed. Strong fire is preferable for drugs with the function of relieving exterior syndrome and promoting diuresis, which are decocted for short time and in relatively small amount of water. However, mild fire is advisable for drugs with nourishing function, which are decocted for longer time and in larger amount of water. In case drugs are burnt, they should be discarded to prevent harmful reaction.

二、煎药用水

除处方有特殊规定者外，煎药用水一般以水质纯净为原则，如自来水、井水、蒸馏水等。前人常用流水、泉水、甘澜水（亦称劳水）、米泔水等。根据药物的特点和疾病的性质，也有用酒或水酒合煎的。用水量应视药量、药物质地及煎药时间而定，由于饮片均为失水后的干品，一旦加水引起药材细胞膨胀时，会吸收大量的水分，因此在煎煮时，一定要加足够量的水。每剂药一般煎煮2次，有的可煎煮3次，第一煎水量可适当多些，一般以漫过药面3～5 cm为宜，第二三煎则可略少，每次煎得量100～200 ml左右。

三、煎药火候

煎药的火候有"武火"与"文火"之分。急火煎煮谓之"武火"，慢火煎煮谓之"文火"。一般先用武火，沸腾后改用文火。另外还要根据药物性味及煎煮所需时间的要求，酌定火候。解表与泻下之剂，宜用武火，煎煮时间应较短，加水量亦较少；补益之剂，宜用文火，煎煮时间应较长，加水量亦较多。如不慎将药煎煮焦枯，则应弃之不用，以防发生不良反应。

1.4.1.4　Methods for Decocting Drugs

The drugs are decocted after they have been thoroughly soaked for 20 - 30 minutes in order that the active elements may be readily decocted out. Special decocting methods should be noted in the prescription.

1.4.1.4.1　Decoct first

Shells and minerals, solid in quality with active constituents difficult to extract, should be broken up and decocted first for about 20 minutes before adding other drugs, e. g. Guiban (*Plasstrum Testudinis*), Biejia (*Carapax Trionycis*), Shijueming (*Concha Haliotidis*), fresh Muli (*Concha Ostreae*), Daizheshi (*Ochra Haematitum*), Longgu (*Os Draconis*), Shigao (*Gypsum Fibrosum*), and Cishi (*Magnetitum*), etc. Some drugs with much sand and mud, such as Zaoxintu (*baked earth*), Nuodaogen (*Radix Oryzae Glutinosae*), and some drugs light but in large dosage, such as Lugen (*Rhizoma Phragmitis*), Xiakucao (*Spica Prunellae*), should all be decocted first to get their clarifying juice, in which other drugs are decocted rather than in water. It should be noted in the prescription.

1.4.1.4.2　Decoct later

Aromatic drugs, which acts by means of their volatile oil, are to be added to the mixture and decocted only for about 3 minutes so that their active elements, which are easy to volatilize, are held up, such as Bohe (*Herba Menthae*), Sharen (*Fructus Amomi*), Doukou (*Amomum Kravanh*) and so on. When Dahuang (*Radix et Rhizoma Rhei*) is chiefly used for purgation, it should be decocted for 5 - 10 minutes. All drugs to be decocted later also need to be soaked first.

1.4.1.4.3　Decoct drugs wrapped

Some drugs should be wrapped in a piece of gauze before they are decocted together with other drugs in case

四、煎药方法

煎药前,先将药物浸泡20～30分钟之后再煎煮,有利于有效成分的煎出。对某些有特殊煎服要求的药物,应在处方中加以注明。

（一）先煎

介壳与矿物类药物,因质地坚实,药力难于煎出,应打碎先煎,煮沸后20分钟左右,再下其他药,如龟版、鳖甲、石决明、生牡蛎、代赭石、生龙骨、生石膏、磁石等。某些泥沙多的药物如灶心土、糯稻根等,以及质轻量大的植物药如芦根、夏枯草等,宜先煎取汁澄清,然后以其药汁代水煎其余药物,处方时注明"煎汤代水"。

（二）后下

气味芳香的药物,用其挥发油取效的,宜在其他药物即将煎好时下,煎3分钟左右即可,以防有效成分的散失,如薄荷、砂仁、豆蔻等。用大黄取其攻下之效时,一般煎5～10分钟即可。对所有后下药物,亦应先进行浸泡再煎。

（三）包煎

某些药物煎煮后可致药液混浊,或对咽喉有刺激作

they may make the decoction turbid, produce irritation to the throat or stick to the pot bottom, such as Chishizhi (*Halloysitum Rubrum*), Huashi (*Talcum*), Cheqianzi (*Semen Plantaginis*), Xuanfuhua (*Flos Inulae*), Pu-huang (*Pollen Typhae*) and so on.

1.4.1.4.4 Simmer or decoct separately

Some rare and expensive drugs should be simmered or decocted separately so as to prevent their active elements from being absorbed by other drugs when decocted together. For example, Rensheng (*Radix Ginseng*) should be cut into small slices and put in a bowl with lid and simmered in the pot for 1 - 2 hours. Other rare drugs whose active elements are difficult to be decocted out, such as Lingyangjiao (*Cornu Antelopis*), Shuiniujiao (*Cornu Bubali*), should be made into thin slices and decocted alone for 2 hours, and taken together with the decoction from other drugs. Otherwise, they can be ground to get fine powder for oral administration together with the decoction from other drugs.

1.4.1.4.5 Melt by heating

Some glutinous, sticky and easily-dissolved drugs, such as Ejiao (*Colla Corii Asini*), Lujiaojiao (*Colla Cornus Cervi*), Guibanjiao (*Colla Plastri Testudinis*), maltose, honey and the like, should be dissolved by heating them separately so as to prevent them from sticking to the pot, burning or adhering to other drugs, and affecting their therapeutic effect. Before taken orally, they should be boiled together with the decoction from other drugs with mild fire or mixed when they are still hot.

1.4.1.4.6 Infuse for oral use

Some aromatic or rare drugs, which are not suitable for heating or boiling, should be smashed into fine powder to be taken after infused in medicinal solution or warm boiled water, such as Niuhuang (*Calculus Bovis*), artificial Shexiang (*Moschus*), Hupo (*Succinum*). Besides

用,或易于粘锅,如赤石脂、滑石、车前子、旋复花、蒲黄等,煎煮时宜用纱布袋将药包好,再放入锅内与其他药物同煎。

(四)另炖或另煎

某些贵重药物,为了保存其有效成分,避免同煎时被其他药物吸附,可另炖或另煎。如人参,应切成薄片,放入加盖碗内,隔水炖1～2小时。对于贵重而又难于煎出气味的羚羊角、水牛角等,应切成薄片另煎2小时取汁和服,亦可磨汁或锉成细粉调服。

(五)溶化(烊化)

胶质、粘性大而且容易溶解的药物,如阿胶、鹿角胶、龟版胶、饴糖、蜂蜜之类,用时应单独加温溶化,再加入去渣的药液中微煮或趁热和匀后服,以免和其他药物同煎时易于粘锅煮焦,且粘附它药,影响疗效。

(六)冲服

某些芳香或贵重药物不宜加热煎煮者,应研为细末,用药液或温开水冲服,如牛黄、人工麝香、琥珀等;散剂、药物的粉末以及药物鲜品的

powder and fresh juice of the herbs should also be taken after infused, e. g. Zixue (*Powder*), Chenxiang (*Lignum Aquilariae Resinatum*) powder, Rougui (*Cortex Cinnamomi*) powder, Shensanqi (*Radix Notoginseng*) powder, fresh lotus root juice and fresh carrot juice, etc.

　　Moreover, the herb dregs should be well pressed to get the left juice after a decoction is made so as to increase the extracting rate of drugs.

自然汁亦需冲服,如紫雪、沉香粉、肉桂末、参三七粉、生藕汁、生萝卜汁等。

　　此外,汤剂煎取药液后,应对药渣进行适当压榨,再收取部分存留药液,如此可以提高药材有效成分的浸出率。

1.4.2　Methods of Taking Drugs

　　It also affects the therapeutic effect if a right method is not carried out. Methods of taking drugs include both the time and the method.

1.4.2.1　Time for Taking Drugs

　　The choice of time depends on the location and condition of illness, the category of drugs and the characteristics of disease. Generally speaking, if a disease focuses on the upper-energizer, it is preferable to take drugs after meals; if on the lower-energizer, before meals. Drugs for acute and serious diseases should be taken at any time, while those for chronic diseases taken regularly. Drugs with tonic or purgative action should be taken with an empty stomach, those with sedatives taken at bedtime, and those irritant to the gastrointestinal tract taken after meals. Drugs for malaria should be taken 2 hours before the onset. Besides special requirements are made for few prescriptions. For example, Shizao Tang needs to be taken at dawn, while Jiming San taken just before dawn.

1.4.2.2　Methods of Taking Drugs

　　Usually one dose is decocted 2 - 3 times and the

第二节　服药法

　　服药是否得法,对疗效也有一定的影响。服药方法包括服药时间以及服用方法。

一、服药时间

　　应当根据病位高下、病情轻重、药物类型以及病证特点来决定药物服用的时间。一般来说,病在上焦,宜食后服药;病在下焦,宜食前服药。急性重病应不拘时服,慢性病则应定时服药。补益药与泻下药,宜空腹时服;安神类药物,宜临卧时服;对胃肠有刺激性的药物,应食后服;治疟药宜在发作前 2 小时服。还有少数方剂的服药时间有特殊要求,如十枣汤应平旦时服,鸡鸣散应五更时服等等。

二、服用方法

　　服药次数,汤剂一般是每

combined decoction is to be taken 2 - 3 times daily. In an emergency case, it is advisable either to take a dose at one draught so as to muster the potency or to take it several times daily as tea in order to achieve lasting effect if necessary, or even to take 2 doses daily to enhance the therapeutic effect. In case of chronic diseases, it is advisable to take 2 - 3 times daily in the form of pill, bolus, powder, extract or medicinal liquor. Generally, decoction is mostly to be taken when it is still warm, but there are exceptions. Decoction for heat syndrome should be taken cool while decoction for cold syndrome taken hot, which is meant to enhance the potency. In case of serious diseases, cold-natured decoction should be taken hot and hot-natured decoction taken cool to prevent patients from vomiting after taking the decoction. When drastic or toxic drugs are applied, they should be taken in a small amount at the beginning and with the amount increased gradually. It must be noted that these drugs should be suspended immediately after they have efficacy, and that they must not be overused to avoid toxin or prevent them from damaging body resistance. What's more, proper amount of ginger juice may be added to the decoction for patients apt to vomit after taking the decoction. Likewise the patient may rub the tongue with fresh ginger or chew a little dried tangerine before taking the decoction, or take it cool in small dosage at frequent intervals. For unconscious patients or patients who have difficulty in swallowing, nasal feeding is recommended.

日 1 剂,将两次或三次煎煮之药液合并,分 2～3 次温服。但对急病重证,可顿服以使药力集中,还可根据病情需要采用一日数服、煎汤代茶频服,以使药力持续,病重者可一日连服 2 剂,以加强疗效。慢性病服用丸、散、膏、酒等剂型时,一般每日服 2～3 次。服用汤药,大多采取温服,但也有例外,如治疗热证可以冷服,治疗寒证可以热服,意在辅助药力;若病情严重时,可能发生服药后呕吐的"拒药"反应,则应寒药热服,或热药冷服,以防邪药格拒。服药剂量,使用峻烈的药物以及有毒性的药物时,宜从小量开始,逐渐加量,取效即止,慎勿过量,以免发生中毒反应或戕伤人体正气。此外,对于服汤药后出现恶心呕吐者,可在药液中加入少量姜汁,或用鲜生姜擦舌,或嚼少许陈皮,然后再服汤药,或采用冷服,小量频饮的方法。对于昏迷或吞咽困难者,可用鼻饲法给药。

2 Specific Discussions　　各　论

2.1 Prescriptions for Relieving Exterior Syndromes

第一章
解表剂

Those that are mainly composed of diaphoretics and can induce diaphoresis, expel pathogenic factors from muscles and skin, promote eruptions, and be used to treat exterior syndromes, fall into this category.

Since exterior syndromes cover two types, namely wind-cold type and wind-heat type, prescriptions for relieving exterior syndromes are divided into prescriptions for relieving exterior syndrome with pungent-warm drugs and those for relieving exterior syndrome with pungent-cool drugs accordingly.

The former mainly comprises drugs with pungent flavor and warm property for relieving exterior syndrome. It is capable of expelling wind and cold and applicable to exterior syndrome due to wind-cold, while the latter, pungent and cool drugs for relieving exterior syndrome, capable of dispelling wind and removing heat and applicable to exterior syndrome caused by wind-heat.

Prescriptions for relieving exterior syndrome cannot be decocted long in order to prevent the drug property from dissipating and influencing the curative effect. Besides the patient should take the decoction warm and pay attention to keeping warm by himself afterwards to ensure mild perspiration over the body. In doing so, the pathogenic factors will be expelled from the exterior.

凡以解表药为主组成,具有发汗、解肌、透疹等作用,用于治疗表证的方剂,统称解表剂。

由于表证主要有风寒表证与风热表证两种证型,因而解表剂相应地分为辛温解表剂与辛凉解表剂两类。

辛温解表剂由辛温解表药为主组成,具有疏散风寒作用,适用于风寒表证。辛凉解表剂由辛凉解表药为主组成,具有疏散风热作用,适用于风热表证。

解表剂入汤剂不宜久煎,以免药性耗散,影响疗效;汤药应温服,服药后注意保暖,使遍身微微出汗以利祛邪。

2.1.1 Prescriptions Pungent in Flavor and Warm in Property for Relieving Exterior Syndromes

Mahuang Tang
(*Ephedra Decoction*)

Source: *Shanghan Lun* (*Treatise on Exogenous Febrile Diseases*).

Ingredients:

No. 1 Mahuang (*Herba Ephedrae*) 9 g;

No. 2 Guizhi (*Ramulus Cinnamomi*) 6 g;

No. 3 Xingren (*Semen Armeniaccae Amarum*) 9 g;

No. 4 Zhigancao (*Radix Glycyrrhizae Praeparatae*) 3 g.

Administration: Decoct the above drugs in water for oral use.

Actions: Inducing perspiration to relieve exterior pathogenic factors, dispersing the lung to relieve asthma.

Clinical Application: This recipe is for exterior-excess syndrome due to exogenous wind-cold, marked by aversion to cold, fever, headache, general aching, dyspnea without perspiration, thin and whitish tongue fur, and superficial and tense pulse. It is applicable to common cold, flu, acute bronchitis, bronchial asthma and other diseases which chiefly manifest aversion to cold without perspiration, cough and dyspnea. If complicated with pathogenic dampness marked by arthralgia, heaviness of the body, add Baizhu (*Rhizoma Atractylodis Macrocephalae*) to eliminate dampness, thus making a new one entitled Mahuang Jiazhu Tang. In case of mild aversion to cold but chiefly asthma, subtract Guizhi (*Ramulus Cinnamoni*) to make a recipe entitled San'ao Tang specially for dispersing the lung to relieve asthma. In case of serious aversion to cold without perspiration and general aching body

第一节 辛温解表剂

麻黄汤

【方源】 《伤寒论》。

【组成】 麻黄9g,桂枝6g,杏仁9g,炙甘草3g。

【用法】 水煎服。

【功用】 发汗解表,宣肺平喘。

【临床应用】 适用于外感风寒表实证。症见恶寒发热,头身疼痛,无汗而喘,舌苔薄白,脉浮紧。感冒、流行性感冒、急性支气管炎、支气管哮喘等以恶寒无汗、咳嗽或气喘为主要表现,属风寒表实证者,可用本方治疗。若兼挟湿邪而见关节疼痛、肢体困重者,可加白术以祛湿,即麻黄加术汤;若恶寒不甚而以咳喘为主者,可去桂枝以专于宣肺平喘,即三拗汤;若恶寒无汗身痛较甚并兼里热烦躁者,可倍用麻黄以加强发汗散邪之力,再加石膏以清泄里热,即

accompanied by dysphoria due to interior heat, double the dosage of Mahuang (*Herba Ephedrae*) to enhance the potency of inducing perspiration for eliminating the pathogenic factors and add Shigao (*Gypsum Fibrosum*) to clear away the interior heat, called Da Qinglong Tang.

Elucidation: The syndrome is due to attack of wind-cold on the exterior, obstruction of defensive qi, stagnation of interstitial space, and failure of pulmonary qi to disperse. It should be treated by inducing perspiration to expel pathogenic factors from the exterior and dispersing the lung to relieve asthma. In this recipe, ingredient No. 1 acts as the monarch drug. It is capable of inducing sweating to dispel exogenous pathogenic factors and dispersing the lung to relieve asthma. Ingredient No. 2, as the minister drug, is capable of dispersing pathogenic cold by warming the meridians. Ingredient No. 3 capable of relieving stagnant lung-qi and No. 1 serve as adjuvant drug to enhance the effect of relieving cough and asthma. The last ingredient serves as the guiding drug, capable of mediating drug properties and invigorating qi and enriching mid-energizer so as to prevent ingredients No. 1 and No. 2 from inducing excessive sweating to impair the vital-qi.

Cautions: The recipe is contraindicated for the exterior syndrome due to wind-cold with sweating because it is drastic in inducing sweating. So patients with general debility, blood deficiency and serious interior heat should use it with great caution.

Guizhi Tang
(*Decoction of Cassia Twig*)

Source: *Shanghan Lun* (*Treatise on Exogenous Febrile Diseases*).

Ingredients:

No. 1 Guizhi (*Ramulus Cinnamoni*) 9 g;

No. 2 Shaoyao (*Radix Paeoniae*) 9 g;

大青龙汤。

【方解】　本方证由风寒束表，卫阳被遏，腠理闭塞，肺气失宣所致，治宜发汗解表，宣肺平喘之法。方中麻黄发汗解表，宣肺平喘，为君药。桂枝温经散寒，助麻黄发汗解表，为臣药。杏仁降肺气，与麻黄配伍，一宣一降，可加强止咳平喘作用，为佐药。炙甘草调和药性，又可益气补中，防止麻黄、桂枝可能发汗太过而耗伤正气，为佐使药。

【注意事项】　本方为辛温发汗峻剂，风寒表证而有汗者禁用；素体阴虚、血虚、内热较重者慎用。

桂枝汤

【方源】　《伤寒论》。

【组成】　桂枝 9 g，芍药 9 g，炙甘草 6 g，生姜 9 g，大枣 3 枚。

No. 3 Zhigancao (*Radix Glycyrrhizae Praeparatae*) 6 g;

No. 4 Shengjiang (*Rhizoma Zingiberis Recens*) 9 g;

No. 5 Dazao (*Fructus Ziziphi Jujubae*) 3 pcs.

Administration: Decoct the above drugs in water for oral use.

Actions: Expelling pathogenic factors from the muscles and skin, and regulating yingqi and weiqi to relieve exterior syndrome.

Clinical Application: This recipe is indicated for exterior deficiency syndrome due to exogenous wind-cold and syndrome with disharmony between yingqi and weiqi, and yin and yang after illness or delivery, marked by headache, fever, perspiration with aversion to wind, thin whitish fur, superficial and moderate pulse. It is applicable to common cold, flu, urticaria, cutaneous pruritus, and unknown low fever and low fever after delivery or illness and others, which pertain to the disorder between yingqi and weiqi, and yin and yang. Ingredient No. 2 is now often substituted for Baishaoyao (*Radix Paeoniae Alba*). If accompanied by stiffness and pain over the neck and back, add Gegen (*Radix Puerariae*) to dispel pathogenic factors from the body surface and promote the production of body fluid, and relaxation of tendons, forming another recipe entitled Guzhi plus Gegen Tang. If concomitant with cough or asthma, add Houpo (*Cortex Magnoliae Officinalis*) and Xingren (*Semen Armeniacae Amarum*) to send down the adversely rising qi for relieving cough and asthma, entitled Guizhi Jia Houpo Xingzi Tang.

Elucidation: The syndrome is caused by exogenous wind-cold, disharmony between yingqi and weiqi, or debility after illness or delivery and disharmony between yingqi and weiqi, and yin and yang. It should be treated by expelling pathogenic factors from the muscles and skin and regulating yingqi and weiqi. Ingredient No. 1 in the

【用法】 水煎服。

【功用】 解肌发表,调和营卫。

【临床应用】 适用于外感风寒表虚证以及病后、产后营卫阴阳失和证。症见头痛发热,汗出恶风,舌苔薄白,脉浮缓。感冒、流行性感冒、荨麻疹、皮肤瘙痒症、原因不明的低热、产后或病后低热等属营卫失调或阴阳失和者,可用本方治疗。方中芍药,现临床多用白芍药。若兼项背强痛,可加葛根以解肌发表,生津舒筋,即桂枝加葛根汤;若兼咳嗽或气喘者,可加厚朴、杏仁以下气止咳平喘,即桂枝加厚朴杏子汤。

【方解】 本方证由外感风寒,营卫失和,或病后、产后体弱,营卫阴阳失和所致,治宜解肌发表,调和营卫之法。方中桂枝解肌散寒,温经助阳,为君药。芍药养阴益津,

recipe is the monarch drug able to expel pathogenic cold from the muscles and skin and warm the meridians for enhancing yang. No. 2 performs the action of nourishing yin to promote the production of body fluid, and astringing yingqi to suppress sweating, functioning as the minister drug. The combination of the first two ingredients in the same dosage ensures removing wind-cold, consolidating yingqi and yin, harmonizing yingqi and weiqi, and yin and yang. Ingredient No. 4 performs, in combination with No. 1, the double action of dispelling cold and regulating the stomach, and No. 5 with No. 2 the action of replenishing yin and reinforcing the spleen. Therefore these two ingredients serve as adjuvant drugs, enhancing the effect of the monarch and minister drugs in regulating yingqi and weiqi, and yin and yang, as well as reinforcing the spleen and stomach to replenish the source of generation and transformation of yingqi and weiqi. Ingredient No. 3, sweet in flavor, plays the part of adjuvant drug on the one hand, replenishing qi and regulating the stomach. When combined with ingredient No. 1 sweet and pungent in flavor, it expels pathogenic factors from the body surface, and with No. 2 sour and sweet in flavor it transforms yin to regulate yingqi. On the other hand, it plays the role of guiding drug, mediating drug properties.

Both Mahuang Tang and Guizhi Tang are used to treat exterior syndrome due to exogenous wind-cold. Mahuang (*Herba Ephedrae*) and Guizhi (*Ramulus Cinnamomi*) plus Xingren (*Semen Armeniaccae Amarum*) in Mahuang Tang are to enhance the effect of inducing sweating and dispelling cold, capable of dispersing the lung and relieving asthma. It is a drastic prescription of inducing sweating with pungent and warm drugs. And it is applicable to the exterior excess syndrome due to exogenous wind-cold, marked by aversion to cold, fever without

敛营止汗，为臣药。桂、芍等量配伍，一散一收，可使风寒外散，营阴内固，营卫和谐，阴阳调和。生姜助桂枝散寒，又能和胃；大枣助芍药益阴，并可补脾，两药既可增强君、臣药调和营卫阴阳之效，又能调补脾胃以充营卫生化之源，共为佐药。炙甘草之功有二：一为佐药，益气和中，合桂枝辛甘化阳以解肌，合芍药酸甘化阴以和营；一为使药，调和药性。

麻黄汤与桂枝汤均可治疗外感风寒表证，但麻黄汤中麻、桂并用，佐以杏仁，发汗散寒力强，又能宣肺平喘，为辛温发汗峻剂，适用于外感风寒，恶寒发热而无汗咳喘之风寒表实证；桂枝汤中桂、芍并用，佐以姜、枣，发汗解表作用不及麻黄汤，但长于调和营卫，适用于外感风寒，发热有

perspiration, cough and asthma. While, Guizhi (*Ramulus Cinnamoni*) and Baishaoyao (*Radix Paeoniae Alba*) plus Shengjiang (*Rhizoma Zingiberis Recens*) and Dazao (*Fructus Ziziphi Jujubae*) are used in Guizhi Tang, its action of relieving the exterior syndrome by means of inducing sweating is not so strong as that of Mahuang Tang, but stronger in regulating yingqi and weiqi. It is applicable to exterior deficiency syndrome due to exogenous wind-cold, marked by fever with perspiration, and aversion to wind.

Cautions: This recipe is mild in its action of inducing sweat, so is called "dispelling pathogenic factors from muscles and skin," and not applicable to patients of exterior syndrome due to exogenous wind-cold but without perspiration. The patient has to take one bowl of hot gruel after administration of the decoction and put on more clothes or quilts to help induce sweat.

Xiangru San
(*Powder of Elsholtziae*)

Source: *Taiping Huimin Hejiju Fang* (*Benevolent Prescription from Taiping Pharmaceutical Bureau*).

Ingredients:

No. 1 Xiangru (*Herba Elsholtziae seu Moslae*) 15 g;

No. 2 Baibiandou (*Semen Dolichoris Album*) 12 g;

No. 3 Houpo (*Cortex Magnoliae Officinalis*) 12 g.

Administration: Grind the above drugs into coarse powder, and then decoct the above drugs in water or water with little liquor, 9 g each time.

Actions: Relieving exterior syndrome and dispelling cold, removing dampness to restore the normal function of the middle-energizer.

Clinical Application: This recipe is indicated for the syndrome of exterior cold with interior dampness

汗而恶风之风寒表虚证。

【注意事项】 本方发汗力量较弱,故称之为"解肌",风寒表证而无汗者不宜使用。服本方后需喝热粥一碗,并增添衣被,以助汗出。

香薷散

【方源】 《太平惠民和剂局方》。

【组成】 香薷15 g,白扁豆12 g,厚朴12 g。

【用法】 共研粗末,每次9 g,水煎服,或加酒少量同煎服。

【功用】 解表散寒,化湿和中。

【临床应用】 适用于夏季外寒内湿证。症见恶寒发

occurring in summer days, marked by aversion to cold, fever without perspiration, headache, abdominal pain, vomiting, diarrhea, chest distress, fatigue, greasy whitish fur, and superficial pulse. It is applicable to common cold and acute gastroenteritis occurring in summer and others, which are marked by aversion to cold without perspiration, headache, heavy sensation of body, chest distress, greasy tongue fur and pertain to external cold and internal dampness. In case of accompanying interior accumulation of summer-heat manifesting thirst, flushed cheeks, superficial and rapid pulse, add Jinyinhua (*Flos Lonicerae*) and Lianqiao (*Fructus Forsythiae*) to clear away summer-heat, which forms another recipe entitled Xinjia Xiangru Yin. In case of serious pathogenic dampness with borborygmus and diarrhea, add Fuling (*Poria*), Baizhu (*Rhizoma Atractylodis Macrocephalae*) to reinforce the spleen and eliminate dampness.

Elucidation: The syndrome is caused by staying in a cool place or having cold drinks in summer, resulting in attack on superficies by cold, stagnated interstitial space, internal impairment due to dampness, and disharmony between the spleen and stomach. It should be treated by relieving exterior syndrome and dispelling cold, and by removing dampness to restore normal function of the middle-energizer. Ingredient No. 1 acted as monarch drug can induce sweat and dispel cold, relieve the exterior syndrome and remove dampness, playing the part of monarch drug. Ingredient No. 3 has the function of promoting qi flow to relieve flatulence, eliminating dampness retention and smoothing the middle energizer, acting as minister drug. Ingredient No. 2, capable of reinforcing the spleen to restore normal function of the middle-energizer and eliminating dampness and summer-heat, is used as adjuvant drug. The small amount of liquor used in decoction is

热,无汗头痛,腹痛吐泻,胸闷身倦,舌苔白腻,脉浮。夏季感冒、急性胃肠炎等以恶寒无汗,头痛身重,胸闷苔腻为主症,属外寒内湿者,可用本方治疗。本方为夏季外感寒邪的常用方剂,若兼暑热内蕴,口渴面赤,脉浮数者,可加金银花、连翘以清热祛暑,即新加香薷饮;若湿邪较甚,肠鸣腹泻者,可加茯苓、白术以健脾渗湿。

【方解】　本方证由暑月乘凉饮冷,外感于寒,腠理闭塞,内伤于湿,脾胃失和所致,治宜解表散寒,化湿和中之法。方中香薷发汗散寒,解表化湿,为君药。厚朴行气除满,燥湿畅中,为臣药。白扁豆健脾和中,化湿消暑,为佐药。入酒少许同煎,意在增强散寒通经之力。

supposed to enhance the effect of expelling cold and activating the meridians.

Cautions: This recipe, which is pungent, warm, bitter and dry, possesses a drastic effect of inducing perspiration. Therefore it is contraindicated for perspiring patients with exterior syndrome due to exogenous wind-cold in summer.

Xingsu San
(*Powder of Almond and Perilla*)

Source: *Wenbing Tiaobian* (*Detailed Analysis of Seasonal Febrile Diseases*).

杏苏散

【方源】 《温病条辨》。

Ingredients:

No. 1 Suye (*Folium Perillae*) 9 g;

No. 2 Xingren (*Semen Armeniacae Amarum*) 9 g;

No. 3 Banxia (*Rhizoma Pinelliae*) 9 g;

No. 4 Fuling (*Poria*) 9 g;

No. 5 Qianhu (*Radix Peucedani*) 9 g;

No. 6 Jiegeng (*Radix Platycodi*) 6 g;

No. 7 Zhike (*Fructus Aurantii*) 6 g;

No. 8 Jupi (*Exocarpium Citri Grandis*) 6 g;

No. 9 Gancao (*Radix Glycyrrhizae*) 3 g;

No. 10 Shengjiang (*Rhizoma Zingiberis Recens*) 3pcs;

No. 11 Dazao (*Fructus Ziziphi Jujubae*) 3pcs.

【组成】 苏叶9 g,杏仁9 g,半夏9 g,茯苓9 g,前胡9 g,桔梗6 g,枳壳6 g,橘皮6 g,甘草3 g,生姜3 片,大枣3 枚。

Administration: Decoct the above drugs in water for oral use.

【用法】 水煎服。

Actions: Eliminating cool-dryness, dispersing the lung and resolving phlegm.

【功用】 轻宣凉燥,宣肺化痰。

Clinical Application: This recipe is indicated for cool-dryness syndrome due to exogenous pathogenic factors, marked by aversion to cold without sweat, slight headache, cough with whitish sputum, nasal obstruction and dryness of throat, thin and whitish fur, taut or superficial pulse. This recipe is also applicable to common cold,

【临床应用】 适用于外感凉燥证。症见恶寒无汗,头微痛,咳嗽痰白,鼻塞咽干,舌苔薄白,脉弦或浮。感冒、流行性感冒、急慢性支气管炎等属外感凉燥证(或外感风寒轻

flu, acute or chronic bronchitis and others, which pertain to exogenous cool-dryness syndrome (or slight wind-cold syndrome). In case of headache and concomitant ache in superciliary arch, add Baizhi (*Radix Angelicae Dahuricae*) to dispel pathogenic wind and relieve headache. If the patient perspires only after the administration but with cough unrelieved, remove ingredient No. 1 and add Sugeng (*Caulis Perillae*) and Pipaye (*Folium Eriobotryae*) so as to enhance the effect of regulating the flow of qi to relieve cough.

Elucidation: The syndrome is due to pathogenic cool-dryness in late autumn days, which results in failure of the lung to disperse and descend, and phlegm due to the accumulation of body fluid. Therefore it should be treated by relieving cool-dryness syndrome with drugs mild in properties, and dispersing the lung to resolve phlegm. Ingredient No. 1, pungent and warm in property with moistening action, can expel pathogenic factors from the surface by means of diaphoresis. Ingredient No. 2, bitter and pungent and warm in property with moistening action, is supposed to disperse the lung to resolve phlegm. The two are combined to treat both the lung and weifen, playing together the part of monarch drug. Minister drug includes ingredient No. 5, No. 6 and No. 7, which function respectively to expel wind and descend adversely rising qi to resolve phlegm, and to regulate qi function. Ingredients No. 3, No. 8 and No. 4 serve as adjuvant drugs, regulating the flow of qi to resolve phlegm. Ingredient No. 9 is meant to mediate drug properties and to resolve phlegm and relieve sore throat in combination with No. 6. Ingredients No. 10 and No. 11 can regulate yingqi and weiqi, and mediate drug properties as well. So the above four ingredients act together as adjuvant and guiding drugs. This recipe, warm but not dry and diaphoretic but not drastic

证)者,可用本方治疗。若头痛兼眉棱骨痛者,可加白芷以祛风止痛;若药后汗出但咳仍不止者,可去苏叶,加苏梗、枇杷叶以加强理气止咳之功。

【方解】　本方证由深秋季节凉燥外袭,肺失宣降,津聚成痰所致,治宜轻宣凉燥,宣肺化痰之法。方中苏叶辛温而润,疏表散邪;杏仁苦辛温润,宣肺止咳,两药配伍,肺卫并治,共为君药。前胡疏风散邪,降气化痰;桔梗、枳壳一升一降,调理气机,同为臣药。半夏、橘皮、茯苓理气化痰,助君、臣药宣肺止咳化痰,为佐药。甘草调和药性,配桔梗宣肺止咳,化痰利咽;生姜、大枣调营卫,和诸药,均为佐使药。本方温而不燥,散而不峻,药性温润平和,因而既是治疗外感凉燥证的代表方,又可用于外感风寒,邪浅病轻之证。

in property, is a representative one in the treatment of cool-dryness syndrome due to exogenous pathogenic factors. Simultaneously it is applicable to slight case of exterior syndrome due to exogenous wind-cold.

Cautions: It is mild in its diaphoretic action and thus not suitable for cases with serious aversion to cold and aching body but without dryness of the nasal cavity and throat.

【注意事项】 本方疏散力轻,恶寒身痛较甚而无鼻咽干燥者不宜使用。

Jiuwei Qianghuo Tang
(*Decoction of Nine Ingredients Containing Notopterygium*)

九味羌活汤

Source: *Prescription developed by Zhang Yuansu, quoted from Cishi Nanzhi (Difficult Medical Problems)*.

【方源】 张元素方,录自《此事难知》。

Ingredients:

No. 1 Qianghuo (*Rhizoma seu Radix Notopterygii*) 6 g;

No. 2 Fangfeng (*Radix Ledebouriellae*) 6 g;

No. 3 Cangzhu (*Rhizoma Atractylodis*) 6 g;

No. 4 Xixin (*Herba Asari*) 3 g;

No. 5 Chuanxiong (*Rhizoma Ligustici Chuanxiong*) 3 g;

No. 6 Baizhi (*Radix Angelicae Dahuricae*) 3 g;

No. 7 Shengdihuang (*Radix Rehmanniae*) 3 g;

No. 8 Huangqin (*Radix Scutellariae*) 3 g;

No. 9 Gancao (*Radix Glycyrrhizae*) 3 g.

【组成】 羌活、防风、苍术各6 g,细辛、川芎、白芷、生地黄、黄芩、甘草各3 g。

Administration: Decoct the above drugs in water for oral use.

【用法】 水煎服。

Actions: Inducing diaphoresis, eliminating dampness, and clearing away interior heat.

【功用】 发汗祛湿,兼清里热。

Clinical Application: This recipe is indicated for syndrome due to the attack of exogenous wind, cold and dampness with interior heat, marked by aversion to cold, fever, absence of perspiration, headache, aching limbs, bitter taste in the mouth with slight thirst, whitish or yellowish fur, and superficial pulse. It is applicable to common cold, flu, rheumatic arthritis, and migraine,

【临床应用】 适用于外感风寒湿邪兼有里热证。症见恶寒发热,无汗头痛,肢体酸楚疼痛,口苦微渴,舌苔白或微黄,脉浮。感冒、流行性感冒、风湿性关节炎、偏头痛等见有上述症状者,属风寒湿

etc. , which have the above symptoms and belong to pathogenic wind, cold and dampness in the exterior with heat in the interior. If there is a sharp pain over the extremities, the dosage of ingredient No. 1 may be doubled to enhance the effect in alleviating arthralgia. In case of slight dampness with mild aching extremities, subtract ingredients No. 3 and No. 4 which are warm and dryness in property. In case of no bitter taste and slight thirst, subtract ingredients No. 7 and No. 8 which are cold in property.

Elucidation：The syndrome is caused by exogenous wind-cold, dampness and interior heat. It should be treated by dispelling wind-cold, removing dampness, relieving the exterior syndrome, and clearing away interior heat. Ingredient No. 1 plays the part of monarch drug, relieving the exterior cold, expelling wind, and removing dampness. The minister drug comprises ingredients No. 2 and No. 3. It acts to remove dampness by inducing perspiration to help the monarch drug dispel pathogenic factors from the exterior. Ingredients No. 4, No. 5 and No. 6 are able to expel wind-cold, promote the circulation of both qi and blood, and alleviate pain, while No. 7 and No. 8 able to eliminate interior heat and prevent pungent, warm, dry and drastic drugs from impairing the body fluid. Thus these five ingredients constitute the adjuvant drug. The last ingredient is supposed to mediate drug properties, acting as guiding drug.

Cautions：This recipe, pungent, warm, dry and drastic in property, is mainly to relieve exterior syndrome. Therefore it is not applicable to cases with excessive interior heat, high fever, thirst, red tongue and rapid pulse.

Xiao Qinglong Tang
（*Small Blue Dragon Decoction*）
Source：*Shanghan Lun*（*Treatise on Exogenous*

邪在表兼有里热者,可用本方治疗。若肢体疼痛较剧者,可倍用羌活以加强通痹止痛之力;若湿邪较轻,肢体酸楚不甚者,可去苍术、细辛以减温燥之性;若无口苦微渴者,可减去寒凉的生地黄、黄芩。

【方解】　本方证由外感风寒湿邪,内有蕴热所致,治宜疏风散寒,祛湿解表,兼清里热之法。方中羌活解表散寒,祛风胜湿,为君药。防风、苍术发汗祛湿,助羌活解表,同为臣药。细辛、川芎、白芷,散风寒,行气血,止疼痛;生地黄、黄芩清泄里热,并防诸辛温燥烈之品伤津之弊,均为佐药。甘草调和药性,为使药。

【注意事项】　本方以解表为主,药性辛温燥烈,若里热偏甚,高热口渴,舌红脉数者禁用。

小青龙汤

【方源】　《伤寒论》。

Febrile Diseases).

Ingredients：

No. 1 Mahuang (*Herba Ephedrae*) 9 g;

No. 2 Shaoyao (*Radix Paeoniae*) 9 g;

No. 3 Xixin (*Herba Asari*) 6 g;

No. 4 Ganjiang (*Rhizoma Zingiberis*) 6 g;

No. 5 Zhigancao (*Radix Glycyrrhizae Praeparatae*) 6 g;

No. 6 Guizhi (*Ramulus Cinnamomi*) 9 g;

No. 7 Banxia (*Rhizoma Pinelliae*) 9 g;

No. 8 Wuweizi (*Fructus Schisandrae*) 6 g.

Administration：Decoct the above drugs in water for oral use.

Actions：Relieving the pathogenic factors from the exterior and expelling cold, warming the lung to resolve retained fluid.

Clinical Application：This recipe is indicated for external cold and interior fluid-retention, marked by aversion to cold, fever without perspiration, headache, cough and asthma with profuse thin sputum, inability to keep horizontal posture if serious, or swollen extremities, smooth whitish fur, and superficial pulse. It is applicable to acute onset of chronic bronchitis, bronchial asthma, and senile pulmonary emphysema, etc., which are marked by aversion to cold, absence of perspiration, cough with profuse sputum and are attributable to exogenous wind-cold and accumulation of cold retention in the lung. Baishaoyao (*Radix Paeoniae Alba*) is now often used as ingredient No. 2. In case of not serious exterior-cold syndrome without obvious aversion to cold, sweating and headache, subtract ingredient No. 6, and replace No. 1 with honey-prepared one so as to weaken the action of relieving pathogenic factors from the exterior. If complicated with thirst, subtract ingredient No. 7 and add Tianhuafen (*Radix Trichosanthis*) to clear away heat and

【组成】 麻黄 9g,芍药 9 g,细辛 6 g,干姜 6 g,炙甘草 6 g,桂枝 9 g,半夏 9 g,五味子 6 g。

【用法】 水煎服。

【功用】 解表散寒,温肺 化饮。

【临床应用】 适用于外 寒内饮证。症见恶寒发热,无 汗头痛,咳嗽气喘,痰多质稀, 甚则不能平卧,或肢体浮肿, 舌苔白滑,脉浮。慢性支气管 炎急性发作、支气管哮喘、老 年性肺气肿等以恶寒无汗,咳 喘痰多为主要表现,属外感风 寒、寒饮伏肺者,可用本方治 疗。方中芍药,现临床多用白 芍药。若表寒不甚,恶寒无汗 头痛不著者,可去桂枝,麻黄 改用蜜炙,以减解表之力;若 兼口渴者,可去半夏之燥,加 天花粉以清热生津;若痰饮化 热,出现烦躁者,可加石膏以 清热除烦,即小青龙加石 膏汤。

promote the production of body fluid. If phlegm retention transforms into heat, manifested as dysphoria, add Shigao (*Gypsum Fibrosum*) to clear away heat and relieve dysphoria, forming another recipe entitled Xiao Qinglong plus Shigao Tang.

Elucidation: The syndrome is the result of wind-cold attack on the exterior, accumulation of cold fluid retention in the lung, and failure of the lung-qi to descend. The treatment should focus on relieving exterior syndrome to dissipate cold as well as warming the lung and resolving fluid-retention. Ingredients No. 1 and No. 6 both act as monarch drugs, inducing diaphoresis to relieve the exterior and dispersing the lung to relieve asthma. No. 3 and No. 4 serve as minister drugs, capable of warming the lung to remove cold and helping yang remove fluid retention. Ingredient No. 2 has the effects of nourishing blood and astringing yin, and No. 8 of astringing the lung to relieve asthma. Both prevent such pungent, warm and dry ingredients as No. 1, No. 3 and No. 4 from impairing body fluid and consuming qi, closing amidst opening, astringing amidst dispersing, and eliminating the pathogenic factors without impairment of vital-qi. Ingredient No. 7 acts as adjuvant drug, drying dampness and resolving phlegm, and No. 5 as guiding drug, replenishing qi and mediating drug properties.

Cautions: This recipe is warm and dry in property, and thus not applicable to cases with cough and asthma with yellowish sputum.

Zhisou San
(*Powder for Relieving Cough*)

Source: *Yixue Xinwu* (*A Summary on Medicine from Clinical Practice*).

Ingredients:

No. 1 Jiegeng (*Radix Platycodi*) 1,000 g;

【方解】　本方证由风寒束表,寒饮伏肺,肺失宣降所致,治宜解表散寒,温肺化饮之法。方中麻黄、桂枝发汗解表,宣肺平喘,共为君药。干姜、细辛温肺散寒,助阳化饮,同为臣药。芍药养血敛阴,五味子敛肺平喘,制约麻黄、细辛、干姜过于辛温燥散可能伤津耗气之偏,可使开中有合,散中寓收,祛邪而不伤正气;半夏燥湿化痰,助干姜、细辛温化寒饮,俱为佐药。炙甘草益气和中,调和药性,为使药。

【注意事项】　本方药性温燥,咳喘痰黄者禁用。

止嗽散

【方源】　《医学心悟》。

【组成】　桔梗、荆芥、紫菀、百部、白前各1 000 g,炙甘

No. 2 Jingjie (*Herba Schizonepetae*) 1,000 g；

No. 3 Ziwan (*Radix Asteris*) 1,000 g；

No. 4 Baibu (*Radix Stemonae*) 1,000 g；

No. 5 Baiqian (*Rhizoma Cynanchi Stauntonii*) 1,000 g；

No. 6 Zhigancao (*Radix Glycyrrhizae Praeparatae*) 375 g；

No. 7 Chenpi (*Pericarpium Citri Reticulatae*) 500g.

Administration：Grind the above ingredients into fine powder for oral administration with water and 9 g each time；for cases that are caused by exogenous wind-cold, they should be taken twice daily after mixed with the decoction of Shengjiang (*Rhizoma Zingiberis Recens*). Or decoct them in water and take it with dosages in proportion to the original recipe.

Actions：Expelling wind and dispersing the lung, relieving cough and eliminating phlegm.

Clinical Application：This is indicated for invasion of the lung by exogenous wind, marked by cough, itching throat, whitish sputum, slight aversion to wind, fever, thin whitish fur, and superficial pulse. It is applicable to upper respiratory tract infection, acute and chronic bronchitis, and pertussis, etc., which have the above symptoms and belong to attack of pathogenic wind on the lung and dysfunction of the lung. In case of attack by exogenous wind-cold, marked by headache, nasal obstruction, marked aversion to cold, and thin whitish fur, add Fangfeng (*Radix Ledebouriellae*), Suye (*Folium Perillae*), Shengjiang (*Rhizoma Zingiberis Recens*) to relieve exterior syndrome and dispel cold. In case of attack by exogenous wind-heat marked by cough with sticky sputum, dryness of the mouth and sore throat, red tongue with yellowish fur, add Niubangzi (*Fructus Arctii*), Jinyinhua (*Flos Lonicerae*), Lianqiao (*Fructus Forsythiae*) to expel wind and clear away heat.

Elucidation：The syndrome is caused by cough due

草375 g,橘皮 500 g。

【用法】 共研细末,每次 9 g,温开水调服,初感风寒者 以生姜汤调服,每日 2 次。亦 可作汤剂,用量按原方比例 酌定。

【功用】 疏风宣肺,止咳 化痰。

【临床应用】 适用于风 邪犯肺证。症见咳嗽咽痒,咯 痰色白,或微有恶风发热,舌 苔薄白,脉浮。上呼吸道感 染、急性支气管炎、慢性支气 管炎、百日咳等见有上述症 状,属风邪犯肺,肺气失宣者, 可用本方治疗。若外感风寒, 头痛鼻塞,恶寒明显,舌苔薄 白者,可加防风、苏叶、生姜以 解表散寒；若外感风热,咳嗽 痰粘,口干咽痛,舌红苔黄者, 可加牛蒡子、金银花、连翘以 疏风清热。

【方解】 本方证为外感

to exogenous pathogenic factors, which is unrelieved after the use of diaphoretic drugs to disperse the lung. It should be treated by means of expelling wind and dispersing the lung as well as relieving cough and resolving phlegm. Ingredients No. 3 and No. 4, bitter, warm but not hot and moist but not greasy, act together as monarch drug, relieving cough and dissolving phlegm. Ingredients No. 1 and No. 5 in combination serve as minister drug, capable of dispersing the lung to descend pulmonary qi and relieving cough and resolving sputum. No. 2, capable of expelling residual pathogenic factors from the superficies, and No. 7, capable of regulating the flow of qi and dissolving phlegm, act together as adjuvant drug. Used as guiding drug, No. 6 can mediate drug properties and relieve sore throat together with No. 1. This recipe is warm, moist and moderate in nature, and thus can be modified to treat protracted cough as the result of the lung being attacked by exogenous pathogenic factors, no matter it belongs to excess cold or heat syndrome.

Cautions: It is not advisable for patients with protracted cough, red tongue and little fur that are associated with deficiency of the lung-yin, or for those with obstruction due to lung-heat marked by cough, dyspnea, and profuse yellowish sputum.

Baidu San
(*Antiphlogistic Powder*)

Source: *Xiao'er Yaozheng Zhijue* (*Key to Therapeutics of Children's Diseases*).

Ingredients:

No. 1 Chaihu (*Radix Bupleuri*) 9 g;

No. 2 Qianhu (*Radix Peucedani*) 9 g;

No. 3 Chuanxiong (*Rhizoma Ligustici Chuanxiong*) 9 g;

No. 4 Zhike (*Fructus Aurantii*) 9 g;

No. 5 Qianghuo (*Rhizoma et Radix Notopterygii*) 9 g;

咳嗽，经服解表宣肺药后而咳仍不止者，治宜疏风宣肺，止咳化痰之法。方中紫菀、百部苦温而润，功专止咳化痰，且皆温而不热，润而不腻，新、久咳嗽均可使用，共为君药。桔梗宣肺化痰，白前降气止咳，两药配伍，宣降肺气，止咳化痰，同为臣药。荆芥疏风散邪，以除在表之余邪；橘皮理气化痰，均为佐药。炙甘草调和药性，合桔梗又可利咽止咳，为使药。本方药性温润平和，故凡外邪犯肺，咳嗽日久不愈，不论偏寒或偏热者，均可加减用之。

【注意事项】　咳嗽日久，舌红少苔，属肺阴不足者，或肺热壅盛，咳喘痰黄者，禁用本方。

败毒散

【方源】　《小儿药证直诀》。

【组成】　柴胡、前胡、川芎、枳壳、羌活、独活、茯苓、桔梗、人参各9 g，甘草5 g。

No. 6 Duhuo (*Radix Angelicae Pubescentis*) 9 g;

No. 7 Fuling (*Poria*) 9 g;

No. 8 Jiegeng (*Radix Platycodi*) 9 g;

No. 9 Renshen (*Radix Ginseng*) 9 g;

No. 10 Gancao (*Radix Glycyrrhizae*) 5 g.

Administration: Grind the drugs into coarse powder. Decoct 6 g of the powder with a small amount of Shengjiang (*Rhizoma Zingiberis Recens*) and Bohe (*Herba Menthae*).

Actions: Replenishing qi and relieving exterior syndrome, expelling cold and dampness.

Clinical Application: This recipe is indicated for qi deficiency due to attack by exogenous pathogenic factors, marked by aversion to cold, fever, headache, aching body, no perspiration, nasal obstruction, cough with whitish sputum, chest distress, pale tongue with whitish fur, superficial and weak pulse. It is applicable to common cold, bronchitis, allergic dermatitis, urticaria, eczema, sores, and ulcer, etc., which have the above symptoms and belong to qi deficiency due to exogenous wind, cold and dampness. In the absence of vital-qi deficiency, subtract ingredient No. 9 or add Jingjie (*Herba Schizonepetae*) and Fangfeng (*Radix Ledebouriellae*) to expel exogenous pathogenic factors and relieving exterior syndrome, forming another recipe entitled Jingfang Baidu San. In case of cutaneous pruritus, add Chantui (*Periostracum Cicadae*) and Kushen (*Radix Sophorae Flavescentis*) to dispel wind, relieve itching, and clear away heat and dampness. At the onset of sores and ulcer, replace ingredient No. 9 with Jinyinhua (*Flos Lonicerae*) and Lianqiao (*Fructus Forsythiae*) to clear away heat and toxins and resolve mass.

Elucidation: The syndrome is the result of weak constitution and attack by pathogenic wind, cold, and

【用法】　共研粗末，每次6 g，入生姜、薄荷少许，水煎服。

【功用】　益气解表，散寒祛湿。

【临床应用】　适用于气虚外感证。症见恶寒发热，头身疼痛，无汗鼻塞，咳嗽痰白，胸闷，舌淡苔白，脉浮而按之无力。感冒、支气管炎、过敏性皮炎、荨麻疹、湿疹、疮疡初起等见有上述症状，属气虚外感风寒湿邪者，可用本方治疗。若正气不虚者，可去人参，或再加荆芥、防风，以专于解表祛邪，即荆防败毒散；若治疗皮疹瘙痒者，可加蝉蜕、苦参以疏风止痒，清热除湿；若用于疮疡初起，可去人参，加金银花、连翘以清热解毒，散结消肿。

【方解】　本方证由正气素虚，外感风寒湿邪，肺失宣

dampness, leading to the lung's failure in dispersing and descending function. The method of replenishing qi and relieving exterior syndrome, and dispelling cold and dampness should be adopted. Ingredients No. 5 and No. 6 act as monarch drugs, dispersing pathogenic wind, cold and dampness. Ingredient No. 3, capable of eliminating pathogenic factors, removing obstruction in meridians and relieving pain, and No. 1, capable of eliminating pathogenic factors from muscles and skin, together play the part of minister drug. Ingredients No. 8, No. 4, No. 2 and No. 7 are meant to disperse the lung-qi, resolve phlegm and relieve cough, and No. 9 has the function of replenishing qi and building up body resistance. These five ingredients together form the adjuvant drug. Ingredient No. 10 serves as guiding drug, mediating drug properties and helping No. 9 carry out its function. Shengjiang (*Rhizoma Zingiberis Recens*) and Bohe (*Herba Menthae*) are supposed to enhance the diaphoretic effect.

2.1.2 Prescriptions Pungent in Flavor and Cool in Property for Relieving Exterior Syndrome

Sangju Yin
(*Decoction of Mulberry Leaf and Chrysanthemum*)

Source: *Wenbing Tiaobian* (*Detailed Analysis of Seasonal Febrile Diseases*).

Ingredients:

No. 1 Sangye (*Folium Mori*) 7.5 g;

No. 2 Juhua (*Flos Chrysanthemi*) 3 g;

No. 3 Xingren (*Semen Armeniacae Amarum*) 6 g;

No. 4 Lianqiao (*Fructus Forsythiae*) 5 g;

No. 5 Bohe (*Herba Menthae*) 2.5 g;

降所致,治宜益气解表,散寒祛湿之法。方中羌活、独活发散一身上下之风寒湿邪,共为君药。川芎散邪通络止痛,柴胡疏风散邪解肌,助君药疏散表邪,同为臣药。桔梗宣开肺气,枳壳行气宽胸,前胡祛痰止咳,茯苓健脾渗湿,四药同用以宣利肺气,化痰止咳;人参益气扶正以驱邪外出,且与辛散药同用,散中有补,不伤元气,皆为佐药。甘草调和药性,并助人参益气和中,为使药。生姜、薄荷为药引,意在取其发散之功以加强解表散邪之效。

第二节 辛凉
解表剂

桑菊饮

【方源】 《温病条辨》。

【组成】 桑叶7.5 g,菊花3 g,杏仁6 g,连翘5 g,薄荷2.5 g,桔梗6 g,生甘草2.5 g,芦根6 g。

No. 6 Jiegeng (*Radix Platycodi*) 6 g;

No. 7 Shenggancao (*Radix Glycyrrhizae*) 2.5 g;

No. 8 Lugen (*Rhizoma Phragmitis*) 6 g.

Administration: Decoct the above drugs in water for oral use.

Actions: Expelling wind and heat, dispersing the lung to relieve cough.

Clinical Application: This recipe is indicated for slight exterior heat syndrome due to exogenous pathogenic wind-warm at the early stage, marked by cough, mild feverish body, slight thirst, red tip and margin of the tongue, superficial and rapid pulse. It is applicable to common cold, flu, acute bronchitis, and acute tonsillitis with the above symptoms and belonging to exterior syndrome due to wind-heat. In case of excessive heat in the lung with rude respiration as if dyspnea, add Shigao (*Gypsum Fibrosum*) and Zhimu (*Rhizoma Anemarrhenae*) to enhance the effect of clearing away heat in the lung. In case of heat in the lung consuming and converting the body fluid into phlegm marked by cough with thick yellowish sputum, add Huangqin (*Radix Scutellariae*) and Sangbaipi (*Cortex Mori Radicis*) to clear the lung to resolve phlegm and relieve cough. In case of excessive impairment of the body fluid marked by thirst with desire to drink, add Tianhuafen (*Radix Trichosanthis*) to clear away heat to promote the production of body fluid. In case of sore throat, add Tuniuxi (*Radix Achyranthes Bidentatae*) and Shandougen (*Radix Sophorae Subprostratae*) to remove pathogenic heat and toxin and relieve sore throat.

Elucidation: This syndrome results from exogenous wind-heat, which invades the lung and leads to stagnated lung-qi. The method to eliminate wind and heat, disperse the lung and relieve cough should be adopted. Ingredients No. 1 and No. 2 act together as monarch drug, expelling

【用法】 水煎服。

【功用】 疏风清热,宣肺止咳。

【临床应用】 适用于风温初起,表热轻证。症见咳嗽,身热不甚,口微渴,舌边尖红,脉浮数。感冒、流行性感冒、急性支气管炎、急性扁桃体炎等见有上述症状,属风热表证者,可用本方治疗。若肺热较重,气粗似喘者,可加石膏、知母以增强清泄肺热之力;若肺热灼津成痰,咳嗽痰黄粘稠者,可加黄芩、桑白皮以清肺化痰止咳;若津伤较甚,口渴欲饮者,可加天花粉以清热生津;若咽喉肿痛者,可加土牛膝、山豆根以清热解毒利咽。

【方解】 本方证由外感风热,邪犯肺络,肺气失宣所致,治宜疏风清热,宣肺止咳之法。方中桑叶、菊花疏风解表,宣肺止咳,共为君药。杏

wind to relieve exterior syndrome, and dispersing the lung to relieve cough. No. 3 and No. 6 function as minister drug, enhancing the effect of the monarch drug. Ingredients No. 4, No. 5 and No. 8 serve as adjuvant drug, functioning respectively to eliminate heat and toxins, dispel wind-heat, clear away heat and promote the production of body fluid. Ingredient No. 7 plays the part of guiding drug, capable of clearing away heat in the lung, relieving cough, and mediating drug properties.

Cautions: This recipe is mild in action and thus should be modified in treating serious cases.

Yinqiao San
(**Powder of Lonicera and Forsythis**)

Source: *Wenbing Tiaobian* (*Detailed Analysis of Seasonal FebrileDiseases*).

Ingredients:

No. 1 Jinyinhua (*Flos Lonicerae*) 30 g;

No. 2 Lianqiao (*Fructus Forsythiae*) 30 g;

No. 3 Jiegeng (*Radix Platycodi*) 18 g;

No. 4 Bohe (*Herba Menthae*) 18 g;

No. 5 Niubangzi (*Fructus Arctii*) 18 g;

No. 6 Zhuye (*Herba Lophatheri*) 12 g;

No. 7 Jingjiesui (*Spica Schizonepetae*) 12 g;

No. 8 Dandouchi (*Semen Sojae Praeparatum*) 15 g;

No. 9 Shenggancao (*Radix Glycyrrhizae Recens*) 15 g.

Administration: These ingredients are ground into powder, each time 18 g is decocted with Xianlugen (*Rhizoma Phragmitis*) decoction for oral administration.

Actions: Relieving exogenous pathogenic factors with drugs pungent in flavor and cool in property, clearing away heat and eliminating toxin.

Clinical Application: This recipe is indicated for seasonal febrile diseases in the early stage and severe

仁降气止咳,桔梗宣肺化痰,两药一宣一降,以加强君药宣肺止咳之功,同为臣药。连翘清热解毒,薄荷疏散风热,芦根清热生津,俱为佐药。生甘草清肺热,止咳嗽,调药性,为佐使药。

【注意事项】 本方药轻力薄,若证重邪甚者需加减使用。

银翘散

【方源】 《温病条辨》。

【组成】 金银花、连翘各30 g,桔梗、薄荷、牛蒡子各18 g,竹叶、荆芥穗各12 g,淡豆豉、生甘草各15 g。

【用法】 共研粗末,每次18 g,以鲜芦根汤煎服。

【功用】 辛凉透表,清热解毒。

【临床应用】 适用于温病初起,表热重证。症见发热

syndrome of exterior heat. The usual symptoms are fever without perspiration, or hindered perspiration, slight aversion to wind-cold, headache, thirst, cough, sore throat, red tip of the tongue, thin whitish or yellowish fur, superficial and rapid pulse. It is applicable to flu, acute tonsillitis, measles of early stage, epidemic encephalitis B, epidemic cerebrospinal meningitis, and parotitis, etc., which belong to the exterior syndrome of wind-heat and are marked by fever, sore throat, and no perspiration. In case of excessive heat marked by high fever with thirst, add Shigao (*Gypsum Fibrosum*), Huangqin (*Radix Scutellariae*) and Daqingye (*Folium Isatidis*) to clear away heat and purge fire. In the absence of perspiration but marked aching body, add Chantui (*Periostracum Cicadae*) and Jiangcan (*Bombyx Batryticatus*) to enhance the effect of relieving the exterior syndrome by expelling wind.

Elucidation: Affection by wind-heat leads to stagnation of defensive qi and failure of the lung in purifying and descending function, for which the method of relieving exterior syndrome by expelling wind, clearing away heat and toxin should be adopted. Ingredients No. 1 and No. 2 in larger amount act as monarch drug, capable of clearing away heat and eliminating toxin as well as expelling exterior pathogenic factors. Ingredients No. 4 and No. 5 pungent in flavor and cool in property, No. 7 and No. 8 pungent in flavor and warm in property, act together as minister drug, enhancing the effect of expelling pathogenic factors, and involving no impairment of the body fluid. Ingredient No. 6 and Lugen (*Rhizoma Phragmitis*) can clear away heat and promote the production of body fluid, and No. 3 disperse the lung to relieve cough, the three constituting adjuvant drug. The last ingredient acts as guiding drug, capable of clearing away heat and toxin,

无汗,或有汗不畅,微恶风寒,头痛口渴,咳嗽咽痛,舌尖红,苔薄白或微黄,脉浮数。流行性感冒、急性扁桃体炎、麻疹初起,以及流行性乙型脑炎、流行性脑脊髓膜炎、腮腺炎等初起属风热表证,见有发热咽痛,表郁无汗者,可用本方治疗。若热毒较重,高热口渴者,可加石膏、黄芩、大青叶以清热泻火解毒;若无汗身痛较著者,可加蝉蜕、僵蚕以增疏风解表之效。

【方解】 本方证为外感风热,卫气被郁,肺失清肃所致,治宜疏风透表,清热解毒之法。方中重用金银花、连翘,清热解毒,并兼透表之功,共为君药。薄荷、牛蒡子辛凉疏散风热,解毒利咽;荆芥穗、淡豆豉辛温发散,且温而不燥,既可加强本方散邪解表之力,又无温燥伤津之弊,四药共助君药以加强解表散邪之力,同为臣药。芦根、竹叶清热生津,桔梗宣肺止咳,皆为佐药。生甘草清热解毒,调和药性,合桔梗擅清利咽喉,为佐使药。

mediating drug property, and being good at soothing the throat together with No. 3.

Both Sangju Yin and Yinqiao San are commonly used prescriptions in treating exterior syndrome due to wind-heat, and both have the ingredients Lianqiao (*Fructus Forsythiae*), Jiegeng (*Radix Platycodi*), Bohe (*Herba Menthae*), Lugen (*Rhizoma Phragmitis*) and Gancao (*Radix Glycyrrhizae*). The former has a better effect in terms of dispersing the lung to relieve cough because it also includes Sangye (*Folium Mori*), Juhua (*Flos Chrysanthemi*), Xingren (*Semen Armeniacae Amarum*). While the latter shows a stronger effect in terms of clearing away heat and relieving the exterior syndrome owing to the ingredients Jinyinhua (*Flos Lonicerae*), Jingjie (*Spica Schizonepetae*), Dandouchi (*Semen Sojae Praeparatum*), Niubangzi (*Fructus Arctii*), Zhuye (*Herba Lophatheri*). Thus they can be selected in the light of clinical needs.

Cautions: It is not applicable to exterior syndrome due to wind-heat with aversion to cold, absence of perspiration, but a mild fever without thirst.

桑菊饮与银翘散均为治疗风热表证的常用方剂,两方中都有连翘、桔梗、薄荷、芦根和甘草,但桑菊饮还有桑叶、菊花、杏仁,宣肺止咳之功较大;银翘散又有金银花、荆芥、淡豆豉、牛蒡子、竹叶,解表清热之力较强。临床可根据所治风热表证的特点酌情选用。

【注意事项】　风热表证虽见有恶寒无汗,但发热不甚、口不渴者,不宜使用本方。

Sangxing Tang
(Decoction of Mulberry Leaf and Almond)

Source: *Wenbing Tiaobian* (*Detailed Analysis of Seasonal Febrile Diseases*).

Ingredients:

No. 1 Sangye (*Folium Mori*) 3 g;

No. 2 Xingren (*Semen Armeniacae Amarum*) 5 g;

No. 3 Shashen (*Radix Adenophorae Strictae*) 6 g;

No. 4 Zhebeimu (*Bulbus Fritillariae Thunbergii*) 3 g;

No. 5 Dandouchi (*Semen Sojae Praeparatum*) 3 g;

No. 6 Zhizipi (*Pericarpium Gardeniae*) 3 g;

No. 7 Lipi (*Exocarpium Pyrus*) 3 g.

桑杏汤

【方源】　《温病条辨》。

【组成】　桑叶3g,杏仁5g,沙参6g,浙贝母3g,淡豆豉3g,栀子皮3g,梨皮3g。

Administration: Decoct the above drugs for oral use.

Actions: Releasing the inhibited lung-qi by dispelling dryness-heat, moistening the lung to relieve cough.

Clinical Application: This recipe is indicated for mild state of exterior syndrome due to dryness, marked by headache, mild feverish body, thirst, dryness of the throat and nasal cavity, cough without sputum or little sticky sputum, red tongue with thin whitish and dry fur, superficial and rapid pulse. It is used to treat upper respiratory tract infection, acute bronchitis, bronchiectasic hemoptysis, and pertussis, etc. occurring in autumn days, which are attributable to exogenous warmness and dryness affecting and burning the lung-yin, and manifested as feverish body, headache, thirst and dryness of the throat. In case of serious dryness of the throat, add Niubangzi (*Fructus Arctii*) and Bohe (*Herba Menthae*) to relieve sore throat. In case of heat scorching the lung collateral marked by expectoration with blood streaks or epistaxis, add Baimaogen (*Rhizoma Imperatae*) and Mudanpi (*Cortex Moutan Radicis*) to cool blood and stop bleeding. In case of excessive heat in the lung with thick yellowish sputum, add Gualoupi (*Pericarpium Trichosanthis*) and Huangqin (*Radix Scutellariae*) to clear away heat and resolve phlegm.

Elucidation: The syndrome is due to attack of warm-dryness in autumn, burning lung-yin and causing lung's failure in its purifying and descending function. It should be treated by releasing stagnated lung-qi with drugs of mild action, and moistening the lung to relieve cough. Ingredient No. 1 expelling dryness-heat and dispersing the lung to relieve cough; No. 2 dispersing the lung and moistening the lung to relieve cough, both of them act as monarch drug. Ingredients No. 5, No. 3 and No. 4 play

【用法】 水煎服。

【功用】 轻宣燥热,润肺止咳。

【临床应用】 适用于外感温燥轻证。症见头痛,身热不甚,口渴,咽干,鼻燥,干咳无痰,或痰少而粘,舌红,苔薄白而干,脉浮数。秋季发生的上呼吸道感染、急性支气管炎、支气管扩张咯血、百日咳等属外感温燥,灼伤肺津,以身热头痛,口渴咽干为主要表现者,可用本方治疗。若咽喉干痛较甚者,可加牛蒡子、薄荷以利咽止痛;若热灼肺络,咳痰带血或鼻衄者,可加白茅根、牡丹皮以凉血止血;若肺热较重,咳痰黄稠者,可加瓜蒌皮、黄芩以清热化痰。

【方解】 本方治证由秋季温燥外袭,灼伤肺津,肺失清肃而致,治宜轻宣燥热,润肺止咳之法。方中桑叶疏散燥热,宣肺止咳;杏仁宣利肺气,润燥止咳,两药配伍,肺卫并治,共为君药。淡豆豉助桑叶宣散表邪,沙参、贝母助杏仁润肺止咳,同为臣药。栀子

together the part of minister drug, capable of helping the monarch drug to clear away heat in the lung and moisten the lung to relieve cough. No. 6, clearing away lung-heat and No. 7 clearing the lung and moistening dryness, serve as adjuvant drug. It is advisable to use this recipe in the mild state of the above syndrome because of its mild action.

Cautions：Since this recipe is mild in action, it is not applicable to serious impairment of the lung-yin by dryness marked by feverish body, cough and dyspnea, dry and red tongue with little fur.

Mahuang Xingren Gancao Shigao Tang
（*Decoction of Ephedra，Almond，Licorice and Gypsum*）

Source：*Shanghan Lun*（*Treatise on Exogenous Febrile Diseases*）.

Ingredients：

No. 1 Mahuang（*Herba Ephedrae*）9 g;

No. 2 Xingren（*Semen Armeniacae Amarum*）9 g;

No. 3 Zhigancao（*Radix Glycyrrhizae Praeparatae*）6 g;

No. 4 Shengshigao（*Gypsum Fibrosum*）18 g（decocted first）.

Administration：Decoct the above drugs for oral use.

Actions：Dispersing heat in the lung, relieving cough and asthma.

Clinical Application：This recipe is indicated for unrelieved exogenous pathogenic factors, cough and asthma due to heat in the lung, marked by fever, thirst, cough and asthma, nares flaring, desire for drinks, perspiration or absence of perspiration, thin whitish or yellowish fur, superficial and rapid pulse. It is applicable to common cold, acute bronchitis, bronchial pneumonia, lobar pneumonia, bronchial asthma, measles complicated

皮清泄肺热,梨皮清肺润燥,均为佐药。本方药轻气薄,故宜于温燥外袭,肺失清肃之轻证。

【注意事项】　本方药轻力薄,燥热灼伤肺阴较重,身热咳喘、舌干红少苔者不宜使用。

麻黄杏仁甘草石膏汤

【方源】《伤寒论》。

【组成】　麻黄9 g,杏仁9 g,炙甘草6 g,生石膏18 g(先煎)。

【用法】　水煎服。

【功用】　宣泄肺热,止咳平喘。

【临床应用】　适用于表邪未解,肺热咳喘证。症见发热口渴,咳嗽气喘,鼻翼扇动,口渴欲饮,有汗或无汗,舌苔薄白或黄,脉浮数。感冒、急性支气管炎、支气管肺炎、大叶性肺炎、支气管哮喘、麻疹合并肺炎等以发热咳喘为主

with pneumonia, etc., main symptoms of which are fever, cough and asthma and belonging to accumulation of pathogenic heat in the lung with unrelieved exogenous pathogenic factors. In case of excessive heat in the lung marked by high fever with perspiration, double the dosage of Shengshigao (*Gypsum Fibrosum*). If accompanied by exterior syndrome marked by aversion to cold without perspiration, add Bohe (*Herba Menthae*) and Suye (*Folium Perillae*) to help bring about the effect of relieving exterior syndrome and releasing the stagnated lung-qi. In case of constipation, add Zhidahuang (*Radix et Rhizoma Rhei Praeparatae*) to remove heat by cathartics.

Elucidation：This syndrome is caused by excessive heat transformed from exogenous wind, which accumulates in the lung and causes its failure in purifying and descending function. It should be treated by dispersing heat and relieving cough and asthma. As monarch drug, ingredient No. 1 is pungent in flavor and warm in property, and No. 4 pungent in flavor and cool in property with larger dosage. They supplement each other in a rational combination to clear away heat in the lung. Ingredient No. 2 acts as minister drug, causing the lung-qi to descend, enhancing the function of relieving cough and asthma. Ingredient No. 3 functions as guiding drug, replenishing qi, regulating the middle-energizer, and mediating drug properties.

Cautions：It is not applicable to cough and asthma due to wind-cold, nor to excessive phlegm-heat.

症,属邪热壅肺,外邪未解者, 可用本方治疗。若肺中热盛, 壮热汗出者,石膏用量可加倍 以增清热之力;若兼有表邪, 无汗而恶寒者,可加薄荷、苏 叶以助解表宣肺之力;若大便 干结者,可加制大黄以通腑导 热下行。

【方解】 本方证由外感 风邪,化热犯肺,热邪壅盛,肺 失清肃而致,治宜宣肺散邪, 清泄肺热,止咳平喘之法。方 中麻黄辛温宣肺散邪,石膏辛 寒清肺泄热,两药合用,一温 一寒,麻黄得石膏则宣肺平喘 而不助热,石膏得麻黄则清泄 肺热而不凉遏,且寒药重于温 药,共奏宣泄肺热之功,并为 君药。杏仁降利肺气,与麻黄 一宣一降,加强止咳平喘作 用,为臣药。炙甘草益气和 中,调和药性,为使药。

【注意事项】 风寒咳喘, 或痰热壅盛者,慎用本方。

2.2 Prescriptions for Clearing away Heat

第二章
清热剂

The prescriptions for clearing away heat chiefly composed of drugs for clearing away heat, purging fire, cooling blood and removing toxin and applied in the treatment of interior heat.

In view of the difference in interior heat syndromes between qifen and xuefen, between warm-heat and summer-heat, between excess and deficiency, between zang and fu organs, prescriptions for clearing away heat are subdivided into prescriptions for clearing away heat from qifen, those for removing heat from yingfen and blood, those for clearing away heat and toxin, those for removing heat from zang-fu organs, those for eliminating asthenic heat, and those for clearing away summer-heat.

Prescriptions for clearing away heat from qifen are chiefly composed of drugs with the effect of clearing away heat from qifen, promoting the production of body fluid, and relieving dysphoria and thirst, which are applicable to the syndrome of excessive heat in qifen. Prescriptions for removing heat from yingfen and blood are chiefly composed of drugs with the effect of clearing away heat from yingfen and nourishing yin, cooling blood and removing stasis, which are applicable to the syndrome of heat accumulating in yingfen and xuefen. Prescriptions for clearing away heat and toxin are chiefly composed of drugs bitter in flavor and cool in property with the effect of purging fire, which are applicable to pestilence and virulent heat pathogen. Prescriptions for removing heat from zang-fu

凡以清热药为主组成,具有清热、泻火、凉血、解毒等作用,适用于治疗里热证的方剂,统称清热剂。

由于里热证有在气、在血之分,有温热、暑热之别,有实热、虚热之异,有脏腑偏胜之殊,因而清热剂相应地分为清气分热剂、清营凉血剂、清热解毒剂、清脏腑热剂、清虚热剂与清暑热剂六类。

清气分热剂由清气分热药为主组成,具有清热生津、除烦止渴作用,适用于气分热盛之证。清营凉血剂由清营凉血药为主组成,具有清营养阴、凉血散瘀作用,适用于邪热传营以及热入血分证。清热解毒剂由清热解毒药为主组成,具有苦寒泻火、直折火毒作用,适用于温疫、温毒等证。清脏腑热剂由针对不同脏腑热证的清热药为主组成,具有清泻脏腑火热的作用,适用于邪热偏盛于某一脏腑而

organs are made up of drugs aimed at clearing away fire-heat from different zang or fu organs, and applicable to the syndrome of heat dominant in a certain zang or fu organ. Prescriptions for clearing away heat of deficiency type are chiefly composed of drugs with the effect of clearing away heat, nourishing yin and expelling pathogenic factors, and applicable to the syndrome of yin impairment due to excessive heat. Prescriptions for clearing away summer-heat are applicable to the syndrome due to attack by pathogenic summer-heat.

Ingredients of the prescriptions for clearing away heat are mostly bitter in flavor and cool in property, therefore they should not be taken for a long time to prevent impairment of the stomach, and yin and yang. And drugs able to reinforce the spleen and stomach should be taken if necessary. Besides great cautions must be paid by patients with constitutional weakness of the spleen and stomach marked by poor appetite and loose stool. In case of excessive interior heat, the phenomenon "Ju Yao" may appear by which is meant the patient vomits immediately when taking decoctions of this kind. To relieve or eliminate this phenomenon, the patient may either take the decoction warm or add to it some ginger juice.

产生的火热证候。清虚热剂由滋阴清热药为主组成,具有清热滋阴透邪作用,适用于热盛阴伤之证。清暑热剂由祛暑药为主组成,具有清热祛暑作用,适用于夏日外感暑热证。

清热剂的组成药物性味大多苦寒,由于苦寒易于败胃,苦燥常致伤阴,寒凉可能伤阳,故不宜久服,必要时配合健脾和胃之药;素体脾胃虚弱,纳少便溏者慎用。若里热炽盛,服凉药入口即吐者,称之"拒药",可采用凉药热服,或加用少量辛温的姜汁以为反佐,以缓解或消除格拒的现象。

2.2.1 Prescriptions for Clearing away Heat from Qifen

Baihu Tang
(*White Tiger Decoction*)

Source: *Shanghan Lun* (*Treatise on Exogenous Febrile Diseases*).

Ingredients:

No. 1 Shigao (*Gypsum Fibrosum*) 50 g;

No. 2 Zhimu (*Rhizoma Anemarrhenae*) 18 g;

第一节 清气分热剂

白虎汤

【方源】《伤寒论》。

【组成】 石膏 50 g,知母 18 g,炙甘草6 g,粳米9 g。

No. 3 Zhigancao (*Radix Glycyrrhizae Praeparatae*) 6 g;

No. 4 Jingmi (*Semen Oryzae Sativae*) 9 g.

Administration: Decoct the above drugs till the rice is well done and take the decoction several times after removal of the residue.

Actions: Clearing away heat and promoting the production of body fluid.

Clinical Application: This recipe is indicated for yangming meridian syndrome, marked by high fever, flushed face, polydipsia, profuse perspiration, aversion to heat, full forceful pulse. It is applicable to infectious diseases such as lobar pneumonia, epidemic encephalitis B, epidemic hemorrhagic fever, and gingivitis with the four characteristics of this syndrome (high fever, polydipsia, profuse perspiration, and full large pulse). In case of impairment of qi and body fluid due to excessive heat marked by full large but weak pulse, thirst not quenched with drink, add Renshen (*Radix Ginseng*) to replenish qi and promote the production of body fluid, forming another recipe entitled Baihu plus Renshen Tang. In case of intense heat in both qifen and xuefen in combination with coma, delirium and skin rashes, add Shengdihuang (*Radix Rehmanniae*) and Shuiniujiao (*Cornu Bubali*) to clear away heat and cool the blood. In case of wind stirring up due to excessive heat concomitant with tic of limbs, add Lingyangjiao (*Cornu Antelopis*) and Gouteng (*Ramulus Uncariae cum Uncis*) to relieve convulsion and spasm. In case of interior heat complicated with dampness, such as damp-warm syndrome with heat prevailing over dampness, or arthritis with reddish, swelling and painful joints, add Cangzhu (*Rhizoma Atractylodis*) to dry pathogenic dampness, constituting another recipe entitled Baihu plus Cangzhu Tang.

Elucidation: This syndrome is the result of exces-

【用法】　水煎至米熟汤成，去渣分服。

【功用】　清热生津。

【临床应用】　适用于阳明经证。症见壮热面赤，烦渴引饮，汗出恶热，脉洪大有力。感染性疾病，如大叶性肺炎、流行性乙型脑炎、流行性出血热、牙龈炎等出现阳明气分热盛的"四大"（大热、大渴、大汗、脉洪大）特征者，可用本方治疗。若热盛耗伤气津，兼见脉大无力，饮不解渴者，可加人参以益气生津，即白虎加人参汤；若温热病气血两燔，兼神昏谵语、身发斑疹者，可加生地黄、水牛角以清热凉血；若热盛动风，兼四肢抽搐者，可加羚羊角、钩藤以熄风止痉；若里热挟湿，如湿温病热重于湿，或风湿热痹，关节红肿疼痛者，可加苍术以燥湿，即白虎加苍术汤。

【方解】　本方证由气分

sive heat in qifen scorching the body fluid, and should be treated by clearing away heat and promoting the production of body fluid. Ingredient No. 1, pungent and sweet in flavor and extremely cold in property, acts as monarch drug, capable of purging away heat without impairing body fluid. Ingredient No. 2, which is bitter in flavor and cold moist in property, serves as minister drug, strengthening the action of the monarch drug and promoting the production of body fluid as well. Ingredients No. 3 and No. 4 function as adjuvant drug that can not only reinforce the stomach and protect body fluid, but also prevent the stomach from being injured by the extremely cold drug as ingredient No. 1. Besides, No. 3 also plays the role of guiding drug, mediating drug properties.

Cautions: This must not be applied to patients with full large but weak pulse when pressed and pale tongue, which are attributable to fever due to blood deficiency.

邪热炽盛,灼伤津液所致,治宜清热生津之法。方中石膏辛甘大寒,清热泻火而不伤津液,为君药。知母苦寒质润,助君药清热泻火,又能滋阴生津,为臣药。粳米、炙甘草益胃护津,又可防石膏大寒伤胃,为佐药。炙甘草兼能调和药性,为使药。

【注意事项】 若脉象洪大而重按无力,且舌质淡者,乃血虚发热,禁用本方。

2.2.2 Prescriptions for Clearing away Heat from Yingfen and Blood

第二节 清营凉血剂

Qingying Tang
(*Decoction for Eliminating Heat in Yingfen*)

Source: *Wenbing Tiaobian* (*Detailed Analysis of Seasonal Febrile Diseases*).

Ingredients:

No. 1 Shuiniujiao (*Cornu Bubali*) 〔originally Xijiao (*Cornu Rhinocerotis*)〕 30 g (decocted first);

No. 2 Shengdihuang (*Radix Rehmanniae*) 15 g;

No. 3 Xuanshen (*Radix Scrophulariae*) 9 g;

No. 4 Zhuyexin (*Herba Lophatheri*) 3 g;

No. 5 Maimendong (*Radix Ophiopogonis*) 9 g;

No. 6 Danshen (*Radix Salviae Miltiorrhizae*) 6 g;

No. 7 Huanglian (*Rhizoma Coptidis*) 5 g;

清营汤

【方源】 《温病条辨》。

【组成】 水牛角(原为犀角)30 g(先煎),生地黄15 g,玄参9 g,竹叶心3 g,麦门冬9 g,丹参6 g,黄连5 g,金银花9 g,连翘6 g。

No. 8 Jinyinhua (*Flos Lonicerae*) 9 g;

No. 9 Lianqiao (*Fructus Forsythiae*) 6 g.

Administration: Decoct the above drugs for oral use.

Actions: Clearing away heat and toxic material and expelling heat and nourishing yin.

Clinical Application: This recipe is indicated for invasion of yingfen by pathogenic heat at the early stage, marked by feverish body which aggravates at night, delirium occurring now and then, thirst or absence of thirst, indistinct skin rashes, deep-red and dry tongue, thready and rapid pulse. It is applicable to epidemic encephalitis B, epidemic cerebrospinal meningitis, hematosepsis, ileotyphus or other epidemic diseases that are attributable to pathogenic heat invading yingfen. In case heat in qifen is not wiped out manifesting high fever and thirst, use Baihu Tang together with this recipe to achieve the effect of clearing away heat from both qifen and yingfen. In case of heat obstructing the heart meridian manifesting delirium, Angong Niuhuang Wan can be taken with this decoction.

Elucidation: This syndrome is the result of pathogenic heat invading yingfen, scorching ying-yin and injuring blood vessels, for which the method of clearing away heat and toxin and nourishing yin should be adopted. Ingredient No. 1 is very good at clearing away heat from yingfen, functioning as monarch drug. Ingredients No. 2, No. 3 and No. 5 act as minister drug, which not only help the monarch drug to purge away heat but also nourish yin and promote the production of body fluid. Ingredients No. 8 and No. 9 are of mild action and, when combined with the above drugs to clear away heat from yingfen and eliminate toxins, can direct heat out of qifen. When combined with ingredient No. 7, they can strengthen the action of the monarch drug. Ingredient No. 6 can cool blood and promote the flow of blood so as to prevent complication of

【用法】 水煎服。

【功用】 清热解毒,透热养阴。

【临床应用】 适用于邪热初入营分证。症见身热夜甚,时有谵语,口渴或不渴,斑疹隐隐,舌绛而干,脉细数。流行性乙型脑炎、流行性脑脊髓膜炎、败血症、肠伤寒或其他热性病属邪热初入营分者,可用本方治疗。若气分之热未尽,高热口渴者,可与白虎汤合用,以收气营两清之功;若兼热闭心包,神昏谵语者,可以清营汤送服安宫牛黄丸。

【方解】 本方证由邪热传入营分,灼伤营阴,扰及血络所致,治宜清热解毒、透热养阴之法。方中水牛角长于清解营分热毒,为君药。生地黄、玄参、麦门冬助君药清营泄热,又能滋阴生津,同为臣药。金银花、连翘轻清透达,与上述清营解毒药配伍,可促使营分之热外透,使邪热转出气分而解;合黄连又可助君药清热解毒之力;丹参凉血活血,以防热与血结,均为佐药。竹叶心清心解毒,又引诸药入心,为使药。

heat with blood, and serves together with the above three ingredients as adjuvant drug. Ingredient No. 4 plays the part of guiding drug, which not only clears away heat in the heart but also directs the other drugs to the heart.

Cautions: Since ingredients No. 2, No. 3 and No. 5 in this recipe are sweet in flavor and cool and moist in nature, it is not applicable to patients manifesting deep-red tongue with whitish glossy fur, which is attributable to syndrome of retained heat due to blockage of dampness.

【注意事项】 方中生地黄、玄参、麦门冬甘凉滋润,若舌绛苔白滑者,是湿遏热伏,禁用本方,以免助湿敛邪。

Xijiao Dihuang Tang
(Decoction of Rhinoceros Horn and Rehmannia)

Source: *Beiji Qianjin Yaofang* (*Valuable Prescriptions for Emergencies*).

Ingredients:

No. 1 Shuiniujiao (*Cornu Bubali*) 〔originally Xijiao (*Cornu Rhinocerotis*)〕30 g (decocted first);

No. 2 Shengdihuang (*Radix Rehmanniae*) 24 g;

No. 3 Shaoyao (*Radix Paeoniae*) 12 g;

No. 4 Mudanpi (*Cortex Moutan Radicis*) 9 g.

Administration: Decoct the above drugs for oral use.

Actions: Clearing away heat and toxin, cooling blood and removing blood stasis.

Clinical Application: This recipe is indicated for syndrome of heat invading xuefen in the course of epidemic febrile diseases, marked by delirium, dark purple color of rashes; or syndrome of heat impairing the blood vessels as the result of miscellaneous diseases marked by haematemesis, epistaxis, hematochezia, hematuria, deep-red tongue with prickle-like fur, thready and rapid pulse. It is applicable to diffuse intravascular coagulation, urinaemia, purpura, acute leukemia, and hematosepsis that are attributable to excessive heat in xuefen. Ingredient No. 3 is now often clinically substituted for Chishaoyao (*Radix Paeoniae Rubra*). If applied for excessive heat and toxin in

犀角地黄汤

【方源】 《备急千金要方》。

【组成】 水牛角(原为犀角)30 g(先煎),生地黄24 g,芍药12 g,牡丹皮9 g。

【用法】 水煎服。

【功用】 清热解毒,凉血散瘀。

【临床应用】 适用于温病热入血分证,症见神昏谵语,斑色紫黑,或杂病热伤血络,症见吐血、衄血、便血、溲血,舌绛起刺,脉细数。弥散性血管内凝血、尿毒症、紫癜、急性白血病、败血症等属血分热盛者,可用本方治疗。方中芍药,现临床多用赤芍药。若用于温病血分证热毒炽盛,神昏发斑者,宜加黄连、栀子、连翘以加强清热解毒之力;若血

xuefen manifesting coma and skin rashes, it is advisable to add Huanglian (*Rhizoma Coptidis*), Zhizi (*Fructus Gardeniae*) and Lianqiao (*Fructus Forsythiae*) to enhance the action of clearing away heat and toxin. In case of blood syndrome complicated with fire in the liver manifesting impetuosity and susceptibility to rage, add Chaihu (*Radix Bupleuri*), Zhizi (*Fructus Gardeniae*) to purge away fire in the liver. In case of heat combined with the accumulation of stagnated blood manifesting mania, add Dahuang (*Radix et Rhizoma Rhei*) and Huangqin (*Radix Scutellariae*) to expel heat and remove stasis.

Elucidation: This syndrome results from heat invading xuefen, causing blood to flow uncontrollably and get stagnated, further giving rise to blood stasis. The method of clearing away heat to cool blood, and promoting the circulation of blood to remove blood stasis should be adopted. Ingredient No. 1 has the function of clearing away heat and toxin, cooling blood and stopping bleeding, acting as monarch drug. Ingredient No. 2 not only helps the monarch drug to carry out its function, but also nourishes yin and promotes the production of body fluid, acting as minister drug. The last two ingredients help the monarch and minister drugs on the one hand, and remove blood stasis and skin rashes on the other hand, serving as adjuvant drug.

2.2.3　Prescriptions for Clearing away Heat and Toxins

Huanglian Jiedu Tang
（*Decoction of Coptis for Detoxification*）

Source：*Cui's Prescriptions from Waitai Miyao* (*Clandestine Medical Essentials from Imperial Library*).

Ingredients：

No. 1 Huanglian (*Rhizoma Coptidis*) 9 g;

证而兼挟肝火,急躁易怒者,可加柴胡、栀子以清泻肝火;若邪热与瘀血相结,蓄血发狂者,可加大黄、黄芩以泻热逐瘀。

【方解】　本方证由热入血分,迫血妄行,热邪煎灼,血滞成瘀所致,治宜清热凉血,活血化瘀之法。方中水牛角清热解毒,凉血止血,为君药。生地黄助君药清热凉血,并能滋阴生津,为臣药。芍药、牡丹皮清热凉血,活血散瘀,既可助君、臣药凉血止血,又能散瘀化斑,并使血止而无留瘀之弊,均为佐药。

第三节　清热解毒剂

黄连解毒汤

【方源】　崔氏方,录自《外台秘要》。

【组成】　黄连9 g,黄芩、黄柏各6 g,栀子9 g。

No. 2 Huangqin (*Radix Scutellariae*) 6 g;

No. 3 Huangbai (*Cortex Phellodendri*) 6 g;

No. 4 Zhizi (*Fructus Gardeniae*) 9 g.

Administration: Decoct the above drugs for oral use.

Actions: Purging pathogenic fire and toxin.

Clinical Application: This recipe is indicated for excess of fire, toxin and heat in the triple energizer, marked by high fever, restlessness, thirst for drink, delirium, insomnia, or dysentery with fever, or sores and carbuncles, red tongue with yellowish fur, rapid and forceful pulse. It is applicable to septicemia, pyosepticemia, dysentery, pneumonia, urinary infection, epidemic cerebrospinal meningitis, epidemic encephalitis B, and other infectious diseases that are attributable to syndrome due to intense fire and toxin. If concomitant with constipation, add Dahuang (*Radix et Rhizoma Rhei*) to promote defecation and cause heat and toxin to descend. If concomitant with hematemesis, epistaxis and skin rashes, add Shengdihuang (*Radix Rehmanniae*), Xuanshen (*Radix Scrophulariae*) and Mudanpi (*Cortex Moutan Radicis*) to clear away heat and cool blood. In case of jaundice, add Yinchenhao (*Herba Artemisiae Scopariae*) and Dahuang (*Radix et Rhizoma Rhei*) to eliminate dampness and jaundice.

Elucidation: The syndrome is the result of heat and toxin accumulating in the three energizer, and should be treated with drugs of extremely cold nature and capable of purging fire and toxin. Ingredient No. 1 specializes in purging away heart-fire and fire in the middle-energizer, acting as monarch drug. Ingredients No. 2, No. 3 and No. 4 function to purge fire respectively in the upper-energizer, the lower-energizer, and triple energizer, and together serve as minister and adjuvant drugs. All the ingredients are extremely bitter in flavor and cold in property, thus

【用法】 水煎服。

【功用】 泻火解毒。

【临床应用】 适用于三焦火毒热盛证。症见高热烦躁,口渴引饮,谵语不眠,或身热下利,或痈肿疔毒,舌红苔黄,脉数有力。败血症、脓毒血症、痢疾、肺炎、泌尿系感染、流行性脑脊髓膜炎、流行性乙型脑炎以及其他感染性疾病属火毒炽盛者,均可用本方治疗。若兼便秘者,可加大黄以通便泻火,导热毒下行;若兼吐血、衄血、发斑者,可加生地黄、玄参、牡丹皮以清热凉血;若出现黄疸者,可加茵陈蒿、大黄以清热祛湿退黄。

【方解】 本方证由热毒壅盛于三焦所致,治宜大寒泻火解毒之法。方中黄连长于泻心火,兼泻中焦之火,为君药。黄芩泻上焦之火,黄柏泻下焦之火,栀子通泻三焦,导热下行,均为臣、佐药。四药皆大苦大寒之品,配伍同用,相得益彰,直折火毒之功颇著。

can achieve a better effect of expelling fire and toxin when combined.

Cautions：This recipe mostly comprises drugs of bitter and cold nature. Since drugs of bitter and dry nature and those of bitter and cold nature are apt to impair respectively yin and the stomach, this recipe is not applicable to patients who do not manifest syndrome of excessive accumulation of fire and toxin. Besides this recipe should be abandoned immediately after it creates the expected result. It must not be applied to patients suffering from a serious impairment of yin with deep-red tongue without fur.

【注意事项】 本方苦寒之药群聚,苦燥劫阴,苦寒败胃,非火毒炽盛者不可服用,且应中病即止。若阴伤较著,舌质光绛者禁用。

Liangge San
(*Powder for Clearing away Heat from the Upper or Middle Energizer*)

凉膈散

Source：*Taiping Huimin Hejiju Fang* (*Benevolent Prescriptions from Taiping Pharmaceutical Bureau*).

【方源】 《太平惠民和剂局方》。

Ingredients：

No. 1 Dahuang (*Radix et Rhizoma Rhei*) 600 g;

No. 2 Mangxiao (*Natrii Sulfas*) 600 g;

No. 3 Zhigancao (*Radix Glycyrrhizae Praeparatae*) 600 g;

No. 4 Zhiziren (*Fructus Gardeniae*) 300 g;

No. 5 Bohe (*Herba Menthae*) 300 g;

No. 6 Huangqin (*Radix Scutellariae*) 300 g;

No. 7 Lianqiao (*Fructus Forsythiae*) 1,250 g.

【组成】 大黄、芒消、炙甘草各 600 g,栀子仁、薄荷、黄芩各 300 g,连翘 1 250 g。

Administration：Grind the above drugs into coarse powder and then take 5 - 12 g at one time to be decocted with 3 g bamboo leaves and a little honey added to it.

【用法】 共研粗末,每次5～12 g,加竹叶3 g,蜜少许,水煎服。

Actions：Purging pathogenic fire and relaxing the bowels, clearing away heat in both the upper and middle energizer.

【功用】 泻火通便,清上泄下。

Clinical Application：This recipe is indicated for fire-heat syndrome in the upper and middle energizers,

【临床应用】 适用于上中二焦火热证。症见烦躁口

marked by dysphoria, thirst, flushed face, parched lips, fever with dysphoria in chest and diaphragm, aphthae, or sore throat, hematemesis, constipation, dark urine, red tongue with yellowish fur, smooth and rapid pulse. It is applicable to pharyngitis, stomatitis, acute tonsillitis, infection of biliary tract, acute icterohepatitis, and other diseases that are attributable to fire-heat syndrome in the upper and middle energizers. It is unnecessary to subtract ingredients No. 1 and No. 2 in the absence of constipation. If smooth defecation or diarrhea occurs with less heat syndrome after the use of drugs, it is advisable to reduce or even subtract the above two ingredients.

Elucidation: The syndrome is due to pathogenic fire or heat accumulating in the upper and middle energizers, and should be treated by clearing away heat and purging fire. Ingredient No. 7 in larger amount acts as monarch drug, capable of clearing away heat and toxins. Ingredients No. 5 and No. 6 are respectively to clear away heat from the heart and the upper energizer, and together act as minister drug, strengthening the effect of the monarch drug. Ingredient No. 4 is meant to purge away heat from the triple energizers, and ingredients No. 1 and No. 2 to descend heat and fire, altogether serving as adjuvant drug. Ingredient No. 3 can not only mediate drug properties, but also relieve the drastic effect of the first two ingredients to clear away heat in the middle energizer with ingredients No. 1 and No. 2, playing the part of adjuvant-guiding drug. Bamboo leaves and honey are helpful in clearing away heat and can promote the production of body fluid because of its sweet in flavor and moist in nature.

Puji Xiaodu Yin
(*Decoction for General Disinfection*)

Source: *Dongyuan Shixiao Fang* (*Effective Prescriptions Tested by Dongyuan*).

渴,面赤唇焦,胸膈烦热,口舌生疮,或咽痛吐衄,便秘溺赤,舌红苔黄,脉滑数。咽炎、口腔炎、急性扁桃体炎、胆道感染、急性黄疸型肝炎等属上、中二焦火热者,可用本方治疗。若无便秘者,大黄、芒消不必减去;若药后大便通畅或腹泻,热象减轻者,大黄、芒消宜减量或去之。

【方解】 本方证由火热之邪郁于上中二焦所致,治宜清热泻火,导热下行之法。方中重用连翘清热解毒,为君药。薄荷辛凉清疏心胸之热,黄芩善清上焦之热,两药共助君药以加强清泄上焦热毒之力,同为臣药。栀子清热解毒,通泄三焦;大黄、芒消泻热降火,导热下行,以加强泻火解毒之力,均为佐药。炙甘草调和药性,与大黄、芒消同用,还可缓其峻泻之力,以利于清泄中焦热邪,为佐使药。煎药时少加竹叶、白蜜,既有助于清热,又可甘润生津。

普济消毒饮

【方源】《东垣试效方》。

Ingredients：

No. 1 Huangqin（*Radix Scutellariae*）（fried with wine）15 g;

No. 2 Huanglian（*Rhizoma Coptidis*）（fried with wine）15 g;

No. 3 Jupi（*Pericarpium Citri Reticulatae*）6 g;

No. 4 Shenggancao（*Radix Glycyrrhizae*）6 g;

No. 5 Xuanshen（*Radix Scrophulariae*）6 g;

No. 6 Chaihu（*Radix Bupleuri*）6 g;

No. 7 Jiegeng（*Radix Platycodi*）6 g;

No. 8 Lianqiao（*Fructus Forsythiae*）3 g;

No. 9 Banlangen（*Radix Isatidis*）3 g;

No. 10 Mabo（*Lasiosphaera seu Calvatia*）3 g;

No. 11 Niubangzi（*Fructus Arctii*）3 g;

No. 12 Bohe（*Herba Menthae*）3 g;

No. 13 Jiangcan（*Bombyx Batryticatus*）2 g;

No. 14 Shengma（*Rhizoma Cimicifugae*）2 g.

Administration：Decoct the above drugs for oral use; or grind them into fine powder and take frequently with boiled water.

Actions：Clearing away heat and toxic material and dispelling wind and other pathogenic factors.

Clinical Application：This recipe is used to treat swollen head due to infection marked by aversion to cold, fever, flushed swollen face and head, sore throat, thirst with preference for drinking, red tongue with yellowish fur, superficial and rapid forceful pulse. It is applicable to parotitis, facial erysipelas, acute tonsillitis, and other diseases due to wind heat and toxins, manifesting chiefly flushed swelling in the face and head and supeficial rapid pulse. In case of complicated orchitis due to parotitis, add Chuanlianzi（*Fructus Meliae Toosendan*）and Longdancao（*Radix Gentianae*）to purge away damp-heat from the liver meridian. In case of constipation, add wine-prepared

【组成】 黄芩（酒炒）、黄连（酒炒）各15 g，橘皮、生甘草、玄参、柴胡、桔梗各6 g，连翘、板蓝根、马勃、牛蒡子、薄荷各3 g，僵蚕、升麻各2 g。

【用法】 水煎服，或研细末，汤调频服。

【功用】 清热解毒，疏风散邪。

【临床应用】 适用于大头瘟证。症见恶寒发热，头面红肿热痛，咽喉疼痛，口渴欲饮，舌红苔黄，脉浮数有力。腮腺炎、颜面丹毒、急性扁桃体炎等属风热毒邪为患，以头面红肿疼痛，脉浮数为主要表现者，可用本方治疗。若腮腺炎并发睾丸炎者，加川楝子、龙胆草以泻肝经湿热；若大便秘结者，加酒大黄以泻火解毒、导热下行。

Dahuang (*Radix et Rhizoma Rhei*) to descend heat.

Elucidation: The syndrome results from exogenous wind-heat and seasonal pathogenic factors accumulating in the upper energizer and further affecting head and face. It should be treated by clearing away heat and toxin and dispelling wind and other pathogenic factors. Ingredients No.1 and No.2, in larger amount and prepared with wine, play the role of monarch drug with the effect of dispelling heat-toxin in the upper energizer. Ingredients No. 11, No.8, No. 12 and No. 13 act together as minister drug, dispelling wind-heat that affects head and face, removing toxin and resolving mass. Ingredients No.5, No. 10, No. 9, No. 7 and No. 4 have the function of removing heat-toxin from the throat, and No. 3 regulating qi to remove obstruction and subdue swelling, all serving as adjuvant drug. Ingredients No. 14 and No. 6 play the part of guiding drug to dispel pathogenic wind-heat and to assist the other drugs in reaching the face and head to remove pathogenic heat there. All the drugs in combination achieve the purpose of clearing away heat and dispelling wind, ascending and descending drugs to the affected site. Thus this recipe is very effective in treating syndromes manifesting excessive accumulation of pathogenic heat and toxin in the upper energizer.

Cautions: Some ointment with the action of clearing away heat and toxin may be applied externally and locally to enhance the effect of subduing swelling and relieving pain as well.

【方解】 本方证由外感风热疫毒之邪，壅于上焦，攻冲头面所致，治宜清热解毒、疏风散邪之法。方中重用黄芩、黄连清热泻火，并酒炒促其上行，以增清上焦热毒之力，共为君药。牛蒡子、连翘、薄荷、僵蚕疏散头面风热，解毒散结，同为臣药。玄参、马勃、板蓝根、桔梗、生甘草清热解毒，兼利咽喉；橘皮理气以疏通壅滞，散结消肿，均为佐药。少加升麻、柴胡以疏散风热，并引诸药上至头面，直达病所，为使药。诸药配伍，清疏并用，升降兼投，因而适宜于治疗上焦热毒壅聚之证。

【注意事项】 服用本方时亦可配合清热解毒药膏局部外敷，以加强消肿止痛之效。

2.2.4 Prescriptions for Removing Heat from Zang-fu Organs

Daochi San
(*Powder for Promoting Diuresis*)
Source: *Xiao'er Yaozheng Zhijue* (*Key to Differ-*

第四节　清脏腑热剂

导赤散

【方源】《小儿药证直

entiation and Therapeutics of Children's Diseases).

Ingredients:

No. 1 Shengdihuang (*Radix Rehmanniae Recens*) 6 g;

No. 2 Mutong (*Caulis Akebiae*) 6 g;

No. 3 Shenggancaoshao (*Radix Glycyrrhizae*) 6 g.

Administration: These ingredients are ground into powder. Each time 9g is decocted with proper amount of Zhuye (*Herba Lophatheri*) for oral administration.

Actions: Removing heart fire and inducing diuresis.

Clinical Application: This recipe is applicable to intense heat syndrome in the heart meridian, manifested as irritability, feverish sensation in the chest, thirst, flushed face, preference for cold drinks, oral ulceration; or dark urine with difficulty and pain in urination, red tongue with thin yellowish fur, and rapid pulse. It can be used to deal with stomatitis, thrush, infantile night cry and infantile urinary infection, which pertain to domination of heat in the heart meridian. In case of excessive fire in the heart manifesting dysphoria and much aphthae, add Huanglian (*Rhizoma Coptidis*) to enhance the action of clearing the heart and purging fire; in case of dark urine with difficulty and burning pain in urination, which is indicative of heat invading the small intestine, add Cheqianzi (*Semen Plantaginis*) and Chifuling (*Poria Rubra*) to promote diuresis; if used for infantile night cry, add Fushen (*Sclerotium Poriae Circum Radicem Pini*) and Suanzaoren (*Semen Ziziphi Spinosae*) to tranquilize the mind.

Elucidation: The syndrome is result of flaming up of the heart-fire due to accumulation of heat in the heart meridian or heat in the heart invading the small intestine. It should be treated by clearing away heat and fire from the heart and promoting diuresis. Ingredient No. 2 is to purge pathogenic fire from the heart, promote urination

诀》。

【组成】 生地黄、木通、生甘草梢各6 g。

【用法】 共研粗末,每次9 g,加竹叶适量,水煎服。

【功用】 清心利水。

【临床应用】 适用于心经热盛证。症见心胸烦热,口渴面赤,渴喜冷饮,口舌生疮,或小便赤涩刺痛,舌红苔薄黄,脉数。口腔炎、鹅口疮、小儿夜啼、小儿泌尿系感染等属心经有热者,可用本方治疗。若心火较盛,心烦口疮重者,可加黄连以助清心泻火之力;若见小便赤涩热痛者,是心热移于小肠,宜加车前子、赤茯苓以增清热利水之功;若用于小儿夜啼,宜加茯神、酸枣仁以宁心安神。

【方解】 本方证由心经蕴热,心火上炎或心热下移小肠所致,治宜清心泻火,利水通淋之法。方中木通清心降火,利水通淋,导心热下行,为君药。生地黄清心滋阴生津,

and induce downward heat in the heart, acting as monarch drug. Ingredient No. 1 is meant to purge away heat from the heart, nourish yin and promote the production of body fluid, and when combined with ingredient No. 2, it can prevent impairment of yin, serving as minister drug. Zhuye (*Herba Lophatheri*) is for reducing heat from the heart, relieving restlessness, inducing heat downward, and plays the part of adjuvant drug. Ingredient No. 3 can clear away heat, relieve painful urination and coordinate the actions of various ingredients in the recipe, acting as guiding drug. All the ingredients in combination achieve the effect of clearing away heat from the heart, promoting urination without impairing yin and nourishing yin without retaining pathogenic factors. Such symptoms as dysphoria, aphthae and painful urination will disappear when heat in the heart is induced downward and out through urination.

This prescription is forbidden to use to treat patients with exuberant heat not in the heart meridian or patients with renal insufficiency since Sanye Mutong (*Radix clematidis Trifolium*), Chu Mutong (*Caulis Clematidis Armandii*) and Guan Mutong (*Caulis Aristolochiae Manshuriensis*) are all used as drugs. But Guan Mutong contains aristolochine. Large dosage of preparation containing Guan Mutong (over 10 g daily) may damage the kidney. So this prescription should not be used for a longer period of time.

Longdan Xiegan Tang
(*Decoction of Gentian for Purging Liver Fire*)

Source: *Yifang Jijie* (*Collection of Prescriptions with Exposition*).

Ingredients:

No. 1 Longdancao (*Radix Gentianae*) (fried with wine) 6 g;

No. 2 Huangqin (*Radix Scutellariae*) (fried with

与木通配伍,则无渗利伤阴之虞,为臣药。竹叶清心除烦,引热下行,加强君药清心利水之效,为佐药。甘草梢清热泻火,通淋止痛,又能调和药性,为佐使药。诸药配伍,清心与利水并施,利水与养阴同用,可使滋阴而不恋邪,利水而不伤阴,心热有下行之路,则烦热、口疮、淋痛等症悉除。

【注意事项】 非心经热盛,或伴有肾功能不全患者,禁用本方。由于木通科的三叶木通、毛茛科的川木通、马兜铃科的关木通均作为"木通"入药,而关木通含有马兜铃酸,大剂量(每日用量超过10 g)或长期服用含有关木通的制剂,有可能造成肾脏损害,因此本方不宜长期服用。

龙胆泻肝汤

【方源】 《医方集解》。

【组成】 龙胆草(酒炒)6 g,黄芩9 g,栀子(酒炒)9 g,泽泻9 g,木通6 g,车前子9 g,当归(酒炒)3 g,生地黄(酒炒)

wine) 9 g;

No. 3 Zhizi (*Fructus Gardeniae*) (fried with wine) 9 g;

No. 4 Zexie (*Rhizoma Alismatis*) 9 g;

No. 5 Mutong (*Caulis Akebiae*) 6 g;

No. 6 Cheqianzi (*Semen Plantaginis*) 9 g;

No. 7 Danggui (*Radix Angelicae Sinensis*) (fried with wine) 3 g;

No. 8 Shengdihuang (*Radix Rehmanniae*) (fried with wine) 6 g;

No. 9 Chaihu (*Radix Bupleuri*) 6 g;

No. 10 Shenggancao (*Radix Glycyrrhizae*) 6 g.

Administration: Decoct the above drugs for oral administration.

Actions: Purging excessive fire from the liver and gallbladder, and removing damp-heat from the lower energizer.

Clinical Application: This recipe is indicated for upward attack of excessive fire in the liver and gallbladder or downward flow of damp-heat from the liver meridian, manifested as headache, conjunctival congestion, hypochondriac pain, bitter taste in the mouth, deafness, pain and bulge of ear; or marked by stranguria with turbid urine, pruritus and swelling of vulva, and leukorrhagia, red tongue with thick yellowish fur, taut and rapid pulse. It is applicable to such diseases with fire of excess type in the liver meridian and damp-heat syndrome as intractable migraine, hypertension, acute conjunctivitis, furuncle of external auditory canal, acute pyelonephritis, acute icterohepatitis, acute cholecystitis, urethritis, vulvitis, bubo, and acute pelvic inflammation. In case of dominance of upward flaming of excess fire in the liver and gallbladder that affects the upper part, ingredients No. 5 and No. 6 should be subtracted and Huanglian (*Rhizoma Coptidis*) added instead to help purge fire from the liver. If downward

6 g,柴胡6 g,生甘草6 g。

【用法】 水煎服。

【功用】 泻肝胆实火,清下焦湿热。

【临床应用】 适用于肝胆实火上炎及肝经湿热下注证。症见头痛目赤,胁痛口苦,耳聋耳肿,或小便淋浊,阴肿阴痒,妇女带下,舌红苔黄腻,脉弦数。顽固性偏头痛、高血压病、急性结膜炎、外耳道疖肿、急性肾盂肾炎、急性黄疸型肝炎、急性胆囊炎、尿道炎、外阴炎、腹股沟淋巴结炎、急性盆腔炎等属肝经实火湿热证者,可以本方治疗。若以肝胆实火上炎为主,病在上部者,宜去木通、车前子,加黄连以助清泄肝火之力;若以肝经湿热下注为主,病在下部者,宜去黄芩、生地黄,加滑石、薏苡仁以增渗利湿邪之

flow of dampness-heat in the liver meridian affects the lower part, ingredients No. 2 and No. 8 should be replaced with Huashi (*Talcum*) and Yiyiren (*Semen Coicis*) to help eliminate dampness. In case of ulceration, swelling and pain at the lower part, ingredient No. 9 can be replaced with Lianqiao (*Fructus Forsythiae*), Pugongying (*Herba Taraxaci*) and Dahuang (*Radix et Rhizoma Rhei*) to purge fire and toxin and relieve swelling.

Elucidation: This syndrome is caused by excess fire in the liver and gallbladder, and upward flaming or downward flow of damp heat along the liver meridian. It should be treated by purging liver-fire and dispelling damp heat. Ingredient No. 1 is used as monarch drug to purge excess fire in the liver and gallbladder and clear away damp heat in the lower-energizer. Ingredients No. 2 and No. 3 are used in combination to reinforce the effect of No. 1, playing the role of minister drug. Functioning together as adjuvant drug, ingredients No. 4, No. 5 and No. 6 have the effect of removing heat and inducing diuresis to dispel damp heat, No. 7 and No. 8 possess the effect of nourishing yin and blood, and No. 9 regulating the function of liver-qi. The last ingredient works as guiding drug with the effect of clearing away heat and coordinating the effect of various ingredients in the recipe so as to prevent the stomach from being hurt by drugs of bitter and cold property. The combination of these drugs produces both purgative and reinforcing, both regulating and nourishing actions, dispelling pathogenic factors without impairing vital-qi, and strengthening vital-qi without retaining damp heat.

Cautions: This recipe should not be applied to those manifesting headache and conjunctival congestion that are attributable to yang excess due to yin deficiency. Stop using the recipe immediately when the expected results

功；若下部湿疮，红肿热痛者，可去柴胡，加连翘、蒲公英、大黄以泻火消肿解毒。

【方解】 本方证由肝胆实火、湿热循经上炎或下注所致，治宜清泻肝火，清利湿热之法。方中龙胆草上清肝胆实火，下泻肝胆湿热，为君药。黄芩、栀子助君药清肝泻火，清热燥湿，同为臣药。车前子、木通、泽泻清热利湿，导湿热下行；当归、生地黄滋阴养血，使苦燥渗利而不伤阴血；柴胡疏畅肝胆之气，均为佐药。甘草清热和中，调和药性，为使药。诸药配伍，泻中兼补，疏中有养，祛邪而不伤正，扶正而不碍邪。

【注意事项】 阴虚阳亢而致头痛目赤者，禁用本方。本方中病即止，不宜长期服用。

have been achieved.

Xiebai San
(*Powder for Purging Lung Heat*)

Source：*Xiao'er Yaozheng Zhijue* (*Key to Differentiation and Therapeutics of Children's Diseases*).

Ingredients：

No. 1 Digupi (*Cortex Lycii Radici*) 30 g；

No. 2 Sangbaipi (*Cortex Mori Radicis*) 30 g；

No. 3 Zhigancao (*Radix Glycyrrhizae Praeparatae*) 3 g.

Administration：Grind the above drugs into coarse powder first and then mix 9 g each time with 20 g Jingmi (*Semen Oryzae Sativae*) and decoct them in water for oral administration.

Actions：Purging pathogenic heat in the lung, relieving cough and asthma.

Clinical Application：This recipe is indicated for mild cases of cough and asthma due to lung-heat in children, manifested as asthma, cough, feverish skin that is aggravated in the afternoon, red tongue with yellowish fur, thready and rapid pulse. It can be used to deal with infantile pneumonia, bronchitis, and early stage of measles, which pertain to cough and asthma due to lung-heat. In case of adverse flow of qi due to lung-heat manifesting dominant fever, cough and asthma, Huangqin (*Radix Scutellariae*) and Zhimu (*Rhizoma Anemarrhenae*) can be added to strengthen the effect of purging lung-heat. For cough with little sputum due to dryness-heat in the lung, Gualoupi (*Pericarpium Trichosanthis*) and Chuanbeimu (*Bulbus Fritillariae Cirhosae*) can be added to help moisten the lung to relieve cough.

Elucidation：The syndrome is due to heat accumulating in the lung and impairing yinfen, further causing lung's failure in purifying and descending function. It should be treated by purging heat in the lung to relieve

泻白散

【方源】 《小儿药证直诀》。

【组成】 地骨皮、桑白皮各 30 g，炙甘草 3 g。

【用法】 共研粗末，每次9 g，再加粳米 20 g，水煎服。

【功用】 清泻肺热，平喘止咳。

【临床应用】 适用于小儿肺热咳喘轻证。症见气喘咳嗽，皮肤蒸热，日晡尤甚，舌红苔黄，脉细数。小儿肺炎、支气管炎、麻疹初期等属肺热咳嗽或气喘者，可以本方治疗。若肺热气逆，发热咳喘较甚者，可加黄芩、知母以助清泄肺热之力；若肺中燥热，干咳痰少者，可加瓜蒌皮、川贝母以增润肺止咳之功。

【方解】 本方证由热郁于肺，伤及阴分，肺失清肃所致，治宜清泻肺热，止咳平喘之法。方中桑白皮清泻肺热，

cough and athma. Ingredient No. 2 has the effect of dispelling lung-heat, and functions as monarch drug. Ingredient No. 1 serves as minister drug, which helps bring about the effect of the monarch drug. Ingredient No. 3 and Jingmi (*Semen Oryzae Sativae*) are used as adjuvant and guiding drug, capable of nourishing the stomach, strengthening the lung by way of reinforcing the spleen, and coordinating the effects of all the ingredients. The four drugs are mild in action and thus can purge heat from the lung without impairing body resistance when applied in children.

Cautions: Simple in ingredients and mild in action, the recipe is not advisable for serious cases of heat accumulation in the lung.

Xiehuang San
(*Powder for Purging Spleen Heat*)

Source: *Xiao'er Yaozheng Zhijue* (*Key to Differentiation and Therapeutics of Children's Diseases*).

Ingredients:

No. 1 Huoxiang (*Herba Agastachis*) 21 g;

No. 2 Zhiziren (*Fructus Gardeniae*) 3 g;

No. 3 Shigao (*Gypsum Fibrosum*) 15 g;

No. 4 Gancao (*Radix Glycyrrhizae*) 90 g;

No. 5 Fangfeng (*Radix Ledebouriellae*) 120 g.

Administration: Grind the above drugs into coarse powder, take 5g each time and decoct it in water for oral administration.

Actions: Purging latent fire in the spleen and stomach.

Clinical Application: This recipe is indicated for latent fire syndrome in the spleen and stomach marked by aphthae, foul breath, excessive thirst, inclination to hunger, dryness of the mouth and lips, as well as unusual movement of the tongue seen in children which is indicative of excessive heat in the spleen, red tongue, and rapid

---

止咳平喘，为君药。地骨皮助君药清热止咳平喘，为臣药。炙甘草、粳米补中益肺，培土生金，兼调药性，为佐使药。四药配伍，寓补于泻，药力平和，施于小儿稚阴之体、娇弱之肺，可使肺热清泄而正气不伤。

【注意事项】 本方药简力轻，药性平和，肺热重证不宜使用。

泻黄散

【方源】 《小儿药证直诀》。

【组成】 藿香21 g，栀子仁3 g，石膏15 g，甘草90 g，防风120 g。

【用法】 共研粗末，每次5 g，水煎服。

【功用】 泻脾胃伏火。

【临床应用】 适用于脾胃伏火证。症见口疮口臭，烦渴易饥，口燥唇干，或小儿脾热弄舌，舌质红，脉数。口腔溃疡、口角炎、舌炎等属脾经伏火者，可用本方治疗。若伏

pulse. It can be used to deal with stomatocace, angular stomatitis and glossitis that pertain to latent fire in the spleen meridians. If body fluid is impaired, manifesting cracked lips and dryness of the tongue, Shanyao (*Rhizoma Dioscoreae*) and Shihu (*Herba Dendrobii*) can be added to nourish the spleen and promote the production of body fluid. If the latent fire causes oral ulceration, swelling and pain, Lianqiao (*Fructus Forsythiae*) and Baihuasheshecao (*Herba Oldenlandiae Diffusae*) can be added to relieve carbuncles.

Elucidation: The syndrome is due to latent fire invading the mouth and lips and should be treated by purging heat from the spleen. Ingredient No. 3, cold in property, acts as monarch drug to purge latent fire in the spleen and stomach. Ingredient No. 2 helps bring about the effect of the monarch drug and induce heat out through urination, while No. 5 is meant to dispel the latent fire from the spleen. Both are used as minister drug. Ingredient No. 1 is used as adjuvant drug for its effect of regulating the spleen, promoting the function of the middle energizer, and reinforcing the effect of No. 5. Acting as guiding drug, No. 4 is supposed to regulate the middle energizer, and coordinate the effect of various ingredients in the recipe. All the drugs together can produce the desirable effects of clearing away heat without retaining pathogenic factors, dispersing without inducing heat, and opposing to and complementing each other.

Cautions: This recipe should not be applied to children suffering from congenital deficiency and cerebral dysgenesis, manifesting pale tongue and unusual movement of the tongue. Nor should it be applied to those with heat due to deficiency of stomach-yin.

Qingwei San
(*Powder for Clearing away Stomach Heat*)
Source: *Lanshi Micang* (*Secret Record of the*

热伤津，唇裂舌燥者，可加山药、石斛以滋脾生津；若郁火生毒，口舌生疮，红肿热痛者，可加连翘、白花蛇舌草以解毒消痈。

【方解】　本方证由脾胃伏火上熏口唇所致，治宜清泻脾热，发越伏火之法。方中石膏大寒以清脾胃伏火，为君药。栀子助石膏清热泻火，并引热邪从小便而出；防风辛温疏散，配石膏以发越脾经郁伏之火，同为臣药。藿香理脾调中，合防风更增疏散郁火之力，为佐药。甘草生用，清热和中，调和药性，为使药。诸药配伍，寓散于清，寓升于降，清凉而不遏邪，升散而不助热，相反而相成。

【注意事项】　小儿先天不足，大脑发育不全，舌色淡白而弄舌者，以及胃阴虚有热者，均禁用本方。

清胃散
【方源】　《兰室秘藏》。

Cabinet of Orchids).

Ingredients:

No. 1 Shengdihuang (*Radix Rehmanniae*) 12 g;

No. 2 Dangguishen (*Radix Angelicae Sinensis*) 6 g;

No. 3 Mudanpi (*Cortex Moutan Radicis*) 9 g;

No. 4 Huanglian (*Rhizoma Coptidis*) 3 – 5 g;

No. 5 Shengma (*Rhizoma Cimicifugae*) 6 g.

Administration: Decoct the above drugs in water for oral administration.

Actions: Purging stomach-heat and cooling blood.

Clinical Application: This recipe is indicated for toothache due to fire in the stomach, marked by headache arising from toothache, feverish cheeks, aversion to heat with preference for cold, or gingival bleeding, or ulceration in the gum, or swelling and soreness of the tongue, lips and cheeks, or hot and foul breath, dryness of mouth and tongue, red tongue with yellowish fur, smooth and rapid pulse. It is applicable to stomatitis, periodontitis, and prosopalgia, etc. with the chief symptoms of toothache and gingival swelling due to the flare-up of stomach-fire. In case of impairment of body fluid due to excessive heat manifesting thirst and preference for cold drinks, Shigao (*Gypsum Fibrosum*) and Zhimu (*Rhizoma Anemarrhenae*) can be added to dispel fire from the stomach and promote the production of body fluid to quench thirst. In case of much gingival bleeding due to excessive fire in the stomach, it is advisable to add Niuxi (*Radix Achyranthis Bidentatae*) to ensure proper downward flow of heat and the blood. If complicated with constipation, Dahuang (*Radix et Rhizoma Rhei*) may be added to relax the bowels for purging heat.

Elucidation: The syndrome is due to upward attack by stomach-heat along yangming meridian of foot. It should be treated by clearing away stomach-fire and cooling

【组成】 生地黄12 g,当归身6 g,牡丹皮9 g,黄连 3～5 g,升麻6 g。

【用法】 水煎服。

【功用】 清胃凉血。

【临床应用】 适用于胃火牙痛证。症见牙痛牵引头痛,面颊发热,其齿喜冷恶热,或牙宣出血,或龈肿溃烂,或唇舌颊腮肿痛,或口气热臭,口舌干燥,舌红苔黄,脉滑数。口腔炎、牙周炎、三叉神经痛等以牙痛龈肿为主症,属胃火上攻者,可用本方治疗。若热甚津伤,口渴饮冷者,可加石膏、知母以清胃泻火,生津止渴;若胃火炽盛,牙龈出血较甚者,宜加牛膝以导热引血下行;若兼便秘者,可加大黄以通腑泻热,导热下行。

【方解】 本方证由胃热循足阳明经脉上攻所致,治宜清胃泻火,凉血消肿之法。方

blood to subdue swelling. Ingredient No. 4 is used as mon-arch drug to clear away fire in the stomach. Ingredients No. 1 and No. 3 are used as minister drug, capable of cool-ing blood and purging heat. While ingredient No. 2, as ad-juvant drug, has the effects of nourishing blood and pro-moting blood circulation, subduing swelling and alleviating pain. Ingredient No. 5 can dispel fire and remove toxin, and functions as guiding drug, leading various ingredients directly to the yangming meridian.

Cautions：It is not fit for toothache due to wind-cold or hyperactivity of fire due to deficiency of the kidney.

Yunü Jian
(*Jade Maiden Decoction*)

Source：*Jingyue Quanshu* (*Jingyue's Complete Works*).

Ingredients：

No. 1 Shigao (*Gypsum Fibrosum*) 15 - 30 g；

No. 2 Shudihuang (*Radix Rehmanniae Praepara-tae*) 9 - 30 g；

No. 3 Maimendong (*Radix Ophiopogonis*) 6 g；

No. 4 Zhimu (*Rhizoma Anemarrhenae*) 5 g；

No. 5 Niuxi (*Radix Achyranthis Bidentatae*) 5 g.

Administration：Decoct the above drugs for oral ad-ministration.

Actions：Clearing away stomach-heat and nouris-hing yin.

Clinical Application：This recipe is suitable for syndromes of stomach-heat and yin deficiency, marked by toothache, odontoseisis, dysphoria with thirst, or diabe-tes, polyorexia, dry and red tongue with yellowish dry fur, thready and rapid pulse. It is applicable to gingivitis, acute stomatitis, glossitis, and diabetes, etc., which be-long to syndromes with stomach-heat and yin deficiency. In case of dominant toothache and thirst due to excessive

中黄连长于清胃泻火，为君药。生地黄、牡丹皮凉血清热，同为臣药。当归养血和血，以利消肿止痛，为佐药。升麻散火解毒，并引诸药入阳明经，为使药。

【注意事项】 属风寒及肾虚火炎牙痛者，禁用本方。

玉女煎

【方源】 《景岳全书》。

【组成】 石膏15～30 g，熟地黄9～30 g，麦门冬6 g，知母、牛膝各5 g。

【用法】 水煎服。

【功用】 清胃滋阴。

【临床应用】 适用于胃热阴虚证。症见牙痛，齿松，牙龈出血，烦热干渴，或消渴，消谷善饥，舌红苔黄而干，脉细数。牙龈炎、急性口腔炎、舌炎、糖尿病等见有牙痛齿松，舌红而干，属阴亏而胃火盛者，可用本方治疗。若胃火

fire in the stomach, Huanglian (*Rhizoma Coptidis*) and Zhizi (*Fructus Gardeniae*) can be added to strengthen the effect of purging fire. In case of dominant heat syndrome of xuefen, manifesting profuse gingival bleeding, ingredient No. 2 can be replaced with Shengdihuang (*Radix Rehmanniae Recens*) and Xuanshen (*Radix Scrophulariae*) to enhance the effect of removing heat from blood.

Elucidation: The syndrome results from flaming up of stomach-fire due to deficiency of kidney-yin, and should be treated by purging fire from the stomach and nourishing kidney-yin. Ingredient No. 1 is used as monarch drug to clear away heat from the stomach. Ingredient No. 2 acts as minister drug with the effect of invigorating kidney-yin. When the two are combined, the desirable effects of clearing away fire and nourishing body fluid can be yielded. Ingredient No. 4 is used to reinforce the effect of No. 1 in purging fire and heat from the stomach, and No. 3 to help No. 2 nourish kidney-yin. Ingredient No. 5 leads heat and blood downward. The above three together serve as adjuvant drug.

Both Qingwei San and Yunü Jian can be applied in the treatment of toothache due to stomach-heat. The former is fit for excess syndrome with upward invasion of stomach-fire, while the latter for excess syndrome of upward invasion of stomach-fire complicated with yin deficiency.

Shaoyao Tang
(*Peony Decoction*)

Source: *Suwen Bingji Qiyi Baoming Ji* (*Basic Questions: Collection on Pathogenesis for Preserving Life*).

Ingredients:

No. 1 Shaoyao (*Radix Paeoniae*) 15 - 20 g;

No. 2 Danggui (*Radix Angelicae Sinensis*) 9 g;

No. 3 Huanglian (*Rhizoma Coptidis*) 5 - 9 g;

炽盛,牙痛口渴较甚者,可加黄连、栀子以助清热泻火之力;若血分热盛,齿衄出血量多者,可去熟地黄,加生地黄、玄参以增清热凉血之功。

【方解】 本方证由肾阴不足,胃火上攻所致,治宜清泻胃火,滋肾养阴之法。方中石膏清泻胃火,为君药。熟地黄益肾滋阴,为臣药。君臣合用,清火而壮水。知母助石膏以清胃泻火,麦门冬助熟地黄以滋补肾阴,牛膝导热并引血下行,同为佐药。

清胃散与玉女煎均可治疗胃热牙痛证,其中清胃散用于胃火上攻,牙龈肿痛的实证;玉女煎用于胃火上攻,兼有阴虚的虚实夹杂证。

芍药汤

【方源】 《素问病机气宜保命集》。

【组成】 芍药 15～20 g,当归9 g,黄连5～9 g,槟榔、木香、炙甘草各5 g,大黄6 g,黄芩9 g,官桂2～5 g。

No. 4 Binglang (*Semen Arecae*) 5 g;

No. 5 Muxiang (*Radix Aucklandiae*) 5 g;

No. 6 Zhigancao (*Radix Glycyrrhizae Praeparatae*) 5 g;

No. 7 Dahuang (*Radix et Rhizoma Rhei*) 6 g;

No. 8 Huangqin (*Radix Scutellariae*) 9 g;

No. 9 Guangui (*Cortex Cinnamomi*) 2 – 5 g.

Administration：Smash the above drugs into coarse powder and decoct 15g each time in water for oral administration.

Actions：Clearing away damp heat and regulating qi and blood.

Clinical Application：This recipe is indicated for dysentery due to damp heat, marked by abdominal pain, pus and blood in the stool, tenesmus, burning sensation in the anus, scanty dark urine, yellowish greasy fur, smooth and rapid pulse. It can be used to treat such diseases with difficult defecation, abdominal pain and tenesmus due to damp heat as bacillary dysentery, amebic dysentery, irritable colitis and acute enteritis, etc. The employment of Chishaoyao (*Radix Paeoniae Rubra*) or Baishaoyao (*Radix Paeoniae Alba*) depends on the actual purpose of removing heat from blood and promoting blood circulation, or of nourishing yin to relieve pain. In case of high fever, pus and blood in the stool, Baitouweng (*Radix Pulsatillae*) and Jinyinhua (*Flos Lonicerae*) can be added to enhance the effects of clearing away heat and toxin to relieve dysentery.

Elucidation：The syndrome is due to accumulation of damp heat and epidemic pathogens in the intestine, leading to incoordination of qi and blood. It should be treated by clearing away heat, eliminating toxin and dampness, and regulating qi and blood. Ingredient No. 3 and No. 8 are capable of clearing away heat and toxin and drying dampness to relieve dysentery, acting as monarch

【用法】　共研粗末,每次 15 g,水煎服。

【功用】　清热燥湿,调和气血。

【临床应用】　适用于湿热痢疾。症见腹痛,便脓血,赤白相兼,里急后重,肛门灼热,小便短赤,舌苔黄腻,脉滑数。细菌性痢疾、阿米巴痢疾、过敏性结肠炎、急性肠炎等见有泻下不畅,腹痛里急,属湿热为患者,可用本方治疗。方中芍药,欲清热凉血活血者,则用赤芍;欲养阴缓急止痛者,则用白芍。若高热,便脓血较甚者,可加白头翁、金银花以助清热解毒止痢之功。

【方解】　本方证由湿热疫毒壅滞肠中,气血失和所致,治宜清热解毒燥湿,调和气血之法。方中黄连、黄芩清热解毒,燥湿止痢,共为君药。大黄苦寒泄降,既可助黄芩、黄连泻火燥湿,又能荡涤肠道

drug. As minister drug, No. 7 is bitter and cold in proper- ty and has purgative and descending actions. It can not only help the monarch drug purge fire and dry dampness, but also remove stagnation in the intestine, which is known as "treating diarrhea with cathartics". No. 1 and No. 2 bear the action of promoting and regulating blood circulation, and No. 4 and No. 5 promoting the flow of qi. With a small dosage No. 9 is meant to prevent drugs of bit- ter and cold property from impairing middle energizer and latent dampness and heat because it is pungent and hot in property. It can also warm and promote the flow of blood and assist No. 1, No. 2, No. 4 and No. 5 in regulating the flow of qi and blood. These five ingredients together play the part of adjuvant drug. No. 6 serves as guiding drug, which mediates the properties of other drugs and can re- lieve spasm and pain when combined with No. 1.

Cautions: This recipe is contraindicated at the onset of dysentery concomitant with exterior syndrome.

Baitouweng Tang
(*Decoction of Pulsatillae*）

Source: *Shanghan Lun* (*Treatise on Febrile Dia- seses*).

Ingredients:

No. 1 Baitouweng (*Radix Pulsatillae*) 15 g;

No. 2 Huangbai (*Cortex Phellodendri*) 12 g;

No. 3 Huanglian (*Rhizoma Coptidis*) 6 g;

No. 4 Qinpi (*Cortex Fraxini*) 12 g.

Administration: Decoct the above drugs in water for oral administration.

Actions: Clearing away heat and toxin, cooling blood and relieving dysentery.

Clinical Application: This recipe is indicated for bloody dysentery due to heat, marked by abdominal pain, tenesmus, burning sensation in the anus, pus and blood in

积滞,有"通因通用"之功,为臣药。芍药、当归行血活血,槟榔、木香行气导滞;少加官桂,取其辛热以避免苦寒伤中或冰伏遏湿热之偏,并可温通血脉,助当归、芍药、槟榔、木香调气和血,均为佐药。炙甘草调和药性,与芍药同用,又能缓急止痛,为使药。

【注意事项】 痢疾初起兼有表证者,禁用本方。

白头翁汤

【方源】 《伤寒论》。

【组成】 白头翁15 g,黄柏12 g,黄连6 g,秦皮12 g。

【用法】 水煎服。

【功用】 清热解毒,凉血止痢。

【临床应用】 适用于热毒血痢证。症见腹痛,里急后重,肛门灼热,下痢脓血,赤多

the stool with blood exceeding pus in amount, thirst with desire for drinking, reddened tongue with yellowish fur, taut and rapid pulse. It is applicable to acute bacillary dysentery, chronic nonspecific ulcerative colitis, acute colitis and other diseases, which belong to excessive-heat syndrome. If functional disorder of qi occurs as the result of excessive accumulation of heat, manifesting severe abdominal pain and tenesmus, add Zhishi (*Fructus Aurantii Immaturus*) and Binglang (*Semen Arecae*) to promote the flow of qi. In case of much blood in stool, add Yinhuatan (*Carbonized Flos Lonicerae*) and Diyu (*Herba Thymi*) to remove toxin and cool blood.

Elucidation: The syndrome is due to dominance of toxic heat in xuefen and should be treated by clearing away heat and removing toxin, cooling blood and relieving dysentery. As monarch drug, ingredient No. 1 is good at removing heat and toxin, cooling blood and relieving dysentery. No. 2 and No. 3 can help the monarch drug eliminate heat and toxin and dry dampness to stop dysentery, functioning as minister drug. No. 4 serves as adjuvant drug, which can clear away heat and dry dampness, and has astringent action.

Shaoyao Tang and this recipe both possess the action of clearing away heat, toxin and relieving dysentery. The former, with a compatibility of drugs able to clear away heat and those to regulate the flow of qi and blood, is fit for dysentery with excessive damp heat manifesting pus and blood in the stool and greasy yellowish fur. The latter, however, is composed totally of drugs with the effects of clearing away heat and toxin, cooling blood and relieving dysentery and fit for dysentery with excessive heat, which is characterized by pus and blood in stool, with blood exceeding pus in amount, and dry yellowish fur. Clinically they can be selected for application in

白少,渴欲饮水,舌红苔黄,脉弦数。急性细菌性痢疾、阿米巴痢疾、慢性非特异性溃疡性结肠炎、急性结肠炎等属热毒炽盛者,可用本方治疗。若热毒壅聚,气机不畅,腹痛里急甚者,可加枳实、槟榔以行气导滞;若大便出血多者,可加银花炭、地榆以解毒凉血。

【方解】 本方证由热毒炽盛,深陷血分,以致纯下血痢,治宜清热解毒,凉血止痢之法。方中白头翁功擅清热解毒,凉血止痢,为君药。黄连、黄柏助君药清热解毒,燥湿止痢,同为臣药。秦皮清热燥湿,收涩止痢,为佐药。

芍药汤与白头翁汤均有清热解毒止痢之功,用于治疗痢疾。芍药汤由清热解毒药配伍调气和血药组成,适用于痢疾湿热较重者,以痢下赤白,赤白相兼,舌苔黄腻为特征;白头翁汤纯由清热解毒凉血治痢药物组成,适用于痢疾热毒较重者,以痢下赤白,赤多白少,舌苔黄燥为特征。临床可根据证情进行选择,或将两方配合使用。

accordance with the actual condition, or used in combination.

Cautions: The syndrome mentioned here is usually severe and critical, therefore it is advisable to use the decoction of this recipe for enema besides oral application so as to enhance the therapeutic effect.

2.2.5 Prescriptions for Clearing away Heat of Deficiency Type

Qinghao Biejia Tang
(*Decoction of Woomwood Artemisia and Soft-shelled Turtle*)

Source: *Wenbing Tiaobian* (*Detailed Analysis of Seasonal Febrile Diseases*).

Ingredients:

No. 1 Qinghao (*Herba Artemisiae*) 6 g;

No. 2 Biejia (*Carapax Trionycis*) 15 g;

No. 3 Shengdihuang (*Radix Rehmanniae*) 12 g;

No. 4 Zhimu (*Rhizoma Anemarrhenae*) 6 g;

No. 5 Mudanpi (*Cortex Moutan Radicis*) 9 g.

Administration: Decoct the above drugs in water for oral administration.

Actions: Nourishing yin and clearing away heat.

Clinical Application: This recipe is suitable for latent pathogenic factors in yinfen at the late stage of seasonal febrile diseases, marked by fever at night and normal temperature in the morning, no perspiration after fever subsides, reddened tongue with little fur, thready and rapid pulse. It is applicable to infantile summer heat, chronic pyelonephritis, postmeasles pneumonia, renal tuberculosis and other diseases with unrelieved low fever for unknown reasons, which pertain to deficiency of yin fluid and latent heat in the interior. In case of dominant heat of

【注意事项】 本方治证病情较重,病势较急,可在内服白头翁汤的同时以本方煎液作保留灌肠,以提高疗效。

第五节 清虚热剂

青蒿鳖甲汤

【方源】 《温病条辨》。

【组成】 青蒿6 g,鳖甲15 g,生地黄12 g,知母6 g,牡丹皮9 g。

【用法】 水煎服。

【功用】 养阴透热。

【临床应用】 适用于温病后期,邪伏阴分证。症见夜热早凉,热退无汗,舌红少苔,脉细数。小儿夏季热、慢性肾盂肾炎、麻疹后肺炎、肾结核以及不明原因的低热不退,属阴液不足,邪热内伏者,可用本方治疗。若虚热较著,兼骨蒸潮热者,可加地骨皮、胡黄连以清退虚热;若阴伤较著,

deficiency type concomitant with steaming sensation in the bones and hectic fever, add Digupi (*Cortex Lycii Radicis*) and Huhuanglian (*Rhizoma Picrorhizae*). In case of severe impairment of yin fluid, thirst and dryness of the lips, add Tianhuafen (*Radix Trichosanthis*) and Maimendong (*Radix Ophiopogonis*) to nourish yin and promote the production of body fluid.

口渴唇燥者,可加天花粉、麦门冬以滋阴生津。

Elucidation: This syndrome results from latent heat accumulating in yinfen at the late stage of epidemic febrile diseases because of the impairment of yin fluid and unsubdued heat. It should be treated by nourishing yin to expel heat from the interior. Ingredient No. 2 is used to nourish yin and clear away heat and No. 1 to expel heat from the interior. Both are used as monarch drug to nourish yin fluid and expel latent heat. Ingredient No. 3, capable of removing heat from blood and nourishing yin, and No. 4, nourishing yin and descending fire, help ingredient No. 2 nourish yin and dispel heat of deficiency type. Both are used as minister drug. Ingredient No. 5 is able to remove heat from blood and help No. 1 expel the remaining heat, acting as adjuvant drug.

【方解】　本方证由温病后期,阴液已伤,邪热未尽,深伏阴分所致,治宜养阴清热透邪之法。方中鳖甲滋阴清热,青蒿清热透邪,两药合用,滋养阴液,清透伏热,共为君药。生地黄凉血滋阴,知母滋阴降火,助鳖甲以养阴退虚热,同为臣药。牡丹皮清热凉血,助青蒿透热清余邪,为佐药。

Cautions: Since Ingredient No. 1 is intolerant of high temperature, it should be soaked in boiling water for oral application, and the rest decocted.

【注意事项】　方中青蒿不耐高温,可用沸水泡服,余药煎服。

Danggui Liuhuang Tang
(*Decoction of Angelica and Six Ingredients with Characters*)

当归六黄汤

Source: *Lanshi Micang* (*Secret Record of the Chamber of Orchids*).

【方源】　《兰室秘藏》。

Ingredients:

No. 1 Danggui (*Radix Angelicae Sinensis*) 6 g;

No. 2 Shengdihuang (*Radix Rehmanniae*) 6 g;

No. 3 Huangqin (*Radix Scutellariae*) 6 g;

No. 4 Huangbai (*Cortex Phellodendri*) 6 g;

【组成】　当归、生地黄、黄芩、黄柏、黄连、熟地黄各6 g,黄芪12 g。

No. 5 Huanglian (*Rhizoma Coptidis*) 6 g;

No. 6 Shudihuang (*Radix Rehmanniae Praeparatae*) 6 g;

No. 7 Huangqi (*Radix Astragali seu Hedysari*) 12 g.

Administration: Grind the above drugs into coarse powder before decocting in water for oral application, 15 g each time.

Actions: Nourishing yin, clearing away heat, consolidating the superficies and arresting perspiration.

Clinical Application: The recipe is indicated for night sweat from hyperactivity of fire due to yin deficiency, marked by fever, night sweat, flushed face, vexation, dryness of the mouth and lips, constipation, reddened tongue and rapid pulse. Clinically such physical signs should be considered as night sweat, flushed face, reddened tongue and rapid pulse. In case of deficiency of yin without dominant fire of excess type, Ingredients No. 5 and No. 3 can be replaced with Zhimu (*Rhizoma Anemarrhenae*) to purge fire without impairing yin. In case of incessant sweating, Fuxiaomai (*Fructus Tritici Levis*) and Duanmuli (*Concha Ostreae*) (calcined) can be added to enhance the effect of arresting perspiration.

Elucidation: The syndrome results from disturbance of fire due to deficiency of yin, leading to the excretion of yin fluid. It should be treated by nourishing yin, purging fire, and consolidating superficial resistance to arrest perspiration. Ingredients No. 1, No. 2 and No. 6 are used as monarch drug to nourish yin and blood, and restrain yang by nourishing yin. Ingredients No. 5, No. 3 and No. 4 function as minister drug to purge fire, and relieve vexation. The doubled dosage of No. 7 is meant to supplement qi to strengthen body resistance, and to arrest perspiration, acting as adjuvant drug.

【用法】 共研粗末,每次15 g,水煎服。

【功用】 滋阴清热,固表止汗。

【临床应用】 适用于阴虚火旺之盗汗证。症见发热盗汗,面赤心烦,口干唇燥,大便干结,舌红脉数。临床使用时以盗汗面赤、舌红脉数为指征。若阴虚而实火不著者,可去黄连、黄芩之苦燥,加知母以使泻火而不伤阴;若汗多不止者,可加浮小麦、煅牡蛎以增收敛止汗之功。

【方解】 本方证由阴虚火扰,阴液外泄所致,治宜滋阴泻火,固表止汗之法。方中当归、生地黄、熟地黄滋阴养血,壮水制火,共为君药。黄连、黄芩、黄柏清热泻火,除烦坚阴,同为臣药。倍用黄芪益气实卫,固表止汗,为佐药。

2.2.6　Prescriptions for Clearing away Summer-heat

Qingshu Yiqi Tang

(*Decoction for Eliminating Summer-heat and Benefiting Qi*)

Source：*Wenre Jingwei* (*Compendium on Seasonal Febrile Diseases*).

Ingredients：

No. 1 Xiyangshen (*Radix Panacis Guinquefolli*) 5 g;

No. 2 Shihu (*Herba Dendrobii*) 15 g;

No. 3 Maimendong (*Radix Ophiopogonis*) 9 g;

No. 4 Huanglian (*Rhizoma Coptidis*) 3 g;

No. 5 Zhuye (*Herba Lophatheri*) 6 g;

No. 6 Hegeng (*Petiolus Nelumbinis*) 6 g;

No. 7 Zhimu (*Rhizoma Anemarrhenae*) 6 g;

No. 8 Gancao (*Radix Glycyrrhizae*) 3 g;

No. 9 Jingmi (*Fructus Oryzae Sativae*) 15 g;

No. 10 Xigua Cuiyi (*Exocarpium Citrulli*) 30 g.

Administration：Decoct the above drugs in water for oral application.

Actions：Clearing away summer-heat and benefiting qi, nourishing yin and promoting production of body fluid.

Clinical Application：This recipe is particularly designed for consumption of qi and fluid by summer-heat, marked by feverish body, profuse perspiration, vexation, thirst, general debility, scanty and dark urine, feeble and rapid pulse. It is applicable to infantile summer fever, polydipsia and tiredness, which pertain to deficiency of qi and body fluid. In case of mild fever due to mild summer-heat, ingredient No. 4 can be subtracted to prevent it from impairing body fluid because of its bitter and dry nature. If complicated with dampness manifesting chest

第六节　清暑热剂

清暑益气汤

【方源】《温热经纬》。

【组成】　西洋参5 g,石斛15 g,麦门冬9 g,黄连3 g,竹叶6 g,荷梗6 g,知母6 g,甘草3 g,粳米15 g,西瓜翠衣 30 g。

【用法】　水煎服。

【功用】　清暑益气,养阴生津。

【临床应用】　适用于暑伤气津证。症见身热汗多,口渴心烦,体倦少气,小便短赤,脉象虚数。小儿夏季热久热不退,烦渴体倦属气津不足者,可以本方治疗。若发热不高,暑热不甚者,可去黄连,以免其苦燥伤津;若兼挟湿邪,胸闷苔腻者,可去麦门冬、知母,以防其滋腻助湿碍邪。

distress and greasy fur, ingredients No. 3 and No. 7 can be subtracted to prevent them from inducing dampness.

Elucidation: The syndrome is due to consumption of qi and body fluid by summer-heat, and should be treated by clearing away summer-heat, supplementing qi and nourishing yin. Ingredients No. 1 and No. 10 act as monarch drug, which supplement qi and promote the production of body fluid, and remove summer-heat respectively. The combined application of both achieves the effect of removing pathogenic factors and strengthening body resistance simultaneously. Ingredient No. 6 helps bring about the effect of No. 10, and No. 2 and No. 3 help No. 1 carry out its function. The three ingredients form minister drug. Ingredients No. 4, No. 5 and No. 7 serve as adjuvant drug, helping subdue summer-heat. Ingredients No. 8 and No. 9 are meant to promote the function of the stomach and mediate drug properties, acting together as guiding drugs.

【方解】 本方证由暑热之邪耗气伤津所致,治宜清热解暑,益气养阴之法。方中西洋参益气生津,西瓜翠衣清热解暑,两药配伍,邪正兼顾,共为君药。荷梗助西瓜翠衣解暑清热;石斛、麦门冬助西洋参养阴生津,同为臣药。黄连、竹叶、知母清热泻火以助祛暑退热之力,均为佐药。甘草、粳米益胃和中,调和药性,为使药。

2.3 Prescriptions for Warming the Interior

第三章 温里剂

Prescriptions for warming the interior refer to those that are mainly made up of drugs of warm nature with the effect of warming the interior, restoring yang, dispelling cold and promoting blood circulation for the treatment of interior-cold syndrome.

Since interior-cold syndrome may affect the viscera, meridians or collaterals, and differ in degrees of severity, prescriptions for warming the interior are accordingly sub-divided into three kinds. They are prescriptions for warming the middle-energizer to dispel cold, those for recuperating depleted yang to rescue the patient from collapse and those for warming the meridians to dispel cold.

Prescriptions for warming the middle-energizer to dispel cold are composed of drugs with the function of warming the middle-energizer and dispersing cold. They are applied in deficiency-cold syndrome of the spleen and stomach. Prescriptions for recuperating depleted yang to rescue the patient from collapse comprise drugs of extreme pungent and heat nature with the functions of warming the interior and dispelling cold, which are applicable to syndrome of excess of yin due to yang deficiency. Prescriptions for warming the meridians to dispel cold mainly consist of drugs capable of warming the meridians to dispel cold and promote blood circulation, which are applicable to syndrome of cold accumulation in the meridians and collaterals.

Prescriptions for warming the interior mostly bear pungent, warm, dry and hot natures, and are apt to

凡以温里药为主组成,具有温里助阳,散寒通脉等作用,用于治疗里寒证的方剂,统称温里剂。

由于里寒证的病位有脏腑经络之别,病情有缓急轻重之异,因而温里剂相应地分为温中祛寒剂、回阳救逆剂与温经散寒剂三类。

温中祛寒剂由温中散寒药为主组成,具有温中补虚作用,适用于脾胃虚寒证。回阳救逆剂由大辛大热的温里祛寒药为主组成,具有回阳救逆作用,适用于阳衰阴盛证。温经散寒剂由温经祛寒药为主组成,具有散寒通脉作用,适用于寒凝经脉证。

温里剂药性多辛温燥热,易于伤阴、助热、动血,故素体

impair yin, induce heat and disturb blood flow. Therefore, great cautions must be taken if they are applied to patients with yin-blood deficiency, or excessive heat in the interior, or women during menstrual period. It is not advisable to use these prescriptions with over-dose in the dog days.

阴血不足、内热偏重者以及妇女经期慎用,炎夏酷暑之时使用温里剂用量不宜过重。

2.3.1 Prescriptions for Warming the Middle-energizer to Dispel Cold

Lizhong Wan
(**Bolus for the Function of Middle Energizer**)

Source: *Shanghan Lun* (*Treatise on Exogenous Febrile Diseases*).

Ingredients:

No.1 Renshen (*Radix Ginseng*) 90 g;

No.2 Ganjiang (*Rhizoma Zingiberis*) 90 g;

No.3 Zhigancao (*Radix Glycyrrhizae Praeparatae*) 90 g;

No.4 Baizhu (*Rhizoma Atractylodis Macrocephalae*) 90 g.

Administration: Grind the above drugs into coarse powder, mix it with honey and make them into boluses, take 6 g orally with warm boiled water each time, three times daily; or decoct them with dosages in proportion to the original ones (it was named Renshen Tang in the book).

Actions: Warming the middle-energizer to dispel cold and replenishing qi to invigorate the spleen.

Clinical Application: This recipe is used to treat deficiency-cold syndrome of the spleen and stomach, marked by epigastric and abdominal pain, preference for warmth and for pressure, aversion to cold, cold limbs, poor appetite, vomiting, diarrhea, or bleeding due to yang deficiency with little dark blood, pale tongue with whitish fur, deep and thready pulse. It is applicable to

第一节 温中祛寒剂

理中丸

【方源】《伤寒论》。

【组成】 人参、干姜、炙甘草、白术各90 g。

【用法】 共研细末,炼蜜为丸,每次6 g,温开水送服,每日3次。亦可作汤剂(原书称之"人参汤"),用量按原方比例酌定。

【功用】 温中祛寒,补气健脾。

【临床应用】 适用于脾胃虚寒证。症见脘腹疼痛,喜温喜按,畏寒肢冷,食欲不振,呕吐腹泻,或阳虚失血,出血不多,血色黯淡,舌淡苔白,脉象沉细。急性胃肠炎、慢性胃肠炎、胃及十二指肠溃疡、慢

such diseases characterized by vomiting, diarrhea, cold and pain as acute or chronic gastroenteritis, gastroduodenal ulcer and chronic colitis, etc., which pertain to deficiency-cold in the stomach and spleen. In case of severe cold syndrome, add the dosage of ingredient No. 2 or add Fuzi (*Radix Aconiti Praeparatae*) to enhance the effect of warming the middle-energizer to dispel cold, which constitutes another recipe known as Fuzi Lizhong Wan. When used in the treatment of bleeding due to yang deficiency, substitute No. 2 with Paojiang (*Rhizoma Zingiberis Praeparatae*). In case of excessive deficiency syndrome, add No. 1 to replenish qi and reinforce the spleen. In case of severe diarrhea, add the dosage of No. 4 to invigorate the spleen and arrest diarrhea. In case of severe vomiting, add Wuzhuyu (*Fructus Evodiae*) and Shengjiang (*Rhizoma Zingiberis Recens*) to warm the stomach and stop vomiting. In case of dysfunction of the spleen in transportation due to deficiency, and phlegm generated from dampness, add Banxia (*Rhizoma Pinelliae*) and Fuling (*Poria*) to resolve phlegm, which constitutes another recipe, entitled Lizhong Huatan Wan.

Elucidation: The syndrome results from yang-deficiency of middle-energizer, and deficiency-cold of the spleen and stomach, leading to dysfunction in digestion and transformation. It should be treated by warming the middle-energizer to dispel cold and replenishing qi to invigorate the spleen. Ingredient No. 2 acts as monarch drug to restore yang of the spleen and stomach by means of warming the middle-energizer to dispel cold. Ingredient No. 1 is used as minister drug for supplementing qi, and strengthening the spleen to promote transportation and transformation. Ingredient No. 4 serves as adjuvant drug, used together with ingredients No. 1 and No. 2 for replenishing qi, strengthening the spleen and eliminating damp-

性结肠炎等以吐、利、冷、痛为特征,属脾胃虚寒者,可用本方治疗。若寒甚者,重用干姜,或加附子以助温中祛寒之力,即附子理中丸;若用于阳虚失血证,宜将干姜改为炮姜;若虚甚者,重用人参以益气补脾;若下利重者,重用白术以健脾助运止利;若呕吐甚者,可加吴茱萸、生姜以温胃止呕;若脾虚不运,聚湿生痰者,可加半夏、茯苓以温化痰饮,即理中化痰丸。

【方解】　本方证由中阳不足,脾胃虚寒,运化失司所致,治宜温中祛寒,补气健脾之法。方中干姜温中助阳祛寒,为君药。人参益气补脾助运,为臣药。白术补气健脾燥湿,合干姜以温运脾阳,配人参可益气补脾,为佐药。炙甘草甘温补中,既可助三药温补脾胃之力,又能调和药性,为佐使药。

ness. Ingredient No. 3, sweet and mild in nature, helps other drugs in the recipe reinforce the spleen and stomach, and mediates other drugs properties, playing the part of guiding drug.

Wuzhuyu Tang
(*Decoction of Evodia*)

吴茱萸汤

Source: *Shanghan Lun* (*Treatise on Exogenous Febrile Diseases*).

【方源】 《伤寒论》。

Ingredients:

No. 1 Wuzhuyu (*Fructus Evodiae*) 9 g;

No. 2 Renshen (*Radix Ginseng*) 9 g;

No. 3 Shengjiang (*Rhizoma Zingiberis Recens*) 18 g;

No. 4 Dazao (*Fructus Ziziphi Jujubae*) 4pcs.

【组成】 吴茱萸9 g,人参9 g,生姜18 g,大枣 4 枚。

Administration: Decoct the above drugs in water for oral administration.

【用法】 水煎服。

Actions: Warming the middle-energizer and invigorating qi, lowering the adverse qi to arrest vomiting.

【功用】 温中补虚,降逆止呕。

Clinical Application: This recipe is indicated for vomiting syndrome due to stomach-cold, marked by nausea, vomiting, cold and pain of the stomach, acid regurgitation; or the liver-cold affecting the stomach, marked by vomiting, headache, pale tongue with thin and whitish fur, deep and thready pulse or taut and slow pulse. It is applicable to chronic gastritis, vomiting from pregnancy, nervous headache, and aural vertigo, etc., which have such chief symptoms as vomiting, pain in the epigastrium and pertain to reversing flow of qi due to stomach-cold. In case of serious vomiting, add Banxia (*Rhizoma Pinelliae*) and Sharen (*Fructus Amomi*) to enhance the effect of sending down the adversely rising qi to stop vomiting. In case of severe headache, add Chuanxiong (*Rhizoma Ligustici Chuanxiong*) and Danggui (*Radix Angelicae Sinensis*) to help bring about the effect of dispersing stagnated liver-qi to relieve pain. In case of dominant re-

【临床应用】 适用于胃寒呕吐证。症见恶心呕吐,胃脘冷痛,吞酸嘈杂,或肝寒犯胃,呕吐头痛,舌淡苔薄白,脉象沉细或弦迟。慢性胃炎、妊娠呕吐、神经性头痛、耳源性眩晕等以呕逆脘痛为主症,属胃寒气逆者,可用本方治疗。若呕吐较甚者,可加半夏、砂仁以加强降逆止呕作用;若头痛较著者,可加川芎、当归以助疏肝止痛之效;若吞酸明显者,可加乌贼骨、煅瓦楞子以增收敛制酸之功。

gurgitation, add Wuzeigu (*Os Sepiellae seu Sepiae*) and Duanwalengzi (*Concha Arcae*) (calcined) to enhance the effect of arresting regurgitation with astringents.

Elucidation: The syndrome results from deficiency-cold in the stomach with turbid yin reversing upwards, for which the method of warming the middle-energizer to restore qi, sending down the reversely ascending qi to arrest vomiting should be adopted. Ingredient No.1 can not only warm the stomach to dispel cold and arrest vomiting, but also warm the liver to send down the reverse flow of qi and relieve pain, functioning as monarch drug. Ingredient No.2 acts as minister drug to supplement and restore qi and nourish the spleen and stomach. Ingredient No.3 has the effect of warming the stomach to arrest vomiting, and No.4 invigorating qi and reinforcing the spleen, which function as adjuvant drug to enhance the effects of the monarch and minister drugs. Besides Ingredient No.4 also serves as guiding drug to mediate the properties of other ingredients.

Cautions: For patients with epigastralgia and acid regurgitation, which are attributable to accumulated heat in the stomach, this recipe is contraindicated.

Xiao Jianzhong Tang
(*Minor Decoction for Strengthening the Middle-energizer*)

Source: *Shanghan Lun* (*Treatise on Exogenous Febrile Diseases*).

Ingredients:

No.1 Shaoyao (*Radix Paeoniae*) 18 g (parched with wine);

No.2 Guizhi (*Ramulus Cinnamomi*) 9 g;

No.3 Zhigancao (*Radix Glycyrrhizae Praeparatae*) 6 g;

No.4 Shengjiang (*Rhizoma Zingiberis Recens*) 9 g;

No.5 Dazao (*Fructus Ziziphi Jujubae*) 12 pcs;

【方解】　本方证由胃中虚寒,浊阴上逆所致,治宜温中补虚,降逆止呕之法。方中吴茱萸既可温胃散寒止呕,又能温肝降逆止痛,为君药。人参益气补虚,滋养脾胃,为臣药。生姜温胃止呕,大枣益气补脾,可加强君、臣药温中补虚,降逆和胃作用,同为佐药。大枣并能调和药性,兼作使药。

【注意事项】　脘痛吞酸属胃中郁热而致者,禁用本方。

小建中汤

【方源】《伤寒论》。

【组成】　芍药(酒炒)18 g,桂枝9 g,炙甘草6 g,生姜9 g,大枣 12 枚 饴糖30 g(烊化)。

No. 6 Yitang (*Saccharum Granorum*) 30 g (melted by heat).

Administration: Decoct the above drugs in water for oral application.

Actions: Warming the middle-energizer to restore qi, relieving spasm and pain, and coordinating yin and yang.

Clinical Application: This recipe is used to treat interior contraction due to consumption, marked by epigastric and abdominal pain relieved by warming and pressing, pale tongue with whitish fur, thready-taut and slow pulse; or palpitation, restlessness, or soreness of the limbs, feverish sensation in the hands and feet, dryness of the mouth and throat. It is applicable to chronic gastritis, gastroduodenal ulcer, neurosism, functional fever and others with the above symptoms attributable to deficiency-cold syndrome of the spleen and stomach. Baishaoyao (*Radix Paeoniae Alba*) is often used clinically as Ingredient No. 1. In case of deficiency of qi in the middle-energizer manifesting lassitude and lack of strength, add Huangqi (*Radix Astragali seu Hedysari*) to invigorate qi and the spleen, namely Huangqi Jianzhong Tang. In case of deficiency of ying blood manifesting sallow complexion, add Danggui (*Radix Angelicae Sinensis*) to nourish the blood and restore qi, namely Danggui Jianzhong Tang.

Elucidation: The syndrome results from pathogenic factors in the liver subjugating the spleen due to deficiency-cold in the middle-energizer and disharmony between yin and yang. It should be treated by warming the middle-energizer to restore qi, relieving spasm and pain, and regulating yin and yang. The last ingredient is used as monarch drug not only to warm the middle-energizer and restore qi but also to relieve spasm and pain. Ingredient No. 2 bears the function of warming yang and dispelling

【用法】 水煎服。

【功用】 温中补虚,缓急止痛,调和阴阳。

【临床应用】 适用于虚劳里急证。症见脘腹疼痛,温按则痛减,舌淡苔白,脉细弦而缓,或心悸虚烦,或四肢酸楚,手足烦热,咽干口燥等。慢性胃炎、胃及十二指肠溃疡、神经衰弱、功能性发热等见有上述症状,属脾胃虚寒者,可用本方治疗。方中芍药,现临床多用白芍药。若中气不足,倦怠乏力者,可加黄芪以益气补脾,即黄芪建中汤;若营血亏虚,面色萎黄者,加当归以养血补虚,即当归建中汤。

【方解】 本方证由中焦虚寒,肝邪乘脾,阴阳失调所致,治宜温中补虚,缓急止痛,调和阴阳之法。方中饴糖温中补脾,缓急止痛,为君药。桂枝温阳祛寒,芍药养阴柔肝,二药既可助君药温里缓急之功,又具有调和营卫阴阳作用,同为臣药。炙甘草甘温益

cold, and No. 1 nourishing yin and the liver. Both act as minister drug and help the monarch drug carry out its function, and regulate yingqi and weiqi as well as yin and yang. Ingredient No. 3 is of sweet and warm nature with the effect of replenishing qi. It can warm the middle-energizer when used together with No. 6 and No. 2 of pungent and sweet nature and relieve spasm and pain when combined with No. 1 of sour and sweet nature. Ingredients No. 4 and No. 5 have respectively the function of warming the stomach and reinforcing the spleen, and serve as adjuvant drug. Their combination is to promote the middle-energizer qi to regulate yingqi and weiqi, and promote the production and transformation of qi and blood. Ingredient No. 3 is meant to mediate the effects of other ingredients and acts as guiding drug.

气,合饴糖、桂枝辛甘养阳,益气温中,合芍药酸甘化阴,缓急止痛;生姜温胃,大枣补脾,合用以升腾中焦生发之气而调营卫,并资气血生化之源,俱为佐药。甘草调和药性,兼作使药。

Cautions: This recipe is sweet in flavor and apt to generate dampness in the middle-energizer, thus is contraindicated for patients with deficiency cold syndrome in the middle-energizer concomitant with flatulence and greasy fur.

【注意事项】　本方味甘助湿满中,中焦虚寒兼有腹胀苔腻者禁用。

2.3.2　Prescriptions for Recuperating Depleted Yang to Rescue the Patient from Collapse

Sini Tang
(Decoction for Resuscitation)

Source: *Shanghan Lun* (*Treatise on Exogenous Febrile Diseases*).

Ingredients:

No. 1 Fuzi (*Radix Aconiti Praeparatae*) 15 g;

No. 2 Ganjiang (*Rhizoma Zingiberis*) 9 g;

No. 3 Zhigancao (*Radix Glycyrrhizae Praeparatae*) 6 g.

Administration: Decoct the above drugs in water

第二节　回阳救逆剂

四逆汤

【方源】　《伤寒论》。

【组成】　附子15 g,干姜9 g,炙甘草6 g。

【用法】　水煎服。

for oral application.

Actions: Recuperating depleted yang to rescue the patient from collapse.

Clinical Application: This recipe is used to treat syndrome of hyperactivity of yin due to yang exhaustion, marked by cold limbs, aversion to cold, lying huddling up, vomiting, absence of thirst, abdominal pain, diarrhea, mental fatigue and sleepiness, whitish and slippery fur, feeble and thready pulse. It is applicable to myocardial infarction, acute cardiac failure, excessive vomiting from acute or chronic gastroenteritis, or to shock as a result of profuse perspiration in some critical cases, which pertain to yin excess due to yang exhaustion, or collapse from yang depletion. In case of predominant yin rejecting yang manifesting flushed face and cold syndrome with pseudo-heat symptoms, add the dosage of the first two ingredients to enhance the effect of recuperating depleted yang and promoting blood circulation, namely Tongmai Sini Tang. In case of dampness accumulating in the interior due to yang deficiency accompanied by edema in the limbs, add Dangshen (*Radix Codonopsis Pilosulae*), Zexie (*Rhizoma Alismatis*) and Fuling (*Poria*) to reinforce the spleen for removing dampness and relieving swelling. This recipe is also made in the form of injection for first aid treatment of shock from various factors.

Elucidation: The syndrome results from depletion of yang-qi and excessive yin-cold in the interior, and should be treated by recuperating yang. Ingredient No.1, extremely pungent and hot in nature, acts as monarch drug to recuperate depleted yang. Ingredient No.2 functions as minister drug, and, in compatibility with No.1, strengthens the efficacy of recuperating depleted yang and dispelling cold. For this reason, there goes the saying "Without Ganjiang (*Rhizoma Zingiberis*), the hot prop-

【功用】 回阳救逆。

【临床应用】 适用于阳衰阴盛证。症见四肢厥冷,恶寒蜷卧,呕吐不渴,腹痛下利,神衰欲寐,舌苔白滑,脉象微细。心肌梗死、急性心功能衰竭、急性或慢性胃肠炎吐泻过多,或某些急证大汗而致休克属阳衰阴盛,甚至亡阳虚脱者,可用本方治疗。若阴盛格阳,面色红赤,真寒假热者,可加重附子与干姜的用量以增回阳通脉之力,即通脉四逆汤;若阳虚水湿内停,兼肢体浮肿者,可加党参、泽泻、茯苓以健脾利湿消肿。本方还被制成注射剂(四逆注射液)用于多种休克的抢救治疗。

【方解】 本方证由机体阳气衰微,阴寒内盛所致,治宜回阳救逆之法。方中附子大辛大热,温里祛寒,回阳救逆,为君药。干姜温中散寒,与附子相配,回阳逐寒之力尤著,故有"附子无姜不热"之说,为臣药。炙甘草益气温中,既助附子、干姜温补之力,

erty of Fuzi (*Radix Aconiti Praeparatae*) can not be brought into play. " The last ingredient is meant to replenish qi and restore yang of the middle-energizer and serves as adjuvant drug, which helps bring about the efficacy of the first two ingredients on the one hand, and reduces the toxic substances of No. 1 on the other hand. It also reduces the side effect of the first two drugs because they are pungent, warm and dry in nature and apt to consume qi and impair body fluid, and mediates the efficacy of various drugs. The three ingredients, simple in compatibility but effective in results, ensure an immediate effect of recuperating depleted yang to rescue the patient from collapse.

Cautions: The syndrome of yang deficiency and yin excess often manifests cold syndrome with pseudo-heat symptoms as seen in predominant yin rejecting yang syndrome or yang-floating syndrome. Prescriptions for clearing away heat should never be used in the above cases. In case of vomiting after application of this recipe, it is advisabe to add in small dosage drugs of cold or cool nature (e.g. pork bile) for the purpose of corrigent, or take the decoction cool to prevent rejection of the drugs.

又能解附子之毒，并可缓附子、干姜辛散温燥耗气伤津之弊，还有调和药性作用，为佐使药。三药配伍，药简效宏，可速达回阳救逆之功。

【注意事项】　阳衰阴盛之证，常可出现阴盛格阳或戴阳的真寒假热征象，切不可误用清热剂；若服本方后出现呕吐，称为"拒药"，可在方中少加寒凉药物（如猪胆汁）作为反佐，或采用热药冷服法以缓解邪盛拒药反应。

2.3.3　Prescriptions for Warming the Meridians to Dispel Cold

Danggui Sini Tang
(*Decoction of Chinese Angelia for Restoring Yang*)

Source: *Shanghan Lun* (*Treatise on Exogenous Febrile Diseases*).

Ingredients:

No. 1 Danggui (*Radix Angelicae Sinensis*) 12 g;

No. 2 Guizhi (*Ramulus Cinnamomi*) 9 g;

No. 3 Shaoyao (*Radix Paeoniae*) 9 g;

第三节　温经散寒剂

当归四逆汤

【方源】　《伤寒论》。

【组成】　当归12 g，桂枝9 g，芍药9 g，细辛3 g，炙甘草6 g，通草6 g，大枣 8 枚。

No. 4 Xixin (*Herba Asari*) 3 g;

No. 5 Zhigancao (*Radix Glycyrrhizae Praeparatae*) 6 g;

No. 6 Tongcao (*Medulla Tetrapanacis*) 6 g;

No. 7 Dazao (*Fructus Ziziphi Jujubae*) 8 pcs.

Administration: Decoct the above drugs in water for oral application.

Actions: Warming the meridians to dispel cold, nourishing blood and promoting blood circulation.

Clinical Application: This recipe is used to treat cold limbs due to cold stagnation with blood deficiency, marked by cold limbs, or local black-and-blue marks, or pain and numbness of the waist, thighs, legs and feet, aversion to cold with preference for warmth, pale tongue with whitish fur, deep thready pulse. It is applicable to thromboangiitis, pulseless disease, Raynaud's disease, and chilblain, etc., which pertain to cold accumulation with blood deficiency and manifest chiefly such symptoms as coldness and pain of the limbs. Baishaoyao (*Radix Paeoniae Alba*) is often used clinically as ingredient No. 3. In case of severe pain of the limbs, add Niuxi (*Radix Achyranthis Bidentatae*), Jixueteng (*Caulis Spatholobi*) and Mugua (*Fructus Chaenomelis*) to promote blood flow and relieve pain. If complicated with cold syndrome of deficiency type in the middle-energizer manifesting abdominal pain and vomiting, add Wuzhuyu (*Fructus Evodiae*) and Shengjiang (*Rhizoma Zingiberis Recens*) to warm the stomach and stop vomiting, namely the recipe entitled Danggui Sini plus Wuzhuyu Shengjiang Tang.

Elucidation: The syndrome is due to constitutional deficiency of blood and yang, causing the meridians to be affected by cold as well as obstructed flow of blood. This should be treated by warming the meridians to dispel cold, nourishing blood to remove obstruction in the meridians. Ingredients No. 1 and No. 2 function as monarch drug, the

【用法】 水煎服。

【功用】 温经散寒,养血通脉。

【临床应用】 适用于血虚寒厥证。症见手足厥冷,或局部青紫,或腰、股、腿、足疼痛麻木,畏寒喜温,舌淡苔白,脉象沉细。血栓闭塞性脉管炎、无脉症、雷诺病、冻疮等属血虚寒凝,以肢体冷、痛为主症者,可用本方治疗。方中芍药,现临床常用白芍药。若肢体疼痛较甚者,可加牛膝、鸡血藤、木瓜以活血通络止痛;若兼中焦虚寒,腹痛呕吐者,可加吴茱萸、生姜以温胃降逆止呕,即当归四逆加吴茱萸生姜汤。

【方解】 本方证由素体血虚阳弱,经脉受寒,血行不畅所致,治宜温经散寒,养血通脉之法。方中当归补血和血,桂枝温经散寒,两药合用,温经养血,散寒通脉,共为君

former with the effect of enriching and regulating blood and the latter warming the meridians to dispel cold. Ingredients No. 3 and No. 4 act as minister drug and help bring about the effects of No. 1 and No. 2. Ingredient No. 6 can promote blood circulation and enhance the effects of the monarch and minister drugs, playing the part of adjuvant drug. Ingredients No. 5 and No. 7, with the effect of replenishing qi to invigorate the spleen, can help No. 1 and No. 3 achieve the purpose of nourishing blood, and help No. 2 and No. 4 activate yang as well.

Cautions：This recipe is contraindicated for patients with cold limbs due to exhaustion of kidney-yang.

药。芍药助当归滋养阴血，细辛助桂枝散寒止痛，同为臣药。通草为古代木通之异名，可通行血脉，加强君、臣药活血通脉的作用，为佐药。甘草、大枣益气补脾，既可资气血生化之源以助当归、芍药养血，与桂枝、细辛配伍又能辛甘化阳以助其通阳。

【注意事项】　若真阳衰微而致四肢厥逆者，禁用本方。

2.4 Purgative Prescriptions

第四章 泻下剂

Purgative prescriptions refer to those that are mainly composed of purgatives with the therapeutic effects of relieving constipation, purging away heat, evacuating retention, and eliminating retained fluid, and used in the treatment of interior syndrome of excess type.

Interior syndrome of excess type may be caused either by the accumulation of heat, or cold, or dryness or fluid, and the human body may differ in the state of healthy qi as being excessive or deficient. Therefore, purgative prescriptions can be subdivided into five categories: purgative prescriptions of cold nature, purgative prescriptions of warm nature, laxatives, prescriptions for eliminating retained fluid and prescriptions for both reinforcement and elimination.

Purgative prescriptions of cold nature mainly consist of cathartics of cold nature with the effect of purging away heat accumulation and are applied in the treatment of excess syndrome of interior heat. Purgative prescriptions of warm nature are usually made up of Dahuang (*Radix et Rhizoma Rhei*) in compatibility with drugs capable of warming the interior, which purge away the accumulated cold and are used in treating excess syndrome of dyspepsia due to interior cold. Laxatives, with the function of relaxing the bowels to relieve constipation, are composed of mild cathartics and applied in the treatment of constipation due to intestinal dryness induced by deficiency of body fluid. Prescriptions for eliminating retained fluid chiefly

凡以泻下药为主组成,具有通便、泻热、攻积、逐水等作用,用于治疗里实证的方剂,统称泻下剂。

由于里实证有热结、寒结、燥结、水结之别,人体正气又有虚实之异,因而泻下剂相应地分为寒下剂、温下剂、润下剂、逐水剂与攻补兼施剂五类。

寒下剂由寒凉攻下药为主组成,具有泻下热结作用,适用于里热积滞实证。温下剂常由大黄配伍温里药为主组成,具有泻下寒积作用,适用于里寒积滞实证。润下剂由润下药为主组成,具有润肠通便作用,适用于肠燥津亏,大便秘结之证。逐水剂由峻下逐水药为主组成,具有攻逐水饮作用,适用于水饮壅盛于里的实证。攻补兼施剂由攻下药配伍补益药为主组成,具

consist of drastic purgatives capable of eliminating retention and are employed in treating excess syndrome of excessive fluid in the body. Prescriptions for both reinforcement and elimination mainly consist of cathartics in compatibility with tonic or restorative drugs. They are expected to achieve the purpose of both purging away the excessive accumulation of pathogenic factor and restoring body resistance and applied in the treatment of excess syndrome of yangming-fu organ with deficiency of the healthy qi.

Purgative prescriptions are likely to impair the middle-energizer, consume body fluid, affect blood flow and cause abortion, and thus should be abandoned immediately when they achieve the expected results. It should be applied with great caution or contraindicated in the aged, the weak, those with blood deficiency from constitutional weakness or after illness, or women during menstruation or pregnancy.

有泻实补虚作用,适用于阳明腑实而兼正气虚弱之证。

泻下剂易于伤中、耗津、动血、堕胎,故使用时应得效即止,慎勿过剂;年老体虚、素体或病后阴血不足、妇女经期以及孕妇等均应慎用或禁用。

2.4.1　Purgative Prescriptions of Cold Nature

第一节　寒下剂

Da Chengqi Tang
(*Decoction for Potent Purgation*)

大承气汤

Source: *Shanghan Lun* (*Treatise on Exogenous Febrile Diseases*).

【方源】《伤寒论》。

Ingredients:

No. 1 Dahuang (*Radix et Rhizoma Rhei*) 12 g;

No. 2 Houpo (*Cortex Magnoliae Officinalis*) 24 g;

No. 3 Zhishi (*Furctus Aurantii Immaturus*) 12 g;

No. 4 Mangxiao (*Natrii Sulphas*) 6 g.

【组成】　大黄12 g,厚朴24 g,枳实12 g,芒消6 g。

Administration: No. 2 and No. 3 are to be decocted prior to No. 1 and the decoction is to be taken after removing the residue and infusing No. 4 in it.

【用法】　枳实、厚朴先煎,大黄后下,汤成去滓,溶入芒消。

Actions: Drastic purgation for eliminating accumu-

【功用】　峻下热结。

lated heat.

Clinical Application: This recipe is used to treat excessive-heat syndrome of yangming-fu organ, manifested as constipation, abdominal pain with tenderness, afternoon fever, thirst with great desire to drink, reddened and prickled tongue with dry yellowish fur or dry blackish fur with fissures, deep and forceful pulse. It is applicable to acute simple ileus, adhesive ileus, acute cholecystitis, acute pancreatitis as well as symptoms of high fever, delirium, coma, convulsion, mania with constipation, yellowish fur and forceful pulse as seen in the course of febrile diseases. In case of consumption of qi due to excessive heat with lassitude, add Renshen (*Radix Ginseng*) to replenish qi and prevent exhaustion of qi induced by drastic purgation. If the accumulating heat impairs yin manifesting extreme thirst with great desire to drink, dry reddened tongue with little fur, add Xuanshen (*Radix Scrophulariae*) and Shengdihuang (*Radix Rehmanniae*) to nourish yin for the production of body fluid and to moisten dryness for relieving constipation.

Elucidation: The syndrome results from pathogenic heat accumulating in the large intestine, leading to obstructed flow of fu-qi. This should be treated by eliminating heat to relax the bowels. Ingredient No.1 acts as monarch drug to eliminate heat and stagnated food and stool in the gastrointestinal tract, and relieve constipation. No.4 possesses the effect of moistening dryness and softening mass, and is used as minister drug to reinforce the effect of the monarch drug. Both No.3 and No.2 are adjuvant drugs, capable of promoting flow of qi and relieving fullness and helping the monarch and minister drugs remove the stagnated food and stool to accelerate discharge of heat and mass. The four drugs in compatibility generates a drastic efficacy in purging heat and mass.

【临床应用】 适用于阳明腑实证。症见大便不通,腹痛拒按,午后热甚,口渴引饮,舌红苔黄燥起刺或焦黑燥裂,脉沉实。急性单纯性肠梗阻、粘连性肠梗阻、急性胆囊炎、急性胰腺炎,以及热病过程中出现高热谵语,神昏惊厥,甚则发狂而见大便不通,苔黄脉实者,均可用本方治疗。若热盛耗气,兼少气倦怠者,可加人参以补气,防止峻下而致气脱;若热结伤阴,大渴引饮,舌干红少苔者,可加玄参、生地黄以滋阴生津,润燥通便。

【方解】 本方证由邪热积滞结于大肠,腑气不通所致,治宜泻下热结,攻积通腑之法。方中大黄泻热通便,荡涤肠胃积滞,为君药。芒消软坚润燥,助大黄以加强泻热通便之功,为臣药。枳实、厚朴行气除满,并助大黄、芒消推荡积滞,加速热结排泄,均为佐药。四药配伍,泻下热结之力颇为峻猛。若减去芒消则成为轻下热结的小承气汤,减去枳实、厚朴,加甘草则成为缓下热结的调胃承气汤,两者

Subtract No. 4 and Xiao Chengqi Tang is formed, which has a mild efficacy. Replace No. 2 and No. 3 with Gancao (*Radix Glycyrrhizae*), and Tiaowei Chengqi Tang is obtained for laxation of heat and mass. The above three share the name of "San Chengqi Tang" and the selective application of them is made clinically in the light of the degrees of severity.

Cautions: It must be applied with great care to those with excess syndrome of yangming-fu organ but without excessive heat, or those with constitutional deficiency of qi and yin, or the aged, those of general asthenia, or pregnant women.

2.4.2 Purgative Prescriptions of Warm Nature

Dahuang Fuzi Tang
(*Decoction of Rhubarb and Aconite*)

Source: *Jingui Yaolue* (*Synopsis of Prescriptions of the Golden Cabinet*).

Ingredients:

No. 1 Dahuang (*Radix et Rhizoma Rhei*) 9 g;

No. 2 Paofuzi (*Radix Aconiti Praeparatae*) baked 9 g;

No. 3 Xixin (*Herba Asari*) 3 g.

Administration: Decoct the above drugs in water for oral application.

Actions: Purging away accumulation of cold and dispelling cold to relieve pain.

Clinical Application: This recipe is used to treat syndrome of interior excess due to cold accumulation, marked by abdominal pain, constipation, hypochondriac pain, fever, cold limbs, whitish and greasy fur, taut and tense pulse. It is applicable to appendicitis, biliary colic, chronic dysentery, acute ileus, and adhesive ileus, etc.,

与上方合称三承气汤,临床常根据阳明腑实证候的轻重缓急酌情选用。

【注意事项】 阳明腑实而热结不甚,或素体气虚阴亏以及年老、体弱、孕妇等慎用本方。

第二节 温下剂

大黄附子汤

【方源】 《金匮要略》。

【组成】 大黄9 g,炮附子9 g,细辛3 g。

【用法】 水煎服。

【功用】 攻下冷积,散寒止痛。

【临床应用】 适用于寒积里实证。症见腹痛便秘,胁下偏痛,发热,手足不温,舌苔白腻,脉弦紧。阑尾炎、胆绞痛、慢性痢疾、急性肠梗阻、粘连性肠梗阻等以腹痛便秘,苔

which chiefly manifest abdominal pain, constipation, whitish fur, taut and tense pulse which pertain to syndrome of cold accumulation in the interior. In case of severe abdominal pain, add Rougui (*Cortex Cinnamomi*) to warm the interior and relieve pain. In case of abdominal distention and fullness with thick greasy fur, which is indicative of excessive accumulation of cold, add Houpo (*Cortex Magnoliae Officinalis*) and Zhishi (*Fructus Aurantii Immaturus*) to promote the flow of qi.

Elucidation: The syndrome is due to accumulated cold leading to functional disorder of yang-qi as well as the obstructed flow of fu-qi. It should be treated by means of dispelling cold and relieving pain. The first two ingredients act as monarch drug, the former capable of removing pathogenic accumulation to relieve constipation, while the latter warming the interior to dispel cold. Ingredient No. 3 functions as adjuvant drug to help No. 2 dispel the interior cold. The cold nature of the first ingredient, when in compatibility with the rest two who are pungent and hot in nature, can be restricted but with the purgative function well preserved. Such compatibility is known as "Restricting the unfavorable property with the favorable preserved."

Cautions: The dosage of drugs with warm nature must be larger than that of those with cold nature. Besides, it is contraindicated for those with syndrome of deficient yang-qi due to internally accumulated cold.

Wenpi Tang
(*Decoction for Warming Spleen*)

Source: *Beiji Qianjin Yaofang* (*Valuable Prescriptions for Emergency*).

Ingredients:

No. 1 Dahuang (*Radix et Rhizoma Rhei*) 12 g (to be decocted later);

白脉弦紧为主症,属寒积内结者,可用本方治疗。若腹痛甚者,可加肉桂以温里止痛;若腹部胀满,舌苔厚腻,积滞较重者,可加厚朴、枳实以行气导滞。

【方解】 本方证由寒积内结,阳气不运,腑气不通所致,治宜攻下冷积,散寒止痛之法。方中大黄攻积通便,附子温里散寒,两药合用,温下并行,荡涤里寒实积,共为君药。细辛散寒止痛,助附子以温散里寒,为佐药。方中大黄性虽寒凉,但与辛热的附子、细辛配伍,则其寒性被制而泻下之功犹存,这种配伍关系称为"去性存用"。

【注意事项】 方中温药用量必须重于寒药。寒积内阻而阳气虚弱者,禁用本方。

温脾汤

【方源】 《备急千金要方》。

【组成】 大黄12 g(后下),附子9 g,干姜6 g,人参6 g,甘草6 g。

No. 2 Fuzi (*Radix Aconiti Praeparatae*) 9 g;

No. 3 Ganjiang (*Rhizoma Zingiberis*) 6 g;

No. 4 Renshen (*Radix Ginseng*) 9 g;

No. 5 Gancao (*Radix Glycyrrhizae*) 6 g.

Administration: Decoct the above drugs in water for oral application.

Actions: Eliminating cold accumulation, warming and invigorating spleen-yang.

Clinical Application: This recipe is used to treat syndrome of cold accumulation due to yang deficiency, marked by abdominal pain, constipation, or protracted diarrhea with pus and blood, cold limbs, pale tongue with thin whitish fur, deep and taut pulse. It is applicable to acute simple ileus, incomplete ileus, chronic dysentery, the acute onset of chronic appendicitis, and other diseases, chief symptoms of which are abdominal pain, constipation, lassitude, aversion to cold with preference for warmth and pertain to the syndrome of interior cold accumulation due to deficiency of yang-qi. In case of severe abdominal pain, add Rougui (*Cortex Cinnamomi*) and Muxiang (*Radix Aucklandiae*) to enhance the effect of warming yang to promote the flow of qi and relieve pain. If concomitant with vomiting, add Zhibanxia (*Rhizoma Pinelliae Praeparatae*) and Sharen (*Fructus Amomi*) to regulate the stomach and relieve vomiting. In case of protracted dysentery with damp heat marked by yellowish greasy fur, add Jinyinhua (*Flos Lonicerae*) and Huangqin (*Radix Scutellariae*) to clear the bowels for arresting dysentery.

Elucidation: The syndrome results from deficiency of spleen-yang, leading to the generation of cold and its accumulation in the intestine. It should be treated by means of purging away cold accumulation and warming and invigorating spleen-yang. The first two ingredients

【用法】 水煎服。

【功用】 攻下冷积,温补脾阳。

【临床应用】 适用于阳虚冷积证。症见腹痛便秘,或久痢赤白,手足不温,舌淡苔薄白,脉沉弦。急性单纯性肠梗阻或不全性肠梗阻、慢性痢疾、慢性阑尾炎急性发作等以腹痛便秘,神倦乏力,畏寒喜温为主症,属阳气不足,冷积内停者,可用本方治疗。若腹痛较甚者,可加肉桂、木香以加强温阳行气止痛之力;若兼见呕吐,可加制半夏、砂仁以和胃降逆;若痢久不愈,兼挟湿热,舌苔黄腻者,可加金银花、黄芩以清肠止痢。

【方解】 本方证由脾阳不足,寒从内生,冷积阻于肠间所致,治宜攻下冷积,温补脾阳之法。方中大黄泻下攻积通便,附子温里助阳散寒,

achieve the results of warming the interior to dispel cold and purging away accumulated mass, and function as monarch drug, with the former relaxing the bowels and the latter strengthening spleen-yang. Ingredient No. 3 helps ingredient No. 2 warm the middle-energizer and dispel cold, acting as minister drug. The last two ingredients, with the functions of replenishing qi and regulating the middle-energizer, and reinforcing the spleen together with ingredients No. 2 and No. 3, are used as adjuvant drug. Besides, the last ingredient also serves as guiding drug to mediate the properties of other drugs.

Dahuang Fuzi Tang and Wenpi Tang are both composed chiefly of Dahuang (*Radix et Rhizoma Rhei*) and Fuzi (*Radix Aconiti Praeparatae*) with the functions of warming the interior to dispel cold and relieving constipation. They are both indicated in such symptoms as abdominal pain with preference for warmth, constipation and cold limbs due to interior accumulation of cold. The former includes also Xixin (*Herba Asari*), which is effective in dispelling cold and relieving pain, and is fit for excess syndrome of interior cold accumulation with quick progress of the disease. While the latter also comprises Renshen (*Radix Ginseng*), Ganjiang (*Rhizoma Zingiberis*) and Gancao (*Radix Glycyrrhizae*), which bear the function of replenishing qi and invigorating the spleen, and is fit for syndrome of deficiency in the root and excess in the branch due to interior cold accumulation with slow progress of the disease.

两药配伍,温里祛寒,攻下寒积,共为君药。干姜助附子温中祛寒,为臣药。人参、甘草益气和中,合附子、干姜以益气温阳补脾,为佐药。甘草调和药性,兼作使药。

大黄附子汤与温脾汤均以附子配伍大黄为主组成,具有温里散寒,泻下通便作用,主治里寒积滞,腹痛喜温,便秘肢冷证候。大黄附子汤中还有细辛,散寒止痛作用较强,适宜于寒积内结的实证,病势较急;温脾汤中还有人参、干姜、甘草,兼具益气补脾作用,适宜于中虚冷积的本虚标实证,病势较缓。

2.4.3 Prescriptions for causing Laxation

Jichuan Jian
(*Blood Replenishing Decoction*)

Source: *Jingyue Quanshu* (*Complete Works of*

第三节　润下剂

济川煎

【方源】《景岳全书》。

Jingyue).

Ingredients：

No. 1 Danggui (*Radix Angelicae Sinensis*) 12 g;

No. 2 Niuxi (*Radix Achyranthis Bidentatae*) 6 g;

No. 3 Roucongrong (*Herba Cistanchis*) 9 g;

No. 4 Zexie (*Rhizoma Alismatis*) 5 g;

No. 5 Shengma (*Rhizoma Cimicifugae*) 3 g;

No. 6 Zhike (*Fructus Aurantii*) 3 g.

Administration：Decoct the above drugs for oral application.

Actions：Warming the kidney and nourishing blood, moistening the intestine to relieve constipation.

Clinical Application：This recipe is used to treat constipation due to deficiency of the kidney, marked by constipation, profuse clear urine, soreness of the waist and knees, pale tongue with whitish fur, and deep, thready and slow pulse. It is applicable to habitual constipation, and senile constipation, which pertain to deficiency of the kidney and body fluid, and dry intestine. If complicated with shortness of breath and lassitude, replace the last ingredient with Renshen (*Radix Gingseng*) to replenish qi and promote the transporting action of the large intestine. In case of excessive deficiency of the kidney essence manifesting dizziness and tinnitus, add Shudihuang (*Radix Rehmanniae Praeparatae*) to reinforce the kidney and replenish kidney essence, as well as nourish yin and loosen the bowels. In case of protracted constipation manifesting dryness of the mouth and tongue, replace ingredient No. 4 with Suoyang (*Herba Cynomorii*) and Huomaren (*Fructus Cannabis*) to enhance the effect of relaxing bowels to relieve constipation.

Elucidation：The syndrome results from deficiency of kidney-qi, leading to disorder in transportation and lack of essence and blood, which further causes lack of nutri-

【组成】　当归12 g，牛膝6 g，肉苁蓉9 g，泽泻5 g，升麻3 g，枳壳3 g。

【用法】　水煎服。

【功用】　温肾养血，润肠通便。

【临床应用】　适用于肾虚便秘证。症见大便秘结，小便清长，腰膝酸软，舌淡苔白，脉沉细迟。习惯性便秘、老年人便秘属肾虚津亏肠燥者，可用本方治疗。若兼气短乏力者，可去枳壳，加人参益气补虚以助大肠传导之力；若肾虚精亏较著，头晕耳鸣者，可加熟地黄以补肾填精，滋阴润肠；若便秘较久，口舌干燥者，可去泽泻，加锁阳、火麻仁以加强润肠通便作用。

【方解】　本方证由肾元亏虚，传导无力，精血不足，肠失濡润所致，治宜温肾养血，

ents in the large intestine. It should be treated by means of warming kidney-yang and enriching blood, as well as moistening the bowels to relieve constipation. Ingredient No. 3 is used as monarch drug to replenish the kidney essence, warm the waist and relax the bowels. Ingredients No. 1 and No. 2 act together as minister drug, the former capable of nourishing blood and moistening the bowels and the latter reinforcing the kidney. Ingredients No. 6 and No. 4 bear the respective function of descending qi and sending down turbid substances, and together promote transporting action of the large intestine. Ingredient No. 5 is meant to ascend the lucid yang and to descend the turbid yin in compatibility with ingredients No. 2, No. 6 and No. 4. The four ingredients together play the role of adjuvant drug. All ingredients in combination achieve the purpose of laxation implied in reinforcement and ascending implied in descending. This recipe can make up deficiency of the kidney, and lack of fluid in the intestine, further promoting the function of the large intestine.

Cautions: It is contraindicated in those with deficiency of kidney-yin and dry intestine, manifesting constipation, dryness of the mouth and reddened tongue.

Maziren Wan
(*Pill of Cannabic Seed*)

Source: *Shanghan Lun* (*Treatise on Exogenous Febrile Diseases*).

Ingredients:

No. 1 Maziren (*Fructus Cannabis*) 500 g;

No. 2 Shaoyao (*Radix Paeoniae*) 250 g;

No. 3 Zhishi (*Fructus Aurantii Immaturus*) 250 g;

No. 4 Dahuang (*Radix et Rhizoma Rhei*) 500 g;

No. 5 Houpo (*Cortex Magnoliae Officinalis*) 250 g;

No. 6 Xingren (*Semen Armeniacae Amarum*) 250 g.

Administration: Grind the above drugs into fine

润肠通便之法。方中肉苁蓉温肾益精,暖腰润肠,为君药。当归养血润肠,牛膝补肾壮腰,同为臣药。枳壳下气,泽泻降浊,助大肠传导之力;少加升麻升举清阳,与牛膝、枳壳、泽泻相配,可使清阳升而浊阴降,俱为佐药。诸药配伍,寓通于补,寄升于降,补肾元之虚损,滋肠津之不足,助肠腑之传导,而成温润通便之剂。

【注意事项】 肾阴不足,肠燥便秘,口干舌红者,禁用本方。

麻子仁丸

【方源】 《伤寒论》。

【组成】 麻子仁500 g,芍药250 g,枳实250 g,大黄500 g,厚朴250 g,杏仁250 g。

【用法】 共研细末,炼蜜

powder and then make them into boluses by mixing them with honey; take 9 g with warm boiled water, twice daily. Or decoct them in water for oral use with an appropriate dosage in proportion to that of the original recipe.

Actions: Moistening the intestine to purge heat and promoting the flow of qi to relieve constipation.

Clinical Application: This recipe is used to treat syndrome of constipation due to intestinal dryness, marked by dry stool, frequent urination, dry mouth and tongue, slight yellowish fur. It is applicable to habitual constipation, senile constipation, postpartum constipation and postoperative constipation from hemorrhoid, which pertain to gastrointestinal dryness and heat syndrome. Presently, Baishaoyao (*Radix Paeoniae Alba*) is often used as ingredient No. 2 in clinical practice. In the absence of excessive dryness and heat, subtract ingredients No. 3 and No. 5 and lessen the dosage of ingredient No. 4.

Elucidation: The syndrome is due to gastrointestinal dryness and heat, deficiency of body fluid, and lack of lubrication in the intestine. It should be treated by means of moistening the bowels to purge heat and promoting the flow of qi to relieve constipation. Ingredient No. 1, mild in nature and abundant in lipid, functions as monarch drug to moisten the large intestine for relieving constipation. Ingredient No. 4 bears the function of purging heat and dryness from the stomach and intestine, No. 6 descending qi and relaxing the bowels, and No. 2 nourishing yin and helping the monarch drug carry out its action. The above three are minister drugs. Ingredients No. 3 and No. 5 promote the flow of qi and dissolve mass, and enhance the effect of No. 4 as well, serving as adjuvant drugs. Honey is meant to further strengthen the effect of moistening dryness and relaxing the bowels.

Cautions: It is contraindicated in constipation due to

为丸,每次9 g,温开水送服,每日 2 次。亦可作汤剂,用量按原方比例酌定。

【功用】　润肠泻热,行气通便。

【临床应用】　适用于肠燥便秘证。症见大便秘结,小便频数,口干舌燥,舌苔微黄。习惯性便秘、老人与产后便秘、痔疮术后便秘等属肠胃燥热者,可用本方治疗。方中芍药,现临床常用白芍药。若燥热不甚者,可去枳实、厚朴,并酌减大黄用量。

【方解】　本方证由肠胃燥热,津液不足,肠失濡润所致,治宜润肠泻热,行气通便之法。方中麻子仁质润多脂,润肠通便,为君药。大黄泻热通便,除肠胃燥热;杏仁降气润肠,芍药养阴和里,助君药滋润肠燥,同为臣药。枳实、厚朴行气破结,并助大黄泻热通便之力,均为佐药。蜂蜜和丸则更增本方润燥滑肠之功。

【注意事项】　便秘因津

exhaustion of body fluid and blood and lack of nutrients in the large intestine without dryness and heat internally.

血亏虚,肠失濡润而内无燥热者禁用。

2.4.4 Prescriptions for Eliminating Fluid Retention

第四节 逐水剂

Shizao Tang
(*Ten Jujube Decoction*)

十枣汤

Source:*Shanghan Lun*(*Treatise on Exogenous Febrile Diseases*).

【方源】《伤寒论》。

Ingredients:

No. 1 Yuanhua (*Flos Genkwa*);

No. 2 Gansui (*Radix Euphorbiae Kansui*);

No. 3 Daji (*Radix Knoxiae*);

Equal in dosage.

【组成】 芫花,甘遂,大戟各等分。

Administration:Grind them into fine powder with 0.5 - 1 g put into a capsule each time and taken with the decoction of Dazao (*Fructus Ziziphi Jujubae*) early in the morning before meal, once daily.

【用法】 共研细末,每次0.5~1 g,装入胶囊,以大枣10~20枚煎汤,于清晨空腹时送服,每日1次。

Actions:Eliminating fluid Retention.

【功用】 攻逐水饮。

Clinical Application:This recipe is used to treat thoracic retention of fluid, marked by cough, shortness of breath, pain in the chest and hypochondrium when coughing, headache, dizziness, deep and taut pulse; or severe edema of the body, abdominal fullness, dyspnea, difficulty in urination and defecation. It is applicable to exudative pleurisy, ascites due to cirrhosis, and chronic nephritic edema, which pertain to strong body resistance with excessive fluid retention.

【临床应用】 适用于悬饮,症见咳嗽气短,胸胁牵引疼痛,头痛目眩,脉沉弦;或水肿重证,症见一身悉肿,腹胀喘满,二便不利。渗出性胸膜炎、肝硬化腹水、慢性肾炎水肿等水饮殊盛而正气尚充者,可用本方治疗。

Elucidation:This syndrome is the result of excessive fluid retaining in the interior, which should be treated by means of eliminating retained fluid by purgation. Ingredient No. 2 is good at eliminating retention of fluid and dampness from meridians, No. 3 excels in eliminating it

【方解】 本方证由水饮壅盛于里所致,治宜攻逐水饮之法。方中甘遂善行经遂络脉之水湿,大戟善泻脏腑肠胃之水湿,芫花善消胸胁伏饮痰

from zang-fu organs, intestine and stomach, and No. 1 removing fluid and phlegm from the chest and hypochondrium. The three ingredients have their respective advantages and can enhance the effect of eliminating retained fluid and relieving edema and fullness when combined. However, they are drastic and toxic in nature and apt to impair body resistance. The decoction of Dazao (*Fructus Ziziphi Jujubae*), therefore, is meant to reinforce the spleen and stomach, and reduce the toxic and drastic properties of the drugs so that they can achieve the purgative result without affecting the healthy qi. It functions as adjuvant drug.

Cautions: This recipe is contraindicated for Pregnant woman for its drastic efficacy. Besides, it is advisable to begin with a small dose and increase or reduce the dose accordingly in the light of the retention after application of drugs and in accordance with the tolerance of the patient. If incessant diarrhea occurs after the use of this recipe, cold porridge is recommended to stop it. If the patient cannot tolerate the drastic purgation because of general debility and excessive pathogenic factors, tonics and this recipe may be used in alteration, either purging away pathogenic factors followed by reinforcement or reinforcing the spleen followed by purgation.

2.4.5 Prescriptions for Purgation Associated with Reinforcement

Huanglong Tang
(*Yellow Dragon Decoction*)

Source: *Shanghan Liushu* (*Six Books on Febrile Diseases*).

Ingredients:

No. 1 Dahuang (*Radix et Rhizoma Rhei*) 9 g;

癖,三药各有所长,合而用之,逐水饮,消肿满之功甚著。但其药性峻猛,又有毒性,易伤正气,故以大枣煎汤送服,意在补脾养胃,并缓和诸药的毒性及峻烈之性,使下不伤正,为佐药。四药合用,共成峻下逐水之剂。

【注意事项】　本方药性十分峻猛,孕妇禁用。服药宜从小量开始,再根据药后水饮消退的情况与患者的耐受性酌情增减用量。若服药后泻下不止,可食冷粥以止之。若体虚邪实不任峻剂攻逐者,可与健脾补益之剂交替使用,或先攻后补,或先补后攻。

第五节　攻补兼施剂

黄龙汤

【方源】　《伤寒六书》。

【组成】　大黄9 g,芒消6 g,枳实9 g,厚朴9 g,甘草3 g,

No. 2 Mangxiao (*Natrii Sulfas*) 6 g;

No. 3 Zhishi (*Fructus Aurantii Immaturus*) 9 g;

No. 4 Houpo (*Cortex Magnoliae Officinalis*) 9 g;

No. 5 Gancao (*Radix Glycyrrhizae*) 3 g;

No. 6 Renshen (*Radix Ginseng*) 6 g;

No. 7 Danggui (*Radix Angelicae Sinensis*) 9 g.

Administration：Add to the above (exclusive of No. 2) 3 g of Jiegeng (*Radix Platycodi*), 3 slices of Shengjiang (*Rhizoma Zingiberis Recens*) and 2 pieces of Dazao (*Fructus Ziziphi Jujubae*) before decocting them in water. Remove the residue from the decoction and dissolve No. 2 in it for oral application.

Actions：Eliminating heat accumulation by purgation, supplementing qi and nourishing the blood.

Clinical Application：This recipe is used to treat syndrome due to deficient qi and blood and excess syndrome in the yangming-fu organs, marked by constipation or watery diarrhea with indigested food, epigastric and abdominal distention and fullness, pain with tenderness, feverish body, thirst, lassitude, dysphoria, even delirium in severe case, parched yellowish or dark fur, feeble pulse. It is applicable to typhoid, paratyphoid, epidemic cerebrospinal meningitis, epidemic encephalitis B and other diseases, which pertain to excess syndrome of the yangming-fu organs with deficiency of qi and blood. In case of severe constipation with abdominal pain, increase the dosage of No. 1 and No. 2; in case of dominant lassitude, increase the dosage of No. 6 and No. 7.

Elucidation：The syndrome is due to excessive heat accumulating in the yangming-fu organs without descending, consuming and impairing qi and blood. It should be treated by purging away heat, supplementing qi and nourishing blood. The first four ingredients (namely those of Da Chengqi Tang) eliminate the excessive heat accumulating

人参6 g,当归9 g。

【用法】 加桔梗3 g,生姜3片,大枣 2 枚,水煎,汤成去滓,溶入芒消。

【功用】 攻下热结,益气养血。

【临床应用】 适用于阳明腑实,气血不足证。症见大便秘结或下利清水,脘腹胀满,疼痛拒按,身热口渴,神倦少气,烦躁,甚则谵语,舌苔焦黄或焦黑,脉虚。伤寒、副伤寒、流行性脑脊髓膜炎、流行性乙型脑炎等疾病见有阳明腑实而兼气血不足之象者,可用本方治疗。若便秘腹痛较甚者,可重用大黄、芒消;若神倦少气明显者,可重用人参、当归。

【方解】 本方证由阳明腑实,应下失下,热结里实,耗伤气血所致,治宜攻下热结,益气养血之法。方中大黄、芒消、枳实、厚朴(即大承气汤)攻下热结,荡涤胃肠实热积

in the stomach and intestine, while the rest three supplement qi and nourish blood. Their combined application can achieve the purpose of strengthening body resistance to eliminate pathogenic factors and purging away heat without impairing healthy qi. Jiegeng (*Radix Platycodi*) is meant to disperse the stagnated lung-qi and eliminate heat from the intestine by purgation, while Shengjiang (*Rhizoma Zingiberis Recens*) and Dazao (*Fructus Ziziphi Jujubae*) are to reinforce the stomach and spleen and prevent them from being impaired by purgation. All the drugs in compatibility ensure the results of purgation with reinforcement, strengthening body resistance with pathogenic factors eliminated.

Zengye Chengqi Tang
(*Purgative Decoction for Increasing Fluid*)

Source: *Wenbing Tiaobian* (*Analysis of Seasonal Febrile Diseases*).

Ingredients:

No. 1 Xuanshen (*Radix Scrophulariae*) 30 g;

No. 2 Maimendong (*Radix Ophiopogonis*) 25 g;

No. 3 Shengdihuang (*Radix Rehmanniae*) 25 g;

No. 4 Dahuang (*Radix et Rhizoma Rhei*) 9 g;

No. 5 Mangxiao (*Natrii Sulfas*) 4.5 g.

Administration: Decoct the first four ingredients in water; dissolve ingredient No. 5 in the decoction after the residue is removed.

Actions: Nourishing yin, increasing fluid, purging heat and inducing defecation.

Clinical Application: This recipe is used to treat syndrome of constipation due to heat accumulation and yin deficiency, marked by feverish body, constipation, epigastric and abdominal distention and fullness, dry mouth and lips, reddened tongue with yellowish fur, thready rapid pulse. It can be modified to treat high fever with

滞;人参、甘草、当归益气养血,扶正达邪,使攻不伤正。煎药时加少许桔梗宣开肺气,以通降肠腑;生姜、大枣养胃补脾,防泻下伤中。诸药配伍,共成攻补兼施,扶正祛邪之剂。

增液承气汤

【方源】 《温病条辨》。

【组成】 玄参30 g,麦门冬25 g,生地黄25 g,大黄9 g,芒消4.5 g。

【用法】 前四药水煎,汤成去滓,溶入芒消。

【功用】 滋阴增液,泄热通便。

【临床应用】 适用于热结阴亏便秘证。症见身热便秘,下之不通,脘腹胀满,口干唇燥,舌红苔黄,脉细数。急性传染病高热便秘,痔疮日久,大便燥结不通属热结未

constipation from acute infectious diseases, and dry stool from protracted hemorrhoid, which is the result of retained heat and impairment of yin fluid with chief symptoms as constipation, dry lips, yellowish and dry fur. If the accumulated heat is not so excessive, lessen the dosage of ingredients No. 4 and No. 5 accordingly,

Elucidation: The syndrome arises when accumulated heat in the stomach burns body fluid and causes it to fail to moisten the intestine. For this the method of relieving constipation by purgation and producing body fluid by nourishing yin should be used. Ingredient No. 1, in larger dosage than other's, is the monarch drug with the effects of nourishing yin for production of body fluid, and purging heat for relieving constipation. Ingredients No. 3 and No. 2 function as minister drug to help bring about the effects of the monarch drug. The last two ingredients are meant to soften and moisten hard mass as adjuvant drug. All Ingredients in compatibility can restore yin fluid and eliminate hard mass so that the disappearance of all symptoms ensues.

Cautions: It should be applied with great caution to those who manifest subdued fever and mild abdominal pain, which pertain to yin deficiency without excessive heat.

去,阴液已伤,以便秘唇燥,苔黄而干为主症者,可用本方加减治疗。若热结不甚者,可酌减大黄、芒消的用量。

【方解】 本方证由热结胃肠,津液受灼,肠腑失润,传导失常所致,治宜泻热通便,养阴生津之法。方中重用玄参滋阴增液,泄热通便,为君药。生地黄、麦门冬助君药滋阴生津,润肠通便,同为臣药。大黄、芒消泻热通便,软坚润燥,均为佐药。诸药配伍,使阴液渐复,热结得下,则诸症可除。

【注意事项】 若身热已退,腹痛不甚,证属阴亏而热结不甚者,慎用本方。

2.5 Prescriptions for Mediation

第五章
和解剂

Those that bear mediating or regulating action and are applied to febrile diseases caused by pathogenic factors in Shaoyang, disharmony between the liver and spleen, intermingling of cold and heat, and coexistent syndrome of both exterior and interior, are known as prescriptions for mediation.

These prescriptions have a wide range of application and, therefore, are subdivided into four classes in accordance with the location of the chief syndromes which these prescriptions treat. They are prescriptions for mediating shaoyang, those for regulating the liver and spleen, those for harmonizing cold and heat syndrome, and those for expelling both exterior and interior pathogenic factors.

Prescriptions for mediating shaoyang are chiefly made up of drugs with the function of mediating the shaoyang meridian. They are used for syndromes of exogenous pathogenic factors in shaoyang. Prescriptions for regulating the liver and spleen are mainly composed of drugs with the function of relieving stagnated liver-qi and invigorating the spleen. They are used for syndromes of attack of the spleen due to depression of the liver and disharmony between the liver and spleen. Prescriptions for harmonizing cold and heat syndrome comprise drugs of pungent and hot nature and drugs of bitter flavor respectively. They possess the effects of subduing pathogenic cold and heat, and relieving stagnation and flatulence and are used to treat simultaneous occurrence of cold and heat

凡具有和解或调和等作用,用于治疗伤寒邪在少阳、肝脾不和、寒热错杂,以及表里同病等证候的方剂,统称和解剂。

由于和解剂的适应范围较广,本章根据其主治证病位的不同分为和解少阳剂、调和肝脾剂、调和寒热剂以及表里双解剂四类。

和解少阳剂由清透少阳之药为主组成,具有和解少阳作用,适用于外感病邪在少阳之证。调和肝脾剂由疏肝理脾药为主组成,具有疏肝解郁,健脾助运作用,适用于肝郁犯脾,肝脾失调之证。调和寒热剂由辛热温中配伍苦降泄热药为主组成,具有平调寒热,开结除痞作用,适用于寒热错杂,气机失调之证。表里双解剂由解表药配伍治里药组成,具有表里同治作用,适用于表里同病证候。

syndromes as well as functional disorder of qi. Prescriptions for expelling both exterior and interior pathogenic factors consist of diaphoresis in compatibility with drugs for relieving interior syndrome and are fit for the syndrome with both exterior and interior pathogenic factors.

Prescriptions for mediation should be applied with care to differentiate what is primary from what is secondary between zang and fu organs, as well as the exterior and the interior. And the proportion of drugs should be weighed carefully to avoid overdose or inadequate dose.

和解剂在使用时应注意分清脏腑、表里的主次轻重，权衡相应治疗药物的比例，以避免太过与不及之弊。

2.5.1 Prescriptions for Treating Shaoyang Disease by Mediation

第一节　和解
少阳剂

Xiao Chaihu Tang
(**Minor Decoction of Bupleurum**)

小柴胡汤

Source：*Shanghan Lun* (*Treatise on Exogenous Febrile Diseases*).

【方源】《伤寒论》。

Ingredients：

No. 1 Chaihu (*Radix Bupleuri*) 24 g;

No. 2 Huangqin (*Radix Scutellariae*) 9 g;

No. 3 Renshen (*Radix Gingseng*) 9 g;

No. 4 Zhigancao (*Radix Glycyrrhizae Praeparatae*) 6 g;

No. 5 Banxia (*Rhizoma Pinelliae*) 9 g;

No. 6 Shengjiang (*Rhizoma Zingiberis Recens*) 9 g;

No. 7 Dazao (*Fructus Ziziphi Jujubae*) 4 pcs.

【组成】　柴胡24 g，黄芩9 g，人参9 g，炙甘草6 g，半夏9 g，生姜9 g，大枣 4 枚。

Administration：Decoct the above drugs in water for oral application.

【用法】　水煎服。

Actions：Treating shaoyang disease by mediation.

【功用】　和解少阳。

Clinical Application：This recipe is used to treat febrile diseases in shaoyang meridian, marked by alternate attacks of chills and fever, fullness in the chest, hypochondriac discomfort, dysphoria, retching, bitter taste in the mouth, dry throat, thin and whitish fur and taut

【临床应用】　适用于伤寒少阳证。症见往来寒热，胸胁苦满，心烦喜呕，口苦咽干，舌苔薄白，脉弦。若有感冒、流行性感冒、慢性肝炎、急性

pulse. It is applicable to common cold, influenza, chronic hepatitis, acute or chronic cholecystitis, pleuritis, pyelonephritis, postpartum infection, gastric ulcer and other diseases, which manifest the above symptoms and pertain to febrile disease in shaoyang meridian. In case of dysphoria without vomiting, which is indicative of heat accumulating in the chest, replace ingredients No. 3 and No. 5 with Gualou (*Fructus Trichosanthis*) to clear away heat and regulate qi for relieving chest fullness. In case of body fluid impaired by heat with manifestation of thirst, replace No. 5 with Tianhuafen (*Radix Trichosanthis*) to produce body fluid for quenching thirst. If the spleen is affected by the stagnated liver-qi with abdominal pain, replace No. 2 with Baishaoyao (*Radix Paeoniae Alba*) to nourish the liver for relieving spasm and pain.

Elucidation: The syndrome is due to pathogenic factors invading shaoyang meridian and fighting against healthy qi in between the exterior and interior. Ingredient No. 1, as monarch drug, dispels the pathogenic factors located in the half exterior and restores the functional activity of shaoyang meridian. Ingredient No. 2 acts as minister drug to purge away heat located in the half interior. They are primary drugs for treating shaoyang disease, one for dispelling pathogenic factor, and the other clearing away the accumulated heat. Ingredients No. 5 and No. 6 can regulate the stomach and relieve vomiting, while ingredients No. 3, No. 4 and No. 7 supplement qi and strengthen body resistance to prevent the pathogenic factors from getting into the interior. These five ingredients play the role of adjuvant drug. Ingredient No. 4 coordinates the actions of various drugs in the recipe and also serves as guiding drug.

Cautions: This recipe should be used with great caution for patients with shaoyang disease but manifesting

胆囊炎、慢性胆囊炎、胸膜炎、肾盂肾炎、产后感染、胃溃疡等上述病症,属伤寒少阳证者,可用本方治疗。若心烦而不呕吐者,为热聚于胸,宜去半夏、人参,加瓜蒌以清热理气宽胸;若热伤津液,兼口渴者,宜去半夏,加天花粉以生津止渴;若肝气乘脾,兼腹痛者,宜去黄芩,加白芍药以柔肝缓急止痛。

【方解】　本方证由邪犯少阳,邪正相争于表里之间所致,治宜和解少阳之法。方中柴胡透达半表之邪,疏畅少阳气机之壅滞,为君药。黄芩清泄半里之热,为臣药。柴胡合黄芩一散一清,共解少阳之邪,为和解少阳的要药。半夏、生姜和胃止呕,人参、炙甘草、大枣益气扶正,实里以防邪气内传,均为佐药。甘草调和药性,兼作使药。

【注意事项】　方中柴胡升散,黄芩、半夏性燥,故少阳

deficiency of yin and blood because Ingredient No. 1 possesses lifting and dispersing action and ingredients No. 2 and No. 5 are of dry nature.

Haoqin Qingdan Tang
(*Decoction of Wormwood and Scutellaria for Clearing away Dampness-heat from the Gallbladder*)

Source: *Chongding Tongsu Shanghan Lun* (*Revised Edition of Popular Treatise on Exogenous Febrile Diseases*).

Ingredients:

No. 1 Qinghao (*Herba Artemisiae Chinghao*) 6 g;

No. 2 Zhuru (*Caulis Bambusae in Taeniam*) 9 g;

No. 3 Banxia (*Rhizoma Pinelliae*) 5 g;

No. 4 Chifuling (*Poria Rubra*) 9 g;

No. 5 Huangqin (*Radix Scutellariae*) 6 g;

No. 6 Zhike (*Fructus Aurantii*) 5 g;

No. 7 Jupi (*Pericarpium Citri Reticulatae*) 5 g;

No. 8 Biyu San (*powder consisting of Talcum, Indigo Naturalis and Radix Glycyrrhizae*) 9 g
　　(to be decocted wrapped).

Administration: Decoct the above drugs in water for oral application.

Actions: Eliminating heat and dampness in the gallbladder, regulating the stomach and resolving phlegm.

Clinical Application: This recipe is used to treat shaoyang syndrome due to damp heat in shaoyang meridian, marked by alternate attacks of chills and fever with the latter severer than the former, bitter taste in the mouth, chest distress, acid regurgitation, or vomiting with sticky yellowish saliva, even retch and hiccup, reddened tongue with greasy whitish fur or with greasy yellowish fur, and taut, smooth and rapid pulse. It is applicable to acute cholecystitis, acute icterohepatitis, acute

证而见阴虚血少者慎用。

蒿芩清胆汤

【方源】《重订通俗伤寒论》。

【组成】 青蒿6 g,竹茹9 g,半夏5 g,赤茯苓9 g,黄芩6 g,枳壳5 g,橘皮5 g,碧玉散(包煎)9 g。

【用法】 水煎服。

【功用】 清胆利湿,和胃化痰。

【临床应用】 适用于湿热少阳证。症见寒热往来,热重寒轻,口苦胸闷,吐酸苦水,或呕黄涎而粘,甚则干呕呃逆,舌红苔白腻或黄腻,脉弦滑数。急性胆囊炎、急性黄疸型肝炎、急性胃肠炎、慢性胃炎、胆汁返流性胃炎、肾盂肾炎、盆腔炎等属少阳证湿热内

gastroenteritis, chronic gastritis, bile-regurgitational gastritis, pyelonephritis, pelvic inflammation and other diseases, which pertain to shaoyang syndrome due to damp heat accumulation in shaoyang meridian. If concomitant with jaundice, add Yinchenhao (*Herba Artemisiae Scopariae*) and Zhizi (*Fructus Gardeniae*) to eliminate damp heat for relieving jaundice. In case of pain over the lower abdomen, add Yanhusuo (*Rhizoma Corydalis*) and Baishaoyao (*Radix Paeoniae Alba*) to regulate the circulation of qi and blood for relieving spasm.

Elucidation: The syndrome results from excessive gallbladder-heat in shaoyang meridian concomitant with phlegm retention caused by damp heat in the middle-energizer. It should be treated by removing dampness from the gallbladder, and regulating the stomach to resolve phlegm. Ingredient No. 1, fragrant in nature, can disperse heat from shaoyang meridian and remove phlegm as well. Ingredient No. 5 has the functions of purging the accumulated fire from the gall bladder meridian and drying dampness. The two play the role of monarch drug. Ingredients No. 2 and No. 3 regulate the stomach to arrest vomiting, and remove phlegm to eliminate dampness, while ingredients No. 6 and No. 7 regulate the stomach and dissolve phlegm, and promote the flow of qi to relieve chest distress. These four in compatibility achieve the purpose of regulating the stomach and flow of qi as well as removing phlegm and descending the adverse flow of qi, acting as minister drug. Ingredients No. 4 and No. 8 are used as adjuvant drug to eliminate damp heat and descend the accumulated heat. Gancao (*Radix Glycyrrhizae*) also functions as guiding drug with the action of mediating the properties of other drugs.

蕴者,可用本方治疗。若兼见黄疸者,可加茵陈蒿、栀子以清利湿热退黄;若少腹疼痛者,可加延胡索、白芍药以行气活血,缓急止痛。

【方解】 本方证由少阳胆热偏重,兼有湿热痰浊中阻所致,治宜清胆利湿,和胃化痰之法。方中青蒿清透少阳邪热,气味芳香又可辟秽化浊;黄芩清泄胆经郁火,并可燥湿,两药相合,内清胆经湿热,外透少阳之邪,共为君药。竹茹、半夏和胃止呕,化痰除湿;橘皮、枳壳和胃化痰,行气宽胸;四药配伍,和胃理气,化痰降逆,同为臣药。赤茯苓、碧玉散(滑石、青黛、甘草)清利湿热,导热下行,俱为佐药。甘草并可调和药性,兼作使药。

2.5.2 Prescriptions for Regulating the Liver and Spleen

Sini San
(*Powder for Treating Cold Limbs*)

Source：*Shanghan Lun* (*Treatise on Exogenous Febrile Diseases*).

Ingredients：

No. 1 Zhigancao (*Radix Glycyrrhizae Praeparatae*) 6 g;

No. 2 Zhishi (*Fructus Aurantii Immaturus*) 6 g;

No. 3 Chaihu (*Radix Bupleuri*) 6 g;

No. 4 Shaoyao (*Radix Paeoniae*) 6 g.

Administration：Grind the above drugs into fine powder, take 3 g twice daily with warm boiled water. Or decoct them with dosages in proportion to those of the original recipe.

Actions：Soothing the liver and regulating the spleen.

Clinical Application：This recipe is used to treat syndrome of disharmony between the liver and spleen, marked by hypochondriac distention and fullness, epigastric and abdominal pain, thin whitish fur, and taut pulse. It is applicable to chronic hepatitis, cholecystitis, cholelithiasis, gastric ulcer, gastritis, gastrointestinal neurosis and other diseases, which pertain to syndrome of stagnated qi in the liver and gallbladder and disharmony between the liver and spleen (or between the gallbladder and stomach). Baishaoyao (*Radix Paeoniae Alba*) is used clinically as ingredient No. 4. In case of severe hypochondriac pain, add Chuanxiong (*Rhizoma Ligustici Chuanxiong*) and Xiangfu (*Rhizoma Cyperi*) to sooth the liver and regulate qi. In case of heat transformed from the stagnated qi manifesting bitter and dry mouth, add Zhizi (*Fructus*

第二节　调和
肝脾剂

四逆散

【方源】《伤寒论》。

【组成】 炙甘草6 g,枳实6 g,柴胡6 g,芍药6 g。

【用法】 共研细末,每次3 g,温开水调服,每日 2 次。亦可作汤剂,用量参照原方比例酌情增减。

【功用】 疏肝理脾。

【临床应用】 适用于肝脾不和证。症见胁肋胀闷,脘腹疼痛,舌苔薄白,脉弦。慢性肝炎、胆囊炎、胆石症、胃溃疡、胃炎、胃肠神经官能症等属肝胆气郁,肝脾(或胆胃)不和者,均可用本方治疗。方中芍药,临床常用白芍药。若胁痛较甚者,可加川芎、香附以疏肝理气止痛;若气郁化热,口苦而干者,可加栀子、川楝子以清肝泄热。

Gardeniae) and Chuanlianzi (*Fructus Meliae Toosen-dan*) to expel heat from the liver.

Elucidation：Originally this recipe is used to treat inward shift of pathogenic heat, accumulation and obstruction of yang-qi, causing cold limbs. Physicians of later generations have expanded its application and used it to deal with various syndromes due to disharmony between the liver and spleen. Ingredient No. 3 is monarch drug with the action of releasing the stagnated liver-qi. The last ingredient functions as minister drug to preserve yin with astringent and nourish blood and the liver. Ingredient No. 2 can regulate liver-qi to remove stagnation and regulate qi movement of the liver and spleen when in compatibility with ingredient No. 3, acting as adjuvant drug. The first ingredient serves as guiding drug, which can relieve spasm in combination with ingredient No. 4, and regulate the middle-energizer in combination with ingredient No. 2, and coordinate the properties of other drugs. The last two in compatibility is meant to regulate the liver, while the first two to regulate the spleen. And all together constitute the result of regulating the middle-energizer as well as the flow of qi.

Sini San, Sini Tang and Danggui Sini Tang are all used in the treatment of cold limbs, but they are different in pathogeneses and therapeutic principles. The syndrome of cold limbs treated with Sini Tang is caused by excessive yin-cold in the interior due to exhaustion of yang-qi with manifestations as coldness extending from hands to elbows and from feet to knees concomitant with deficiency cold syndrome of the body. For this reason, the recipe focuses on recuperating the depleted yang. As for Danggui Sini Tang, deficient yang and blood cause cold to retain in the vessels, which manifests milder coldness compared with that in Sini Tang and is accompanied by such symptoms

【方解】　本方在《伤寒论》中原治伤寒邪热传里，郁遏阳气而致四肢厥逆，故以"四逆"名方。后世对本方的应用有较大发展，目前多用于治疗肝脾不和诸证。方中柴胡疏肝行气解郁，为君药。芍药敛阴养血柔肝，为臣药。枳实理气解郁，与柴胡配伍一升一降，调畅肝脾气机，为佐药。炙甘草合芍药缓急止痛，配枳实和中理脾，并可调和药性，为佐使药。方中柴胡、芍药相伍以调肝，枳实、甘草合用以调脾，四药配伍，共奏疏肝理脾，行气和中之效。

四逆散与四逆汤、当归四逆汤均可治疗"四逆"，但其病机与立法各异。四逆汤证之四肢厥逆是由于阳气衰微，阴寒内盛，不能温养四肢所致，其手冷过肘，足冷过膝，并伴有全身虚寒之象，故方以回阳救逆为法；当归四逆汤证之四肢厥逆是由于阳虚血弱，寒凝经脉所致，其肢冷程度较之四逆汤证为轻，并伴肢体疼痛、舌淡脉细等血虚经脉不利之

showing deficiency and obstructed circulation of blood as pain of the limbs, pale tongue and thready pulse. That's why the principle of warming the meridians to dispel cold and nourishing the blood to remove obstruction is adopted in this case. In terms of Sini San, cold limbs are the result of heat invading inward and causing yang-qi to be stagnated and fail in warming the limbs. This is characterized by coldness of only the fingers and toes with feverish body and taut pulse. Thus the therapeutic principle aims at dispersing heat to relieve stagnancy.

Xiaoyao San
(*Ease Powder*)

Source：*Taiping Huimin Hejiju Fang* (*Benevolent Prescriptions from Taiping Pharmaceutical Bureau*).

Ingredients：

No. 1 Zhigancao (*Radix Glycyrrhizae Praeparatae*) 15 g;

No. 2 Danggui (*Radix Angelicae Sinensis*) 30 g;

No. 3 Fuling (*Poria*) 30 g;

No. 4 Shaoyao (*Radix Paeoniae*) 30 g;

No. 5 Baizhu (*Rhizoma Atractylodis Macrocephalae*) 30 g;

No. 6 Chaihu (*Radix Bupleuri*) 30 g.

Administration：Grind the above drugs into fine powder, take 6 g twice daily with the decoction of a small amount of roasted ginger and peppermint; or prepare into decoction with doses in proportion to the original recipe.

Actions：Soothing the liver, nourishing blood and invigorating the spleen.

Clinical Application：This recipe is used to treat stagnation of liver-qi and deficiency of blood and spleen, marked by hypochondriac pain, headache, dizziness, dry mouth and throat, mental fatigue and poor appetite, or

象,故方以温经散寒,养血通脉为法;四逆散证之四肢厥逆是由于邪热入里,阳气内郁不能达于四肢所致,因其阳气不虚,亦非寒邪致病,仅表现为指、趾不温,并伴身热、脉弦等症,故方以透邪解郁为法。

逍遥散

【方源】 《太平惠民和剂局方》。

【组成】 炙甘草15 g,当归、茯苓、芍药、白术、柴胡各30 g。

【用法】 共研细末,每次6 g,以煨姜、薄荷少许煎汤冲服,每日 2 次。亦可作汤剂,用量按原方比例酌定。

【功用】 疏肝解郁,养血健脾。

【临床应用】 适用于肝郁血虚脾弱证。症见两胁作痛,头痛目眩,口燥咽干,神疲食少,或往来寒热,或月经不

alternate attacks of chills and fever, or irregular menstru-ation, distension in the breast, reddish tongue, taut and thready pulse. It is applicable to chronic hepatitis, choleli-thiasis, gastroduodenal ulcer, chronic gastritis, gastroin-testinal neurosis, premenstrual tension, hyperplasia of lobule of mammary gland, menopausal syndrome, and chronic pelvic inflammation, whose symptoms are stagna-tion of liver-qi with deficiency of blood as well as failure of the spleen in transportation and transformation with chief manifestations as hypochondriac distention and pain, mental fatigue and poor appetite. Baishaoyao (*Radix Paeoniae Al-ba*) is often used clinically as ingredient No. 4. In case of heat converted from stagnated liver-qi manifesting dry and bitter mouth, add Mudanpi (*Cortex Moutan Radicis*) and Zhizi (*Fructus Gardeniae*) to purge heat from the liver, namely Jiawei Xiaoyao San. In case of excessive deficien-cy of blood with pale complexion, dizziness and pale tongue, add Shudihuang (*Radix Rehmanniae Praepara-tae*) to nourish yin and blood, namely Hei Xiaoyao San.

Elucidation: The syndrome is due to protracted stagnation of liver-qi consuming blood, liver-wood depres-sion subjugating spleen-earth and dysfunction of the spleen in transportation and transformation. It should be treated by dispersing the liver-qi and nourishing blood, invigorat-ing the spleen to promote transportation and transforma-tion. The last ingredient is the monarch drug in the reci-pe, used to disperse stagnated liver-qi. Ingredients No. 2 and No. 4 are used as minister drugs to nourish blood for retaining yin, nourish the liver to relieve spasm. As adju-vant drugs, ingredients No. 3, No. 5 and No. 1 can supple-ment qi, strengthen the middle-energizer, reinforce the spleen to prevent the liver from subjugating it, and com-plement the source of qi and blood. Ingredient No. 1 also mediates the effects of other ingredients, and acts as

调,乳房胀痛,舌淡红,脉细弦。慢性肝炎、胆石症、胃及十二指肠溃疡、慢性胃炎、胃肠神经官能症、经前期紧张症、乳腺小叶增生、更年期综合征、慢性盆腔炎等属肝郁血虚,脾运失健,以胁肋胀痛、神疲食少为主症者,可用本方治疗。方中芍药,现临床常用白芍药。若肝郁化热,口苦口干者,可加牡丹皮、栀子以清肝泄热,即加味逍遥散;若血虚较甚,面色无华,头晕舌淡者,可加熟地黄以滋阴养血,即黑逍遥散。

【方解】　本方证由肝郁日久,暗耗阴血,木郁乘土,脾失健运所致,治宜疏肝养血,健脾助运之法。方中柴胡疏肝解郁,为君药。芍药、当归养血敛阴,柔肝缓急,同为臣药。茯苓、白术、炙甘草益气补中,健脾助运,实脾以防肝乘,并资气血生化之源,均为佐药。甘草兼以调和药性,又作使药。服药时少加薄荷、生姜,前者可助柴胡疏肝解郁,后者可协茯苓、白术温中和胃。诸药配伍,疏中有养,治肝顾脾,使肝郁得舒,肝血得

guiding drug. The peppermint and ginger respectively assist ingredient No. 6 to disperse the stagnated liver-qi, and help ingredients No. 3 and No. 5 warm and regulate the middle-energizer. All the drugs are used together to disperse the stagnated liver-qi and enrich liver blood on the one hand, and restore the normal function of the spleen on the other so that the patient gets fully recovered.

充,脾运复健,则诸症可愈。

Tongxie Yaofang
(*Recipe for Diarrhea with Pain*)

Source：*Liu Caochuang's recipe from Yixue Zhengzhuan (Orthodox Medical Records)*.

Ingredients：

No. 1 Baizhu (*Rhizoma Atractylodis Macrocephalae*) 90 g (baked);

No. 2 Baishaoyao (*Radix Paeoniae Alba*) 60 g (baked);

No. 3 Chenpi (*Pericarpium Citri Reticulatae*) 45 g (baked);

No. 4 Fangfeng (*Radix Ledebouriellae*) 60 g.

Administration：Grind the above drugs into coarse powder, take 9 g once and decoct in water for oral use.

Actions：Purging liver fire and invigorating the spleen, relieving pain and diarrhea.

Clinical Application：This recipe is used to treat painful diarrhea due to disharmony between the liver and spleen marked by borborygmus, abdominal pain, diarrhea with abdominal pain, thin whitish fur, taut and slow pulse. It is applicable to acute enteritis, chronic colitis, neurotic diarrhea and other diseases, which pertain to syndrome of hyperfunctioning liver restricting the spleen, and are characterized by diarrhea with abdominal pain and relieved pain after defecation. In case of protracted diarrhea, add Huangqi (*Radix Astragali seu Hedysari*) and

痛泻要方

【方源】 刘草窗方,录自《医学正传》。

【组成】 炒白术90 g,炒白芍药60 g,炒陈皮45 g,防风60 g。

【用法】 共研粗末,每次9 g,水煎服。

【功用】 泻肝补脾,止痛止泻。

【临床应用】 适用于肝脾失调之痛泻证。症见肠鸣腹痛,大便泄泻,泻必腹痛,舌苔薄白,脉弦缓。急性肠炎、慢性结肠炎、神经性腹泻等属肝木乘脾,具有泻必腹痛,泻后痛缓特征者,可用本方治疗。若泄泻日久不愈者,可加黄芪、炒升麻以补气升阳止泻;若兼挟湿热,舌苔黄腻者,

Shengma (*Rhizoma Cimicifugae*) (baked) to supplement qi and lift yang to relieve diarrhea. If concomitant with damp heat manifesting yellowish greasy fur, add Huanglian (*Rhizoma Coptidis*) and Huangqin (*Radix Scutellariae*) to dispel pathogenic factors from the intestine and dry dampness to relieve diarrhea.

Elucidation：The syndrome is due to excess of the liver and deficiency of the spleen, leading to abnormal transportation and transformation. It should be treated by purging liver-fire and invigorating the spleen to relieve pain and diarrhea. The first ingredient is monarch drug with the function of benefiting qi and reinforcing the spleen, drying dampness and relieving diarrhea. Ingredient No. 2 can nourish the liver and blood, and relieve spasm and pain, used as minister drug. Ingredient No. 3 bears the effect of regulating the flow of qi and drying dampness, invigorating the spleen and regulating the stomach. The last ingredient is pungent and warm in nature with lifting and dispersing functions, which helps ingredient No. 2 disperse the stagnated liver-qi and ingredient No. 1 lift yang and regulate the spleen. So ingredients No. 3 and No. 4 play the role of adjuvant drugs. Besides the last ingredient also serves as guiding drug, which leads other ingredients to the spleen.

可加黄连、黄芩以清肠燥湿止泻。

【方解】　本方证由肝旺脾虚，木郁乘土，运化失常所致，治宜泻肝补脾，止痛止泻之法。方中白术益气健脾，燥湿止泻，为君药。白芍药柔肝养血，缓急止痛，为臣药。陈皮理气燥湿，醒脾和胃；防风辛温升散，合白芍药以疏肝解郁，合白术升阳舒脾，均为佐药。防风又可引诸药入脾，兼作使药。

2.5.3　Prescriptions for Harmonizing Cold-heat Syndrome

Banxia Xiexin Tang
(**Pinellia Decoction for Purging Stomach Fire**)

Source：*Shanghan Lun* (*Treatise on Exogenous Febrile Diseases*).

Ingredients：
No. 1 Banxia (*Rhizoma Pinelliae*) 12 g;

第三节　调和寒热剂

半夏泻心汤

【方源】　《伤寒论》。

【组成】　半夏12 g，黄芩、干姜、人参各9 g，黄连3 g，大

No. 2 Huangqin (*Radix Scutellariae*) 9 g;

No. 3 Ganjiang (*Rhizoma Zingiberis*) 9 g;

No. 4 Renshen (*Radix Ginseng*) 9 g;

No. 5 Huanglian (*Rhizoma Coptidis*) 3 g;

No. 6 Dazao (*Fructus Ziziphi Jujubae*) 4 pcs;

No. 7 Zhigancao (*Radix Glycyrrhizae Praeparatae*) 9 g.

Administration: Decoct the above drugs in water for oral application.

Actions: Regulating cold and heat, and dispersing accumulation to relieve fullness.

Clinical Application: This recipe is used to treat syndrome of abdominal fullness due to intermingling of cold and heat, marked by epigastric fullness without pain, retching or vomiting, borborygmus and diarrhea, thin yellowish and greasy fur, taut and rapid pulse. It is applicable to acute or chronic gastroenteritis, chronic colitis, neurotic gastritis, chronic hepatitis, chronic cholecystitis and other diseases, which pertain to intermingling syndrome of cold and heat, and deficiency and excess as well with chief manifestations as abdominal fullness and distention, vomiting, and diarrhea. In case of fullness and vomiting with mild state of qi deficiency of the middle-energizer, replace ingredients No. 4 and No. 6 with Zhishi (*Fructus Aurantii Immaturus*) and Shengjiang (*Rhizoma Zingiberis Recens*) to regulate qi and the stomach for relieving vomiting.

Elucidation: The syndrome is due to deficient yang in the middle energizer, intermingling of cold and heat, and disorder of ascending and descending. It should be treated by regulating cold and heat, and dispersing accumulation to relieve fullness. Ingredients No. 2 and No. 5 are monarch drugs, bitter and cold in nature with the function of clearing away heat. Ingredients No. 1 and No. 3 are used as minister drugs with pungent and warm

枣 4 枚,炙甘草 9 g。

【用法】 水煎服。

【功用】 平调寒热,开结除痞。

【临床应用】 适用于寒热互结之痞证。症见心下痞满不痛,干呕或呕吐,肠鸣下利,舌苔薄黄而腻,脉弦数。急性胃肠炎、慢性胃肠炎、慢性结肠炎、神经性胃炎、慢性肝炎、慢性胆囊炎等属寒热虚实错杂,以痞、呕、利为主症者,可用本方治疗。若痞满呕吐而中虚不甚者,可去人参、大枣,加枳实、生姜以理气和胃止呕。

【方解】 本方证由中阳不足,寒热互结,升降失常所致,治宜平调寒热,开结除痞之法。方中黄连、黄芩苦寒降泄以清热,共为君药。半夏、干姜辛温开结以祛寒,同为臣药。人参、炙甘草、大枣益气补虚,合干姜可温中补虚,益

nature to dispel cold. Ingredients No. 4, No. 7 and No. 6 replenish qi and strengthen the middle-energizer and serve as adjuvant drugs to warm the middle-energizer and regulate the stomach and spleen in combination with ingredient No. 3. The last ingredient also acts as guiding drug with the effect of mediating the properties of other drugs. All ingredients together regulate both cold and heat and restore normal ascending and descending functions to relieve fullness, vomiting and dysentery by simultaneously using warming and clearing methods, descending and opening with drugs bitter and pungent in flavor for both reinforcement and purgation.

Cautions：This recipe is contraindicated for those with epigastric fullness due to qi stagnation or retention of indigested food.

脾养胃,均为佐药。甘草兼能调和药性,又作使药。诸药配伍,温清并用,补泻兼施,辛开苦降,使寒热去而升降复常,则痞满可消,呕吐、下利自止。

【注意事项】　心下痞满因气滞或食积而致者,禁用本方。

2.5.4　Prescriptions for Expelling both Exterior and Interior Pathogenic factors

第四节　表里双解剂

Da Chaihu Tang
(*Major Bupleurum Decoction*)

大柴胡汤

Source：*Jingui Yaolue* (*Synopsis of Prescriptions of the Golden Cabinet*).

【方源】　《金匮要略》。

Ingredients：

No. 1 Chaihu (*Radix Bupleuri*) 15 g;

No. 2 Huangqin (*Radix Scutellariae*) 9 g;

No. 3 Shaoyao (*Radix Paeoniae*) 9 g;

No. 4 Banxia (*Rhizoma Pinelliae*) 9 g;

No. 5 Zhishi (*Fructus Aurantii Immaturus*) 12 g;

No. 6 Dahuang (*Radix et Rhizoma Rhei*) 6 g;

No. 7 Shengjiang (*Rhizoma Zingiberis Recens*) 12 g;

No. 8 Dazao (*Fructus Ziziphi Jujubae*) 5 pcs.

【组成】　柴胡15 g,黄芩9 g,芍药9 g,半夏9 g,枳实12 g,大黄6 g,生姜12 g,大枣5枚。

Administration：Decoct the above drugs in water

【用法】　水煎服。

for oral application.

Actions: Mediating shaoyang and purging heat accumulation.

Clinical Application: This recipe is used to treat combined disease of shaoyang and yangming, marked by alternate attack of chill and fever, fullness in the chest and hypochondrium, vomiting, bitter mouth, epigastric fullness and pain or stuffiness and fullness, constipation or diarrhea, thick yellowish fur, taut rapid and forceful pulse. It is applicable to acute cholecystitis, cholelithiasis, acute pancreatitis, gastroduodenal ulcer and other diseases, which pertain to combined disease of shaoyang and yangming and are characterized by alternate attack of chill and fever and abdominal pain with constipation. Ingredient No. 3 should be selected according to clinical needs, that is, Baishaoyao (*Radix Paeoniae Alba*) is recommended for relieving spasm or pain and Chishaoyao (*Radix Paeoniae Rubra*) for clearing away heat and cooling blood. If concomitant with jaundice, add Yinchenhao (*Herba Artemisiae Scopariae*) and Zhizi (*Fructus Gardeniae*) to relieve jaundice by clearing away heat and promoting diuresis. In case of sharp hypochondriac and epigastric pain, add Chuanlianzi (*Fructus Meliae Toosendan*) and Yanhusuo (*Rhizoma Corydalis*) to promote the circulation of both qi and blood for relieving pain. In case of incessant vomiting, add Zhuru (*Caulis Bambusae in Taeniam*) (prepared with ginger decoction), Huanglian (*Rhizoma Coptidis*) and Daizheshi (*Ochra Haematitum*) to descend the adverse rising qi and regulate the stomach for relieving vomiting. In case of biliary duct calculi, add Yujin (*Radix Curcumae*), Jinqiancao (*Herba Lysimachiae*) and Haijinsha (*Spora Lygodii*) to disperse stagnated liver-qi, promote discharge of bile, and remove stones.

【功用】　和解少阳,泻下热结。

【临床应用】　适用于少阳与阳明合病。症见往来寒热,胸胁苦满,呕吐,口苦,心下满痛或痞硬,便秘或下利,舌苔黄厚,脉弦数有力。急性胆囊炎、胆石症、急性胰腺炎、胃及十二指肠溃疡等属少阳阳明合病,往来寒热、腹痛便秘并见者,可用本方治疗。方中芍药,宜根据临床证候酌定:若欲缓急止痛则用白芍药,欲清热凉血则用赤芍药。若兼黄疸者,可加茵陈蒿、栀子以清热利湿退黄;若胁脘疼痛较剧者,可加川楝子、延胡索以行气活血止痛;若呕吐不止者,可加姜竹茹、黄连、代赭石以降逆和胃止呕;若胆管结石者,可加郁金、金钱草、海金沙以疏肝利胆化石。

Elucidation: The syndrome is due to unrelieved pathogenic factors in shaoyang that affect yangming and cause excessive accumulation of heat and indigested food in the intestine. It should be treated with mediating method to purge away heat accumulation from shaoyang. The first ingredient in larger dosage is meant to dispel pathogenic factors and ingredient No. 2 to purge heat from shaoyang, both being the primary drugs for treating shaoyang disease and acting as monarch drug in this recipe. Ingredient No. 6 in smaller dosage and ingredient No. 5 are the primary drugs for purging away heat accumulation and serve as minister drug, the former for purging away heat to relieve constipation and the latter removing stagnation of qi. Used as adjuvant drug, ingredient No. 3 bears the function of relieving spasm or pain, and ingredients No. 4 and No. 7 regulating the stomach and descending the adverse rising qi. The last ingredient serves as guiding drug to regulate the properties of other drugs. This recipe is actually prepared on the basis of Xiao Chaihu Tang and Da Chengqi Tang with modification, the combination of which generates the result of removing pathogenic factors from shaoyang in the exterior and purging away heat accumulated in yangming in the interior.

Cautions: Since this recipe, with a larger dosage of the first ingredient, is expected mainly to treat shaoyang disease, it is unfit for the case of both shaoyang and yangming disease with the latter prevailing.

Gegen Huangqin Huanglian Tang
(*Decoction of Pueraria*,
Scutellariae and Coptis)

Source: *Shanghan Lun* (*Treatise on Exogenous Febrile Diseases*).

Ingredients:

No. 1 Gegen (*Radix Puerariae*) 15 g;

【方解】 本方证由少阳之邪不解,内传阳明,以致邪热与肠中积滞相结成实,治宜和解少阳,泻下热结之法。方中重用柴胡疏散少阳之邪,黄芩清泄少阳之热,两者配伍,为和解少阳要药,共为君药。轻用大黄泻热通便,枳实破气除满,两者配伍,为泻下热结要药,同为臣药。芍药缓急止痛,半夏、生姜和胃降逆,均为佐药。大枣调和药性,为使药。本方实为小柴胡汤与大承气汤加减变化而成,合而用之,故外可解少阳之邪,内可泻阳明热结。

【注意事项】 由于本方重用柴胡,故以和解少阳为主,若少阳阳明合病而阳明证较著者不宜使用。

葛根黄芩黄连汤

【方源】《伤寒论》。

【组成】 葛根15 g,炙甘草6 g,黄芩9 g,黄连9 g。

No. 2 Zhigancao (*Radix Glycyrrhizae Praeparatae*) 6 g;

No. 3 Huangqin (*Radix Scutellariae*) 9 g;

No. 4 Huanglian (*Rhizoma Coptidis*) 9 g.

Administration: Decoct the above drugs in water for oral application.

Actions: Dispelling pathogenic factors from the exterior and clearing away heat from the interior.

Clinical Application: This recipe is used to treat diarrhea due to heat in the exterior and interior, marked by feverish body with diarrhea, dysphoria, thirst, perspiration, reddened tongue with yellowish fur, and rapid pulse. It is applicable to acute enteritis, bacillary dysentery, gastrointestinal cold and other diseases, which have the chief manifestation as diarrhea and pertain to unrelieved exterior symptoms with excessive interior heat. In case of sharp abdominal pain, add Baishaoyao (*Radix Paeoniae Alba*) (baked) to nourish the liver and relieve pain. In case of dysentery due to damp heat with tenesmus, add Muxiang (*Radix Aucklandiae*) and Binglang (*Semen Arecae*) to promote the circulation of qi and relieve tenesmus.

Elucidation: The syndrome is the result of unrelieved exterior heat invading the interior and affecting the large intestine. It should be treated by means of eliminating both exterior and interior heat. The first ingredient acts as monarch drug with the action of clearing away exterior heat and lifting yang to relieve diarrhea. The last two act as minister drug to clear away heat and toxic substances and relieve diarrhea by drying dampness. Ingredient No. 2 is meant to coordinate the properties of other drugs and plays the role of guiding drug. All ingredients in combination aim to treat both the exterior and interior symptoms but focus on expelling interior heat. Since the monarch drug bears a pungent and cool nature with the

【用法】 水煎服。

【功用】 解表清里。

【临床应用】 适用于表里俱热之泄泻证。症见身热下利,胸脘烦热,口渴汗出,舌红苔黄,脉数。急性肠炎、细菌性痢疾、胃肠型感冒等以腹泻为主要表现,属表证未解,里热较甚者,可用本方治疗。若腹痛甚者,可加炒白芍药以柔肝缓急止痛;若湿热痢疾里急后重者,可加木香、槟榔以行气而除后重。

【方解】 本方证为表证未解,邪热入里,下迫大肠而致下利,治宜解表清里之法。方中葛根解表清热,升阳止利,为君药。黄芩、黄连清热解毒,燥湿止利,同为臣药。炙甘草调和药性,为使药。诸药合用,表里同治而以清里热为主。由于葛根性味辛凉,功能清热止利,故本方亦可用于下利外无表证而纯属里热引起者。

function of clearing away heat and relieving diarrhea, this recipe can also be used to treat diarrhea caused completely by interior heat without any exterior syndrome.

Cautions: This recipe is contraindicated for patients with diarrhea that is concomitant with aversion to cold, pale tongue and thready pulse.

【注意事项】　下利而伴见畏寒，舌淡脉细者，禁用本方。

2.6 Tonic Prescriptions

第六章
补益剂

Tonic prescriptions refer to those composed chiefly of tonic drugs, which act to invigorate qi, blood, yin and yang of the human body, and are indicated for various deficiency syndromes.

Since syndromes of deficiency include four types, namely qi deficiency, blood deficiency, yin deficiency, and yang deficiency, and the first two types are concomitant to each other, tonic prescriptions are accordingly subdivided into five categories. They are prescriptions for invigorating qi, those for nourishing blood, those for invigorating both qi and blood, those for invigorating yin and those for invigorating yang.

Prescriptions for invigorating qi are made up of tonics with the effects of benefiting qi and invigorating deficiency, and applicable to qi deficiency of the spleen and lung. Prescriptions for invigorating blood comprise drugs of nourishing blood and invigorating deficiency, and are suitable for blood deficiency of the heart and liver. Prescriptions for reinforcement of both qi and blood consist of drugs with the effects of benefiting qi and nourishing blood and are applied to deficiency syndrome of both qi and blood. Prescriptions for invigorating yin are mainly composed of drugs able to nourish yin and benefit essence, and used to treat yin deficiency of the liver, kidney and lung. Prescriptions for invigorating yang are mainly composed of drugs capable of warming and reinforcing kidney-yang and used to treat yang deficiency of the kidney.

凡以补益药为主组成,具有补养人体气、血、阴、阳等作用,用于治疗各种虚证的方剂,统称补益剂。

由于虚证主要有气虚、血虚、阴虚、阳虚四种证型,气虚与血虚又常常并见,因而补益剂相应地分为补气剂、补血剂、气血双补剂、补阴剂与补阳剂五类。

补气剂由补气药为主组成,具有益气补虚作用,适用于脾肺气虚证。补血剂由补血药为主组成,具有养血补虚作用,适用于心肝血虚证。气血双补剂由补气药配伍补血药组成,具有益气养血作用,适用于气血两虚证。补阴剂由补阴药为主组成,具有滋阴益精作用,适用于肝肾肺阴虚证。补阳剂由补阳药为主组成,具有温补肾阳作用,适用于肾阳亏虚证。

Tonic prescriptions should not be applied for long time because they are mostly strong and greasy and apt to affect the stomach. Besides they should be used carefully in cases with usual deficiency of the spleen and stomach, or with poor appetite and loose stool. In such a case, it is necessary to add some drugs capable of strengthening the spleen and stomach and regulating qi to promote transportation and transformation. For patients with deficiency syndrome and intolerance of tonics, it is advisable to regulate the spleen and stomach before tonic prescriptions are given. These prescriptions should be decocted for a longer period with mild fire and taken before meals or with an empty stomach to promote the absorption of the drugs.

补益方剂多味厚滋腻,易于碍胃,不宜久服;素体脾胃虚弱,食少便溏者慎用,或适当加入健脾和胃,理气助运之品,以资运化。对于虚不受补的患者,应先调理脾胃。本类方剂入汤剂时须文火久煎,并于饭前或空腹时服用,以利药物的吸收。

2.6.1　Prescriptions for Invigorating Qi

Sijunzi Tang

(*Decoction of Four Noble Ingredients*)

Source：*Taiping Huimin Hejiju Fang* (*Benevolent Prescriptions from Taiping Pharmaceutical Bureau*).

Ingredients：

No. 1 Renshen (*Radix Ginseng*) 9 g;

No. 2 Baizhu (*Rhizoma Atractylodis Macrocephalae*) 9 g;

No. 3 Fuling (*Poria*) 9 g;

No. 4 Zhigancao (*Radix Glycyrrhizae Praeparatae*) 6 g.

Administration：Decoct the above drugs in water for oral application.

Actions：Replenishing qi and strengthening the spleen.

Clinical Application：This recipe is used to treat qi deficiency syndrome of the spleen and stomach marked by pale complexion, low and weak voice, shortness of breath and lassitude, poor appetite, watery stool, pale tongue with whitish fur, thready and weak pulse. It is applicable

第一节　补气剂

四君子汤

【方源】　《太平惠民和剂局方》。

【组成】　人参、白术、茯苓各9 g,炙甘草6 g。

【用法】　水煎服。

【功用】　益气健脾。

【临床应用】　适用于脾胃气虚证。症见面色萎白,语声低微,气短乏力,食少便溏,舌淡苔白,脉细弱。慢性胃炎、胃及十二指肠溃疡等见有

to chronic gastritis, gastroduodenal ulcer and other diseases, which have the above symptoms and pertain to qi deficiency of the spleen and stomach. If concomitant with qi stagnation manifesting chest and epigastric fullness, add Chenpi (*Pericarpium Citri Reticulatae*) to promote the flow of qi, which forms another recipe entitled Yigong San. If concomitant with phlegm and dampness retaining in the interior and cough with profuse sputum, add Chenpi (*Pericarpium Citri Reticulatae*) and Banxia (*Rhizoma Pinelliae*) to remove phlegm by drying dampness, which constitute another recipe entitled Liujunzi Tang. If concomitant with cold-dampness retaining in the middle-energizer, functional disorder of the stomach-qi and obstructed circulation of qi, add Muxiang (*Radix Aucklandiae*), Sharen (*Fructus Amomi*), Chenpi (*Pericarpium Citri Reticulatae*) and Banxia (*Rhizoma Pinelliae*) to promote the flow of qi of the middle-energizer and regulate the stomach to relieve vomiting. This forms a new recipe named Xiangsha Liujunzi Tang.

Elucidation: The syndrome is due to qi deficiency of the spleen and stomach, leading to disorder of transportation and transformation. It should be treated by means of replenishing qi and strengthening the spleen. Ingredient No.1 possesses the effect of invigorating qi, and acts as monarch drug to strengthen the spleen and nourish the stomach. Used as minister drug, No. 2 is effective in invigorating the spleen and eliminating dampness. Ingredient No. 3 serves as adjuvant drug to eliminate dampness and strengthen the spleen. The last ingredient acts to invigorate qi, reinforce the middle-energizer and mediate the Properties of other drugs as guiding drug. The combination of ingredients No. 1, No. 2 and No. 4 brings about the effects of invigorating qi, reinforcing the spleen and stomach, while that of ingredients No. 2 and No. 3 invig-

上述症状,属脾胃气虚者,可用本方治疗。若兼气滞而胸脘满闷者,可加陈皮以行气化滞,即异功散;若兼痰湿内阻,咳嗽痰多者,可加陈皮、半夏以燥湿化痰,即六君子汤;若兼寒湿中阻,胃气失和,气机不畅者,可加木香、砂仁、陈皮、半夏以行气畅中,和胃止呕,即香砂六君子汤。

【方解】 本方证由脾胃气虚,运化乏力所致,治宜益气健脾之法。方中人参益气健脾养胃,为君药。白术益气健脾燥湿,为臣药。茯苓渗湿健脾助运,为佐药。炙甘草益气补中,调和药性,为使药。方中人参、白术、甘草合用以益气补脾养胃;白术、茯苓相伍以健脾祛湿助运。四药配伍,补而不滞,温而不燥,共成甘温平补脾胃之剂。

orating the spleen and eliminating dampness to promote transportation and transformation. The four ingredients in compatibility constitute the recipe. For reinforcing the spleen and stomach with sweat and warm drugs, which has the characteristics of reinforcement without stagnancy and warming without dryness.

Shenling Baizhu San
(Powder of Ginseng, Poria and Bighead Atractylodes)

Source: *Taiping Huimin Hejiju Fang* (*Benevolent Prescriptions from Taiping Pharmaceutical Bureau*).

Ingredients:

No. 1 Lianzirou (*Semen Nelumbinis*) 500 g;

No. 2 Yiyiren (*Semen Coicis*) 500 g;

No. 3 Sharen (*Fructus Amomi*) 500 g;

No. 4 Jiegeng (*Radix Platycodi*) 500 g;

No. 5 Biandou (*Semen Dolichoris Album*) 750 g;

No. 6 Fuling (*Poria*) 1,000 g;

No. 7 Renshen (*Radix Ginseng*) 1,000 g;

No. 8 Zhigancao (*Radix Glycyrrhizae Praeparatae*) 1,000 g;

No. 9 Baizhu (*Rhizoma Atractylodis Macrocephalae*) 1,000 g;

No. 10 Shanyao (*Rhizoma Dioscoreae*) 1,000 g.

Administration: Grind the above drugs into fine powder, take 6 g each time and twice daily with the decoction of Dazao (*Fructus Ziziphi Jujubae*). Or prepare them into a decoction with the dosage in proportion to the original recipe.

Actions: Benefiting qi and strengthening the spleen, eliminating dampness and relieving diarrhea.

Clinical Application: This recipe is used to treat qi deficiency of the spleen and stomach concomitant with dampness, marked by lassitude of the extremities, general

参苓白术散

【方源】《太平惠民和剂局方》。

【组成】 莲子肉500 g,薏苡仁500 g,砂仁500 g,桔梗500 g,扁豆750 g,茯苓1 000 g,人参1 000 g,炙甘草1 000 g,白术1 000 g,山药1 000 g。

【用法】 共研细末,每次6 g,大枣煎汤调服,每日 2 次。亦可作汤剂,用量按原方比例酌定。

【功用】 益气健脾,渗湿止泻。

【临床应用】 适用于脾胃气虚挟湿证。症见四肢无力,形体消瘦,饮食不化,或吐

debility, dyspepsia, vomiting or diarrhea, chest distress and epigastric fullness, sallow complexion, pale tongue with whitish and greasy fur, feeble and moderate pulse. It is applicable to chronic gastroenteritis, infantile dyspepsia, anemia, chronic bronchitis, chronic nephritis, leukorrhea and other diseases, which pertain to deficiency of the spleen with dampness. If concomitant with interior cold manifesting abdominal pain with preference for warmth, add Ganjiang (*Rhizoma Zingiberis*) and Rougui (*Cortex Cinnamomi*) to warm the middle-energizer and dispel cold. For infantile dyspepsia with poor appetite and flatulence, add Maiya (*Fructus Hordei Germinatus*) (baked), Shanzha (*Fructus Crataegi*) (charred) and Shenqu (*Massa Fermentata Medicinalis*) (baked) to promote digestion. In case of phlegm induced by dampness and cough with productive whitish sputum, add Banxia (*Rhizoma Pinelliae*) and Chenpi (*Pericarpium Citri Reticulatae*) to remove phlegm by eliminating dampness.

Elucidation:The syndrome results from disorder in transportation and transformation, and generation of dampness in the interior due to deficiency of the spleen and stomach. It should be treated by means of replenishing qi, strengthening the spleen and eliminating dampness to remove diarrhea. Ingredients No. 7 and No. 9 act together as monarch drugs to benefit qi, strengthen the spleen and eliminate dampness. Ingredients No. 10 and No. 1 help No. 7 replenish qi and strengthen the spleen, while No. 5, No. 2 and No. 6 help No. 9 reinforce the spleen and promote diuresis. These five ingredients together are used as minister drug. Ingredient No. 3 can regulate the stomach and invigorate the spleen, and No. 4 disperse the lung-qi, promote diuresis and lead other drugs upwards to the lung. Ingredient No. 8 is effective in supplementing qi and reinforcing the spleen and capable of

或泄,胸脘闷胀,面色萎黄,舌淡苔白腻,脉虚缓。慢性胃肠炎、小儿消化不良、贫血、慢性支气管炎、慢性肾炎及妇女带下病等属脾虚挟湿者,可用本方治疗。若兼里寒而腹痛喜温者,可加干姜、肉桂以温中祛寒止痛;若小儿消化不良食少腹胀者,可加炒麦芽、焦山楂、炒神曲以消食和胃助运;若脾湿生痰而咳痰量多、色白者,可加半夏、陈皮以燥湿化痰和中。

【方解】 本方证由脾胃虚弱,运化失常,湿自内生所致,治宜益气健脾,渗湿止泻之法。方中人参、白术益气补虚,健脾渗湿,共为君药。山药、莲子肉助人参益气补脾;扁豆、薏苡仁、茯苓助白术健脾渗湿,同为臣药。砂仁和胃醒脾,行气化滞;桔梗宣利肺气,通调水道以助祛湿,又载药上行,以益肺气;炙甘草益气补脾,调和药性,均为佐使药。

mediating the properties of other drugs. These three ingredients serve as guiding drug.

Buzhong Yiqi Tang
(Decoction for Reinforcing
Qi in the Middle Energizer)

Source：*Neiwaishang Bianhuo Lun* (*Differentiation on Endogenous and Exogenous Diseases*).

Ingredients：

No. 1 Huangqi (*Radix Astragali seu Hedysari*) 18 g;

No. 2 Zhigancao (*Radix Glycyrrhizae Praeparatae*) 9 g;

No. 3 Renshen (*Radix Ginseng*) 6 g;

No. 4 Danggui (*Radix Angelicae Sinensis*) 3 g;

No. 5 Jupi (*Pericarpium Citri Reticulatae*) 6 g;

No. 6 Shengma (*Rhizoma Cimicifugae*) 6 g;

No. 7 Chaihu (*Radix Bupleuri*) 6 g;

No. 8 Baizhu (*Rhizoma Atractylodis Macrocephalae*) 9 g.

Administration：Decoct the above drugs in water for oral application.

Actions：Invigorating middle-energizer and replenishing qi, elevating the spleen-yang to improve the functional activities of qi and viscera.

Clinical Application：This recipe is indicated for prolapse due to deficient qi, marked by poor appetite, lassitude, loose stool, fever with perspiration, thirst with preference for hot drinks, or prolapse of the rectum, prolapse of the uterus, protracted diarrhea, protracted dysentery, metrorrhagia and metrostaxis, pale and large tongue with thin whitish fur. It is applicable to visceral ptosis, chronic gastroenteritis, chronic dysentery, myasthenia gravis, chronic hepatitis, long-term low fever from unknown reasons, hypermenorrhea, and chyluria, which pertain to qi collapse due to deficiency of the middle-energizer. For visceral ptosis and myasthenia gravis, it is necessary to add Zhishi (*Fructus Aurantii Immaturus*) to

补中益气汤

【方源】《内外伤辨惑论》。

【组成】 黄芪18 g,炙甘草9 g,人参6 g,当归3 g,橘皮6 g,升麻6 g,柴胡6 g,白术9 g。

【用法】 水煎服。

【功用】 补中益气,升阳举陷。

【临床应用】 适用于气虚下陷证。症见食少体倦,纳差便溏,发热自汗,渴喜热饮,或脱肛,子宫脱垂,久泻,久痢,崩漏,舌质淡胖,苔薄白。脏器下垂、慢性肠胃炎、慢性痢疾、重症肌无力、慢性肝炎、不明原因的长期低热不退、月经过多、乳糜尿等属中虚气陷者,可用本方治疗。若内脏下垂或重症肌无力者,可加枳实以助补气药升提之力;若气不摄血而月经过多者,可加仙鹤

lift qi of the middle-egergizer. If qi fails to control blood with the manifestation as hypermenorrhea, add Xianhecao (*Herba Agrimoniae*) and Haipiaoxiao (*Os Sepiellae seu Sepiae*) to arrest bleeding. In case of turbid urine, add Qianshi (*Semen Eurgales*) and Yizhiren (*Fructus Alpiniae Oxyphyllae*) to arrest discharge of nutrient substances.

Elucidation: The syndrome results from qi deficiency of the spleen and stomach, causing yang's failure in ascent or even prolapse of middle-energizer qi. It should be treated by means of supplementing qi and lifting yang. The first ingredient, in larger dosage, reinforces qi of middle-energizer and lifts yang to strengthen the superficial resistance as monarch drug. Ingredients No. 3, No. 8 and No. 2 are used as minister drugs to replenish qi and strengthen the spleen, and combined with No. 1 to get better such effects. Ingredient No. 4 help No. 3 and No. 1 invigorate qi and nourish blood, and No. 5 can regulate qi and the stomach and make other drugs perform tonic action without stagnancy. Both serve as adjuvant drug. Ingredients No. 6 and No. 7, as guiding drug, bear the function of lifting collapsed middle-energizer qi.

Cautions: This recipe is contraindicated for cases concomitant with dampness and manifesting greasy fur and smooth pulse, or those with fever due to yin deficiency.

Yupingfeng San
(*Jade-screen Powder*)

Source: *Yifang Leiju* (*Classified Prescriptions*).

Ingredients:

No. 1 Fangfeng (*Radix Ledebouriellae*) 50 g;

No. 2 Zhihuangqi (*Radix Astragali seu Hedysari Praeparatae*) 100 g;

No. 3 Baizhu (*Rhizoma Atractylodis Macrocephalae*) 100 g.

草、海螵蛸以收敛止血;若小便混浊者,可加芡实、益智仁以固涩精微。

【方解】 本方证由脾胃气虚,清阳不升,甚则中气下陷所致,治宜补气升阳之法。方中重用黄芪补中益气,升阳固表,为君药。人参、白术、炙甘草益气健脾,与黄芪配伍则益气补中之效益佳,同为臣药。当归养血补虚,协人参、黄芪以补气养血;陈皮理气和胃,使诸药补而不滞,均为佐药。再配少量升麻、柴胡升阳举陷,与补气药合用以升提下陷之中气,为佐使药。

【注意事项】 若兼挟湿邪,苔腻脉滑者,以及阴虚发热者,禁用本方。

玉屏风散

【方源】 《究原方》,录自《医方类聚》。

【组成】 防风50 g,炙黄芪、白术各100 g。

Administration：Grind the above drugs into coarse powder, take 9 g each time for making decoction.

Actions：Replenishing qi, consolidating the superficies and arresting perspiration.

Clinical Application：This recipe is indicated for lowered superficial resistance due to deficiency, marked by perspiration with aversion to wind, pale complexion, or general debility subjective to pathogenic wind, pale tongue with whitish fur, superficial and feeble pulse. It is applicable to rhinallergosis, and upper respiratory tract infection, which pertain to syndrome of invasion by pathogenic wind due to lowered superficial resistance, as well as bronchial asthma, glomerulonephritis and other diseases, the recurrence of which is often induced by common cold. In case of polyhidrosis with aversion to wind, add Fuxiaomai (*Fructus Tritici Levis*), Duanmuli (*Concha Ostreae*) (calcined) and Mahuanggen (*Radix Ephedrae*) to enhance the effect of strengthening superficial resistance for arresting perspiration. In case of sneeze and nasal discharge, add Xinyi (*Flos Magnoliae*) and Cang'erzi (*Fructus Xanthii*) to relieve stuffy nose.

Elucidation：The syndrome arises when deficient wei-qi fails to consolidate body superficies. It should be treated by means of supplementing qi and consolidating the superficies to arrest perspiration. The second ingredient is good at replenishing qi and consolidating the superficies and used as monarch drug. The last ingredient, with the function of invigorating the spleen and supplementing qi, acts as minister drug to help bring about the effect of the monarch drug. The first ingredient can dispel wind and, when in compatibility with the rest two, build up body resistance and eliminate pathogenic factors as adjuvant drug. Combination of the three has the characteristics of reinforcing the superficies with pathogenic factors

【用法】　共研粗末,每次 9 g,水煎服。

【功用】　益气固表止汗。

【临床应用】　适用于表虚不固证。症见汗出恶风,面色㿠白,或体虚易感风邪,舌淡苔白,脉浮而虚。过敏性鼻炎、上呼吸道感染等属表虚不固而外感风邪者,以及支气管哮喘、肾小球肾炎等易因伤风感冒而诱致病情反复者,均可用本方治疗。若汗多恶风较著者,可加浮小麦、煅牡蛎、麻黄根以加强固表止汗之效;若打喷嚏流清涕者,可加辛夷、苍耳子以宣通鼻窍。

【方解】　本方证由卫气虚弱,不能固表所致,治宜益气固表止汗之法。方中黄芪长于益气固表止汗,为君药。白术健脾益气,加强黄芪益气固表之力,为臣药。防风疏风散邪,配黄芪、白术有扶正祛邪之功,为佐药。三药配伍,固表而不留邪,散邪而不伤正,表虚自汗者服之,有益气固表止汗之功;虚人易感风邪者服之,则有益气固表御风之效。

eliminated and eliminating pathogenic factors without impairing the body resistance. Therefore, it is good for patients with spontaneous perspiration because it replenishes qi, strengthens superficial resistance and arrests perspiration. As for those with general debility and apt to be attacked by wind, it can reinforce the body resistance to wind.

Cautions: It is contraindicated for spontaneous perspiration due to exogenous pathogenic factors, or night sweating due to yin deficiency, or general debility attacked by exogenous pathogenic factors.

Shengmai San
(*Pulse-activating Powder*)

Source: *Yixue Qiyuan* (*The Origin of Medicine*).

Ingredients:

No. 1 Renshen (*Radix Gingseng*) 9 g;

No. 2 Maimendong (*Radix Ophiopogonis*) 9 g;

No. 3 Wuweizi (*Fructus Schisandrae*) 6 g.

Administration: Decoct the drugs in water for oral application.

Actions: Benefiting qi and promoting the production of body fluid, astringing yin and arresting perspiration.

Clinical Application: This recipe is indicated for impairment of both qi and yin, marked by lassitude, polyhidrosis, shortness of breath, mental fatigue, dry throat and thirst, or protracted cough with little but sticky sputum, dry reddened tongue with little fur, feeble rapid pulse. It is applicable to chronic bronchitis, tuberculosis, cardiac arrhythmia and other diseases, which have such chief symptoms as lassitude, shortness of breath, dry throat, and reddened tongue, and pertain to deficiency of both qi and yin. The first ingredient in the recipe is sweet and warm in nature and could be replaced by Xiyangshen (*Radix Panacis Quinquefolii*) in cases of qi and yin

【注意事项】 外感自汗或阴虚盗汗,以及虚人外感邪多虚少者,禁用本方。

生脉散(又名生脉饮)

【方源】 《医学启源》。

【组成】 人参9 g,麦门冬9 g,五味子6 g。

【用法】 水煎服。

【功用】 益气生津,敛阴止汗。

【临床应用】 适用于气阴两伤证。症见体倦汗多,气短神疲,咽干口渴,或久咳不愈,痰少而粘,舌干红少苔,脉虚数。慢性支气管炎、肺结核、心脏病心律不齐等以体倦气短,咽干舌红为主症,属气阴两虚者,可用本方治疗。方中人参性味甘温,若属气阴不足,阴虚有热者,可用西洋参代替;病情急重者,全方剂量宜加重。本方制成的注射液

deficiency wiht heat. For critical cases the dosage of all the ingredients should be enlarged. Injection prepared on the basis of this recipe (Shengmai Injection) is commonly used to treat acute myocardiac infarction, cardiogenic shock, toxic shock, hemorrhagic shock, coronary heart disease and endocrinopathy, which pertain to deficiency of both qi and yin.

Elucidation: The syndrome results from impairment of yin by warm-heat and summer-heat, or impairment of qi and yin due to impairment of the lung by protracted cough. It should be treated by means of invigorating qi and nourishing yin, and concurrently arresting perspiration and relieving cough. The first ingredient acts as monarch drug to replenish qi and promote the production of body fluid for invigorating the lung. Ingredient No. 2 is used as minister drug to nourish yin and clear away heat for moistening the lung. The last ingredient can not only astringe yin and arrest perspiration, but also astringe the lung and relieve cough, acting as adjuvant drug. Respectively with tonic, moist and astringent effect, the three ingredients are together used to achieve the results of invigorating qi and nourishing yin, preserving yin to arrest perspiration, moistening the lung to stop cough, and promoting the production of body fluid to quench thirst.

Cautions: This recipe is contraindicated for cases with unsubdued heat or for those with cough and profuse sputum.

（生脉注射液）常用于治疗急性心肌梗死、心源性休克、中毒性休克、失血性休克以及冠心病、内分泌等疾病属气阴两虚证者。

【方解】 本方证由温热、暑热之邪耗伤气阴，或久咳伤肺，气阴不足所致，治宜益气养阴为主，兼以敛汗止咳。方中人参益气生津以补肺，为君药。麦门冬养阴清热以润肺，为臣药。五味子既可敛阴以止汗，又能敛肺以止咳，为佐药。三药配伍，一补一润一敛，共收益气养阴，敛阴止汗，润肺止咳，生津止渴之功。

【注意事项】 热邪未清或咳嗽痰多者，禁用本方。

2.6.2 Prescriptions for Nourishing Blood

Siwu Tang
（*Decoction of Four Ingredients*）

Source: *Xianshou Lishang Xuduan Mifang* (*Clandestine Prescriptions for Wounds and Bone-*

第二节 补血剂

四物汤

【方源】《仙授理伤续断秘方》。

setting Handed down by the Fairy).

Ingredients：

No. 1 Shudihuang (*Radix Rehmanniae Praeparatae*) 12 g;

No. 2 Danggui (*Radix Angelicae Sinensis*) 9 g;

No. 3 Baishaoyao (*Radix Paeoniae Alba*) 9 g;

No. 4 Chuanxiong (*Rhizoma Ligustici Chuanxiong*) 6 g.

Administration：Grind the drugs into coarse powder, decoct 9 g each time in water for oral application.

Actions：Nourishing and regulating blood.

Clinical Application：This recipe is indicated for syndrome of deficiency and stagnation of nutrient qi and blood, marked by palpitation, insomnia, dizziness, pale complexion, or menstrual disorder, scanty menstruation, or amenia with vague pain of the lower abdomen, pale tongue and thready pulse. It is applicable to menstrual disorder, chronic dermatosis, chronic eczema, urticaria, orthopedic and traumatic diseases, allergic purpura, and nervous headache and others, which pertain to deficiency and stagnation of nutrient qi and blood. If concomitant with deficiency of qi manifested as lassitude and shortness of breath, add Renshen (*Radix Gingseng*) and Huangqi (*Radix Astragali seu Hedysari*) to supplement qi for generating blood, which forms another recipe entitled Shengyu Tang. In case of dominant blood stasis manifested as sharp abdominal pain during menstruation, replace the third ingredient with Chishaoyao (*Radix Paeoniae Rubra*) and add Taoren (*Semen Perisicae*) and Honghua (*Flos Carthami*) to enhance the action of promoting blood circulation to remove blood stasis, which is known as Taohong Siwu Tang. In case of blood deficiency complicated with cold syndrome manifesting abdominal pain with preference for warmth, add Rougui (*Cortex Cinnamomi*), Paojiang (*Rhizoma Zingiberis Praeparatae*)

【组成】 熟地黄12 g,当归9 g,白芍药9 g,川芎6 g。

【用法】 上研粗末,每次9 g,水煎服。

【功用】 补血和血。

【临床应用】 适用于营血虚滞证。症见心悸失眠,头晕目眩,面色无华,或妇人月经不调,量少或经闭不行,脐腹隐痛,舌淡,脉细。妇女月经不调,慢性湿疹、荨麻疹等慢性皮肤病,骨伤科疾病,过敏性紫癜,神经性头痛等属营血虚滞者,均可用本方治疗。若兼气虚,神倦气短者,可加人参、黄芪以补气生血,即圣愈汤;若血瘀明显,经行腹痛较甚者,可将白芍药改为赤芍药,再加桃仁、红花以加强活血祛瘀之力,即桃红四物汤;若血虚有寒,腹痛喜温者,可加肉桂、炮姜、吴茱萸以温通血脉;若血虚有热,口干咽燥者,可将熟地黄改为生地黄,再加黄芩、牡丹皮以清热凉血。

and Wuzhuyu (*Fructus Evodiae*) to warm and dredge the vessels. In case of blood deficiency with heat syndrome manifesting dry mouth and throat, replace the first ingredient with Shengdihuang (*Radix Rehmanniae*) and add Huangqin (*Radix Scutellariae*) and Mudanpi (*Cortex Moutan Radixis*) to clear away heat and cool blood.

Elucidation: The syndrome results from deficiency of nutrient qi and blood, and obstructed blood circulation. It should be treated by nourishing and regulating blood. The first ingredient is capable of nourishing yin and blood and used as monarch drug. Ingredient No. 2 acts as minister drug with effects of nourishing blood and the liver and regulating menstruation. The last two ingredients function as adjuvant drug, the former nourishing blood and the liver and the latter promoting circulation of both qi and blood. Ingredients No. 1 and No. 3 are designed for nourishing blood, while No. 2 and No. 4 for nourishing and regulating blood. The compatibility of this recipe aims to nourish blood without inducing stasis, promote blood circulation without impairing it. Therefore they also have the function of regulating menstruation.

Cautions: This recipe is unfit for women with menstrual disorder manifesting stabbing abdominal pain due to blood stagnation, or qi exhaustion concomitant with metrorrhagia.

Danggui Buxue Tang
(*Chinese Angelica Decoction for Enriching Blood*)

Source: *Neiwaishang Bianhuo Lun* (*Differentiation on Endogenous and Exogenous Diseases*).

Ingredients:

No. 1 Huangqi (*Radix Astragali seu Hedysari*) 30 g;

No. 2 Danggui (*Radix Angelicae Sinensis*) 6 g.

Administration: Decoct the drugs in water for oral

【方解】 本方证由营血亏虚,血行不畅所致,治宜补血和血之法。方中熟地黄滋阴养血,为君药。当归补血养肝,和血调经,为臣药。白芍药养血柔肝和营,川芎活血行气,为佐药。方中熟地黄、白芍药专于滋补阴血,当归、川芎补中有行,四药配伍,补中有行,补血而不滞血,行血而不伤血,既有养血补虚之功,又具和血调经之效。

【注意事项】 妇女月经不调而瘀滞较甚,腹痛如刺,或血崩气脱者,不宜使用本方。

当归补血汤

【方源】 《内外伤辨惑论》。

【组成】 黄芪30 g,当归6 g。

【用法】 水煎服。

application.

Actions: Invigorating qi to promote blood generation.

Clinical Application: This recipe is indicated for syndrome of fever due to blood deficiency marked by feverish body and flushed face, polydipsia with desire for drink, large but weak pulse when pressed. It can be modified to treat menstrual and postpartum fever and headache, long and unhealed carbuncles and ulcers, anemia, allergic purpura and others, which pertain to deficiency of blood and qi.

Elucidation: The syndrome is caused by floating yang due to blood deficiency, and yin failing to keep yang well, which should be treated by replenishing qi and promoting blood production. Used as monarch drug, the first ingredient in larger dosage is capable of invigorating spleen and lung qi, enriching the source of blood and consolidating superficial resistance to astringe the floating yang. The second ingredient acts as minister drug with the effect of nourishing blood. The two ingredients promote generation of yang and growth of yin, abundance of qi and generation of blood. When they are taken by patients with fever due to blood deficiency, the abundance of ying blood may enrich yang. When they are taken by patients with blood and qi deficiency, the abundance of primordial qi ensures blood generation.

Cautions: This recipe is contraindicated for patients of yin deficiency with hectic fever.

2.6.3 Prescriptions for Nourishing both Qi and Blood

Bazhen Tang
(*Decoction of Eight Precious Ingredients*)

Source: *Zhengti Leiyao* (*Classification and*

【功用】 补气生血。

【临床应用】 适用于血虚发热证。症见肌热面赤,烦渴欲饮,脉洪大而重按无力。妇女经期、产后发热头痛、疮疡溃后久不收口、贫血、过敏性紫癜等属血虚气弱者,可用本方加减治疗。

【方解】 本方证由血虚阳浮,阴不维阳所致,治宜补气生血之法。方中重用黄芪大补脾肺之气,既可资生血之源,又能固表而挽回浮阳,为君药。当归养血和营,为臣药。两药配伍,可使阳生阴长,气旺血生。血虚发热者服之,则营血充以涵阳;血虚气弱者服之,则元气旺而血生。

【注意事项】 阴虚潮热者,禁用本方。

第三节 气血双补剂

八珍汤

【方源】 《正体类要》。

Treatment of Traumatic Diseases）.

Ingredients：

No. 1 Danggui（*Radix Angelicae Sinensis*）9 g；

No. 2 Chuanxiong（*Rhizoma Ligustici Chuanxiong*）6 g；

No. 3 Baishaoyao（*Radix Paeoniae Alba*）9 g；

No. 4 Shudihuang （ *Rhizoma Rehmanniae Praeparatae*）12 g；

No. 5 Renshen（*Radix Gingseng*）6 g；

No. 6 Baizhu（*Rhizoma Atractylodis Macrocephalae*）9 g；

No. 7 Fuling（*Poria*）6 g；

No. 8 Zhigancao（*Radix Glycyrrhizae Praeparatae*）3 g.

Administration：Add 2 slices of Shengjiang（*Rhizoma Zingiberis Recens*）and 3 pieces of Dazao（*Fructus Ziziphi Jujubae*）into the above ingredients and decoct all the drugs in water for oral application.

Actions：Invigorating qi and nourishing blood.

Clinical Application：This recipe is indicated for deficiency syndrome of both qi and blood, marked by pale or sallow complexion, dizziness, lassitude, shortness of breath, dislike for talking, poor appetite, pale tongue with thin whitish fur, thready and weak pulse. It can be modified to treat deficiency syndrome of qi and blood as seen after serious diseases or in various chronic diseases or menstrual disorder with chief manifestations as shortness of breath, weakness, dizziness, pale tongue and thready pulse. For severe cases, add Huangqi（*Radix Astragali seu Hedysari*）and Rougui（*Cortex Cinnamomi*）to enhance the effect of restoring qi and blood, namely Shiquan Dabu Tang. If concomitant with palpitation and insomnia due to deficient cultivation of cardiac spirit, add Fushen（*Sclerotium Poriae Circum Radicem Pini*）and Suanzaoren（*Semen Ziziphi Spinosae*）to tranquilize mind.

Elucidation：The syndrome is mostly caused by prolonged duration of disease, disorder after disease or

【组成】　当归9 g，川芎6 g，白芍药9 g，熟地黄12 g，人参6 g，白术9 g，茯苓6 g，炙甘草3 g。

【用法】　加生姜2片，大枣3枚，水煎服。

【功用】　益气补血。

【临床应用】　适用于气血两虚证。症见面色苍白或萎黄，头晕目眩，四肢倦怠，气短懒言，食欲不振，舌质淡，苔薄白，脉细弱。大病之后、各种慢性病以及妇女月经不调属气血不足，以气短乏力，头晕目眩，舌淡脉细为主症者，可用本方加减治疗。若气血虚弱较甚者，可加黄芪、肉桂以加强补益虚损之功，即十全大补汤；若兼心神失养，心悸失眠者，可加茯神、酸枣仁以宁心安神。

【方解】　本方证多由久病、病后失调或失血过多，气

excessive hemorrhage and insufficiency of qi and blood. It should be treated by means of nourishing qi and blood. Ingredients No. 5 and No. 4 are respectively to invigorate the primordial qi and blood and function as monarch drug. Ingredients No. 6, No. 7, No. 1 and No. 3 act as minister drug to help bring about the effect of the monarch drug. Ingredient No. 2 with the action of promoting the circulation of qi and blood is used as adjuvant drug. And the last ingredient serves as guiding drug to regulate the middle-energizer and mediate the properties of other drugs. Shengjiang (*Rhizoma Zingiberis Recens*) and Dazao (*Fructus Ziziphi Jujubae*) added while decocting the drugs are meant to supplement qi, regulate the spleen and stomach. This compatibility is actually the combination of two prescriptions, Sijunzi Tang and Siwu Tang, thus achieving the result of nourishing both qi and blood.

Guipi Tang
(*Decoction for strengthening the Heart and Spleen*)

Source: *Jisheng Fang* (*Prescriptions for Life Saving*).

Ingredients:

No. 1 Baizhu (*Rhizoma Atractylodis Macrocephalae*) 9 g;

No. 2 Fushen (*Sclerotium Poriae Circum Radicem Pini*) 9 g;

No. 3 Huangqi (*Radix Astragali seu Hedysari*) 12 g;

No. 4 Longyanrou (*Arillus Longan*) 12 g;

No. 5 Suanzaoren (*Semen Ziziphi Spinosae*) 12 g;

No. 6 Renshen (*Radix Ginseng*) 6 g;

No. 7 Muxiang (*Radix Aucklandiae*) 6 g;

No. 8 Zhigancao (*Radix Glycyrrhizae Praeparatae*) 3 g;

No. 9 Danggui (*Radix Angelicae Sinensis*) 9 g;

No. 10 Yuanzhi (*Radix Polygalae*) 6 g.

Administration: Grind the above drugs into fine

血不足所致,治宜益气补血之法。方中人参大补元气,熟地黄补血益精,共为君药。白术、茯苓助人参补气,当归、白芍药助熟地养血,同为臣药。川芎活血行气,使补而不滞,为佐药。炙甘草益气和中,调和药性,为使药。煎药加生姜、大枣调补脾胃,以资生化。诸药配伍,乃四君子汤与四物汤合方,故有气血双补之效。

归脾汤

【方源】 《济生方》。

【组成】 白术9 g,茯神9 g,黄芪12 g,龙眼肉12 g,酸枣仁12 g,人参6 g,木香6 g,炙甘草3 g,当归9 g,远志6 g。

【用法】 共研粗末,每次

powder, decoct 12 g each time with 6 g of Shengjiang (*Rhizoma Zingiberis Recens*) and 3 pieces of Dazao (*Fructus Ziziphi Jujubae*) in water for oral application.

Actions: Replenishing qi and nourishing blood, invigorating the spleen and heart.

Clinical Application: This recipe is indicated for deficiency syndrome of both qi and blood of the spleen and heart and syndrome of failure of the spleen to control blood, marked by palpitation or severe palpitation, amnesia, insomnia, poor appetite and lassitude, sallow complexion, or metrorrhagia, hemafecia, advanced menstruation in large amount and light color, or dribbling menstruation, pale tongue with thin whitish fur, thready and weak pulse. It is applicable to neurosis and angiocardiopathy which pertain to deficiency of both the spleen and heart, as well as gastroduodenal ulcer bleeding, dysfunctional uterine bleeding, thrombocytopenic purpura and others, which pertain to failure of the spleen to control blood. In case of excessive deficiency of blood, add Shudihuang (*Rhizoma Rehmanniae Praeparatae*) to enhance the function of nourishing blood, which is called Hei Guipi Wan when made into pills. If the bleeding syndrome belongs to cold type, add charcoals of Aiye (*Folium Artemisiae Argyi*) and Paojiang (*Rhizoma Zingiberis Praeparatae*) to warm the meridians for stopping bleeding. If the bleeding syndrome belongs to heat type, add charcoals of Shengdihuang (*Radix Rehmanniae*), Ejiao (*Colla Corii Asini*) and Zonglu (*Petiolus Trachycarpi*) to remove heat from the blood for arresting bleeding.

Elucidation: The syndrome is caused by impairment of the heart and spleen due to excessive contemplation, leading to deficiency of qi and blood and further giving rise to failure of the spleen in transportation and deficient cultivation of cardiac spirit. This should be treated by replenishing

12 g,加生姜6 g,大枣 3 枚,水煎服。

【功用】 益气补血,健脾养心。

【临床应用】 适用于心脾气血两虚证及脾不统血证。症见心悸怔忡,健忘失眠,食少体倦,面色萎黄,或妇女崩漏,便血,月经超前,量多色淡,或淋漓不止,舌质淡,苔薄白,脉细弱。神经衰弱、心血管系统疾病属心脾气血两虚者,以及胃及十二指肠溃疡出血、功能性子宫出血、血小板减少性紫癜等属脾不统血者,均可用本方治疗。若血虚较著者,可加熟地黄以加强滋补阴血之功,如制成丸剂名为黑归脾丸;若出血证偏寒者,可加艾叶炭、炮姜炭以温经止血;若出血证偏热者,可加生地黄炭、阿胶珠、棕榈炭以凉血止血。

【方解】 本方证由思虑过度,劳伤心脾,气血不足,脾失健运,心神失养所致,治宜益气补血,健脾养心之法。方中黄芪益气补脾,龙眼肉养血

qi and nourishing blood, and reinforcing the spleen and heart. Ingredient No. 3 can replenish qi and invigorate the spleen, and No. 4 nourish blood and tranquilize mind. Both play the role of monarch drug and can nourish qi and blood simultaneously. Ingredients No. 6, No. 1 and No. 9 function as minister drugs to help bring about the effect of monarch drugs. Ingredient No. 2, No. 5, No. 10 and No. 7 act as adjuvant drugs, of which the first three possess the action of tranquilizing mind and the last regulating qi and invigorating the spleen. Ingredient No. 8 is used as guiding drug to supplement qi, regulate the middle-energizer and mediate the properties of other drugs. Shengjiang (*Rhizoma Zingiberis Recens*) and Dazao (*Fructus Ziziphi Jujubae*) are meant to regulate the spleen and stomach.

Zhigancao Tang (Also Called Fumai Tang) (*Baked Licorice Decoction*)

Source: *Shanghan Lun* (*Treatise on Exogenous Febrile Diseases*).

Ingredients:

No. 1 Zhigancao (*Radix Glycyrrhizae Praeparatae*) 12 g;

No. 2 Shengjiang (*Rhizoma Zingiberis Recens*) 9 g;

No. 3 Renshen (*Radix Ginseng*) 6 g;

No. 4 Shengdihuang (*Radix Rehmanniae*) 30 g;

No. 5 Guizhi (*Ramulus Cinnamomi*) 9 g;

No. 6 Ejiao (*Colla Corii Asini*) 6 g;

No. 7 Maimendong (*Radix Ophiopogonis*) 10 g;

No. 8 Humaren (*Fructus Cannabis*) 10 g;

No. 9 Dazao (*Fructus Ziziphi Jujubae*) 10 pcs.

Administration: Mix and decoct all except ingredient No. 6; then add 10ml rice wine to the decoction with residue removed; stew No. 6 separately till it melts and divide it into two portions; mix one portion well with half decoction for oral application.

Actions: Replenishing qi to enrich blood, nourishing

安神,两药同用,气血并补,共为君药。人参、白术助黄芪补气;当归助龙眼肉养血,同为臣药。茯神、酸枣仁、远志宁心安神,木香理气醒脾,俱为佐药。炙甘草补气和中,调和药性,为使药。煎药时少加生姜、大枣调和脾胃,以资生化。

炙甘草汤(又名复脉汤)

【方源】 《伤寒论》。

【组成】 炙甘草12 g,生姜9 g,人参6 g,生地黄30 g,桂枝9 g,阿胶6 g,麦门冬10 g,胡麻仁10 g,大枣 10 枚。

【用法】 上药除阿胶外,其余各药混合煎煮,取汁倒出,加入清酒10 ml。另将阿胶炖化,分 2 次入药汁和匀服。

【功用】 益气养血,滋阴

yin to restore pulse.

Clinical Application: This recipe is indicated for palpitation or severe palpitation from deficiency of qi and blood, marked by intermittent pulse, lassitude, shortness of breath, dry reddened tongue with little fur; or deficiency of qi and yin due to protracted cough. It is applicable to coronary atherosclerotic cardiopathy, rheumatic heart disease, viral myocarditis, hyperthyroidism, functional arrhythmia and others, which manifest palpitation, shortness of breath, and intermittent pulse and pertain to deficiency of qi and blood. It can also be used to treat chronic bronchitis and protracted cough from tuberculosis, which pertain to impairment of both qi and yin. Clinically Shudihuang (*Radix Rehmanniae Praeparatae*) is often used. In case of severe palpitation, add Suanzaoren (*Semen Ziziphi Spinosae*) and Baiziren (*Semen Platycladi*) or Longchi (*Fossilia Dentis Mastodi*) and Cishi (*Magnetitum*) to tranquilize mind for arresting palpitation. For protracted cough due to deficiency of the lung, it is advisable to subtract No. 5 and No. 2 to prevent the impairment of body fluid by the warm and dry nature of the drugs. Instead, add Chuanbeimu (*Bulbus Fritillariae Cirhosae*) and Maimendong (*Radix Ophiopogonis*) to nourish the lung for arresting cough.

Elucidation: The syndrome is caused by yin-blood deficiency of the meridians and deficiency of yang-qi and blood. It should be treated by means of replenishing qi to nourish blood, nourishing yin to restore pulse. With larger dosages, ingredients No. 1 and No. 4 act as monarch drugs, one invigorating qi and heart and the other nourishing yin and blood. Used as minister drugs, ingredients No. 3 and No. 9 help No. 1 in supplementing qi, and No. 6, No. 7 and No. 8 assist No. 4 in nourishing blood. Ingredients No. 5 and No. 2 function as adjuvant drugs with the

复脉。

【临床应用】 适用于气血不足之心悸怔忡,脉结或代,体倦少气,舌红少苔而干;亦可治疗久咳肺虚,气阴不足。冠状动脉粥样硬化性心脏病、风湿性心脏病、病毒性心肌炎、甲状腺功能亢进、功能性心律不齐等见有心悸气短、脉结代属气虚血少者,以及慢性支气管炎、肺结核久咳不愈,属气阴两伤者,均可用本方治疗。方中生地黄,现临床多改用熟地黄。若心悸较甚者,可加酸枣仁、柏子仁或龙齿、磁石以加强安神定悸之功;若用于肺虚久咳,宜去桂枝、生姜以防温燥伤津,加川贝母、麦门冬以润肺止咳。

【方解】 本方证由阴血不足,血脉失于充盈,加之阳气虚弱,无力鼓动血脉所致,治宜益气养血,滋阴复脉之法。方中重用炙甘草益气补心,生地黄滋阴养血,共为君药。人参、大枣助炙甘草补气,阿胶、麦门冬、胡麻仁助生地黄养血,同为臣药。桂枝、生姜温心阳,通血脉,为佐药。

effects of warming the heart-yang and promoting blood flow. Besides the first ingredient also mediates the properties of other drugs and is used as guiding drug. All drugs in compatibility enrich the meridians with sufficient blood, restore pulse and relieve palpitation.

炙甘草调和药性,兼作使药。诸药配伍,使阴血足而血脉充,阳气旺而心脉通,则心悸自止,脉象可复。

2.6.4 Prescriptions for Nourishing Yin

Liuwei Dihuang Wan
(*Pill of Six Ingredients with Rehmanniae*)

Source: *Xiao'er Yaozheng Zhijue* (*Key to Therapeutics of Children's Diseases*).

Ingredients:

No. 1 Shudihuang (*Rhizoma Rehmanniae Praeparatae*) 24 g;

No. 2 Shanzhuyu (*Fructus Corni*) 12 g;

No. 3 Shanyao (*Rhizoma Dioscoreae*) 12 g;

No. 4 Zexie (*Rhizoma Alismatis*) 9 g;

No. 5 Mudanpi (*Cortex Moutan Radicis*) 9 g;

No. 6 Fuling (*Poria*) 9 g.

Administration: Grind the drugs into fine powder and mix with honey to make boluses; take 6 -9 g each time and three times daily with warm boiled water or light salty water. Or decoct the above drugs with dosages in proportion to the original recipe.

Actions: Nourishing yin and invigorating the kidney.

Clinical Application: This recipe is indicated for deficiency syndrome of kidney-yin, marked by soreness and weakness of the waist and knees, vertigo, tinnitus, deafness, night sweat, seminal emission, diabetes, steaming sensation in the bones, hectic fever, feverish sensation in the palms and soles, dry tongue and sore throat, gomphiasis, pain in heels, dribbling urination,

第四节 补阴剂

六味地黄丸

【方源】 《小儿药证直诀》。

【组成】 熟地黄24 g,山茱萸、山药各12 g,泽泻、牡丹皮、茯苓各9 g。

【用法】 共研细末,炼蜜为丸,每次 6~9 g,每日 3 次,温开水或淡盐汤送服。亦可作汤剂,用量按原方比例酌定。

【功用】 滋阴补肾。

【临床应用】 适用于肾阴虚证。症见腰膝酸软,头晕目眩,耳鸣耳聋,盗汗,遗精,消渴,骨蒸潮热,手足心热,舌燥咽痛,牙齿动摇,足跟作痛,小便淋漓,以及小儿囟门不合,舌红少苔,脉细数。慢性

persistent opening of fontanel, reddened tongue with little fur, thready and rapid pulse. It is applicable to chronic nephritis, hypertension, diabetes, tuberculosis, renal tuberculosis, hyperthyroidism, central retinitis, anovulatory dysfunctional uterine bleeding, menopausal syndrome and other diseases, which pertain to the syndromes of kidney-yin deficiency. In case of hyperactivity of fire due to yin deficiency, add Zhimu (*Rhizoma Anemarrhenae*) and Huangbai (*Cortex Phellodendri*) to enhance the action of clearing away heat, which constitute another recipe entitled Zhibai Dihuang Wan. If concomitant with deficiency of the liver-yin manifesting blurring of vision, add Gouqizi (*Fructus Lycii*) and Juhua (*Flos Chrysanthemi*) to nourish the liver, forming another recipe entitled Qiju Dihuang Wan. If concomitant with deficiency of the lung-yin manifesting cough and dyspnea, add Maimendong (*Radix Ophiopogonis*) and Wuweizi (*Fructus Schisandrae*) to preserve the lung-yin, forming another recipe entitled Maiwei Dihuang Wan.

Elucidation: The syndrome is caused by deficiency of kidney-yin and flaring up of deficiency fire. It should be treated by nourishing yin and invigorating the kidney. The first ingredient in larger dosage is the monarch drug, meant to enrich the kidney essence. Ingredients No. 2 and No. 3 act as minister drugs, the former bearing the functions of nourishing the liver and kidney and retaining kidney essence, and the latter reinforcing the spleen and kidney and consolidating kidney essence. Ingredient No. 4 can promote diuresis to eliminate dampness and prevent the first ingredient from generating dampness. Ingredient No. 5 possesses the functions of clearing away heat from the liver and inhibiting the warm property of No. 2. While the last ingredient, mild in its action of eliminating dampness from the spleen, helps No. 3 promote transportation

肾炎、高血压病、糖尿病、肺结核、肾结核、甲状腺功能亢进、中心性视网膜炎、无排卵性功能性子宫出血、更年期综合征等属肾阴亏虚为主者，可用本方治疗。若阴虚而火旺者，可加知母、黄柏以加强清热降火之功，即知柏地黄丸；若兼肝阴不足，视物模糊者，可加枸杞子、菊花以养肝明目，即杞菊地黄丸；若兼肺阴不足，咳嗽气喘者，可加麦门冬、五味子以滋阴敛肺，即麦味地黄丸。

【方解】　本方证由肾阴亏损，虚火上炎所致，治宜滋阴补肾之法。方中重用熟地黄滋阴补肾，填精益髓，为君药。山茱萸补养肝肾而涩精，山药补益脾肾而固精，俱为臣药。泽泻利湿泄浊，并防熟地黄之滋腻；牡丹皮清肝泄火，并制山茱萸之温；茯苓淡渗脾湿，以助山药之健运，均为佐药。诸药配伍，"三补"与"三泻"并用，以补益为主；肝脾肾三阴并补，以补肾阴为主，共成补通开合，补中寓泻，平补肾阴之剂。

and transformation of the spleen. These three ingredients play the role of adjuvant drug. The combination of all ingredients achieves "three tonic effects and three purgative effects", focusing on the former. With yin of the liver, spleen and kidney reinforced, this recipe is mainly aimed at nourishing the kidney-yin, thus forming the recipe for promoting opening and closing, reinforcement with purgation and reinforcing kidney-yin.

Zuogui Wan
(*Bolus for Tonifying Kidney-yin*)

Source: *Jingyue Quanshu* (*Complete Works of Zhang Jingyue*).

Ingredients:

No. 1 Shudihuang (*Rhizoma Rehmanniae Praeparatae*) 240 g;

No. 2 Shanyao (*Rhizoma Dioscoreae*) 120 g (baked);

No. 3 Gouqizi (*Fructus Lycii*) 120 g;

No. 4 Shanzhuyu (*Fructus Corni*) 120 g;

No. 5 Chuanniuxi (*Radix Cyathulae*) 90 g;

No. 6 Tusizi (*Semen Cuscutae*) 120 g;

No. 7 Lujiaojiao (*Colla Cornus Cervi*) 120 g (parched into pearls);

No. 8 Guibanjiao (*Colla Plastri Testudinis*) 120 g (parched into pearls).

Administration: Decoct the first ingredient into ointment, which is then mixed well with the fine powder of the rest and made into boluses by adding honey; take 9 g each time and twice daily with warm boiled water or with light salty water. Or prepare them into decoction with dosages in proportion to the original recipe.

Actions: Nourishing yin and reinforcing the kidney, replenishing essence to benefit the marrow.

Clinical Application: This recipe is indicated for syndrome of deficiency of genuine yin, marked by vertigo,

左归丸

【方源】 《景岳全书》。

【组成】 熟地黄240 g,炒山药120 g,枸杞子120 g,山茱萸120 g,川牛膝90 g,菟丝子120 g,鹿角胶(炒珠)120 g,龟版胶(炒珠)120 g。

【用法】 先将熟地黄煎煮成膏,余药共研细末,与膏和匀,加炼蜜为丸,每次9 g,温开水或淡盐汤送服,每日 2次。亦可作汤剂,用量按原方比例酌定。

【功用】 滋阴补肾,填精益髓。

【临床应用】 适用于真阴不足证。症见头晕目眩,腰

soreness of the waist and knees, seminal emission or spermatorrhea, night sweat, spontaneous perspiration, dry mouth and tongue, reddened tongue with little fur, thready pulse. It is applicable to chronic nephritis, hypertension, infertility, osteoporosis, diabetes and others, which pertain to the syndrome of deficiency of genuine yin. In case of upward flaming of fire, subtract No. 3 and No. 7 and add Nüzhenzi (*Fructus Ligustri Lucidi*) and Maimendong (*Radix Ophiopogonis*) to nourish yin and clear away heat. In case of steaming sensation in bones and hectic fever, add Digupi (*Cortex Lycii Radicis*) to clear away heat of deficiency type. In case of dry stool, subtract No. 6 and add Roucongrong (*Herba Cistanchis*) instead to moisten the intestine for relieving constipation.

Elucidation: The syndrome results from deficiency of kidney-yin, consumption of essence and marrow. It should be treated by nourishing kidney-yin to replenish essence and supplement marrow. With a larger dosage, the first ingredient is meant to replenish kidney essence and used as monarch drug. Acting as minister drug, ingredients No. 4 and No. 3 invigorate the liver and kidney, and preserve essence and improve eyesight. Ingredients No. 7 and No. 8 are miracle drugs for replenishing essence and marrow. Besides, No. 7 is capable of invigorating the kidney-yang and, when in compatibility with drugs for nourishing yin, enhancing such effect. This is known as "treating yin within yang". Ingredient No. 2 possesses the actions of reinforcing the spleen and kidney and consolidating essence, No. 6 invigorating the kidney and liver and improving eyesight, and No. 5 invigorating the liver and kidney and strengthening the waist and knees. The above five ingredients play the role of adjuvant drugs. All ingredients together greatly reinforce genuine yin and kidney essence without any purgative effect.

膝酸软,遗精滑泄,自汗盗汗,口燥舌干,舌红少苔,脉细。慢性肾炎、高血压病、不育症、骨质疏松症、糖尿病等属真阴不足者,可用本方治疗。若真阴不足,虚火上炎者,可去枸杞子、鹿角胶,加女贞子、麦门冬以养阴清热;若潮热骨蒸者,可加地骨皮以清虚热,退骨蒸;若大便燥结者,可去菟丝子,加肉苁蓉以润肠通便。

【方解】 本方证由肾阴不足,精髓亏损所致,治宜滋补肾阴,填精益髓之法。方中重用熟地黄滋肾益精以填真阴,为君药。山茱萸、枸杞子滋养肝肾,涩精明目,同为臣药。龟、鹿两胶,为血肉有情之品,峻补精髓,鹿角胶又可补肾壮阳,与滋阴药配伍可加强补阴作用,即"阳中求阴"之意;山药补脾益阴,滋肾固精;菟丝子补肾固精,养肝明目;川牛膝补肝肾,强腰膝,均为佐药。诸药纯补无泻,为大补真阴,填精益髓之剂。

Cautions: This recipe should not be used frequently or constantly because the ingredients are likely to generate dampness.

Dabuyin Wan
(*Pill for Replenishing Yin*)

Source: *Danxi Xinfa* (*Danxi's Experiential Therapy*).

Ingredients:

No. 1 Shudihuang (*Rhizoma Rehmanniae Praeparatae*) 180 g;

No. 2 Zhiguiban (*Plastrum Testudinis Praeparatae*) 180 g;

No. 3 Huangbai (*Cortex Phellodendri*) 120 g (parched);

No. 4 Zhimu (*Rhizoma Anemarrhenae*) 120 g (parched).

Administration: Grind the above drugs into fine powder, then mix the powder with steamed pork spinal cord and honey to make boluses; take 9 g each time and twice daily with warm boiled water or with light salty water. Or prepare them into decoction with dosages in proportion to the original recipe.

Actions: Nourishing yin and purging fire.

Clinical Application: This recipe is indicated for syndrome of hyperactivity of fire due to yin deficiency marked by steaming sensation in bones, hectic fever, night sweat, seminal emission, cough, hemoptysis, vexation, irritability, feverish and sore knees and feet, reddened tongue with little fur, rapid and forceful chi pulse. It is applicable to hyperthyroidism, tuberculosis, renal tuberculosis, bone tuberculosis, diabetes and others attributable to hyperactivity of fire due to yin deficiency. In case of deficiency of the lung-yin with cough, add Tianmendong (*Radix Asparagi*) and Maimendong (*Radix Ophiopogonis*) to nourish yin by moistening pathogenic dryness. In case of severe hemoptysis and hematemesis,

【注意事项】 本方药性偏于滋腻,脾虚、气滞、湿热者不宜。

大补阴丸

【方源】《丹溪心法》。

【组成】 熟地黄、炙龟版各180 g,炒黄柏、炒知母各120 g。

【用法】 共研细末,将猪脊髓蒸熟,炼蜜为丸,每次9 g,温开水或淡盐汤送下,每日2次。亦可作汤剂,用量按原方比例酌定。

【功用】 滋阴降火。

【临床应用】 适用于阴虚火旺证。症见骨蒸潮热,盗汗遗精,咳嗽咯血,心烦易怒,足膝疼热,舌红少苔,尺脉数而有力。甲状腺功能亢进、肺结核、肾结核、骨结核、糖尿病等属阴虚火旺者,可用本方治疗。若肺阴虚干咳较著者,可加天门冬、麦门冬以润燥养阴;若咯血、吐血较甚者,可加仙鹤草、白茅根以凉血止血;若阴虚火旺,盗汗较重者,可加地骨皮、煅牡蛎以清退虚

add Xianhecao (*Herba Agrimoniae*) and Baimaogen (*Rhizoma Imperatae*) to arrest bleeding by removing heat from the blood. In case of severe night sweat caused by hyperactivity of fire due to yin deficiency, add Digupi (*Cortex Lycii Radicis*) and Duanmuli (*Concha Ostreae*) (calcined) to dispel fire of deficiency type and strengthen the superficial resistance for stopping sweating. In case of severe seminal emission, add Jinyingzi (*Fructus Rosne Laevigatae*) and Sangpiaoxiao (*Ootheca Mantidis*) to consolidate kidney essence for arresting emission.

Elucidation: The syndrome is caused by upward flaming of deficiency fire due to yin deficiency of the liver and kidney, which should be treated by nourishing yin and purging fire. The first two ingredients act as monarch drug to nourish yin and suppress yang. While the last two, cold in nature and bitter in flavor, are used as minister drug to purge away heat and preserve yin. Pork spinal cord and honey are sweet and moist in nature and used as adjuvant drug, which can help the monarch drug in replenishing essence and inhibit the bitter and dry nature of Ingredient No. 3.

Huqian Wan
(*Huqian Pill*)

Source: *Danxi Xinfa* (*Danxi's Experiential Therapy*).

Ingredients:

No. 1 Huangbai (*Cortex Phellodendri*) 150 g;

No. 2 Zhiguiban (*Plastsum Testudinis Praeparatae*) 120 g;

No. 3 Chaozhimu (*Rhizoma Anemarrhenae*) 60 g (baked);

No. 4 Shudihuang (*Rhizoma Rehmaniae Praeparatae*) 60 g;

No. 5 Chenpi (*Pericarpium Citri Reticulatae*) 60 g;

火,固表止汗;若遗精较甚者,可加金樱子、桑螵蛸以固精止遗。

【方解】　本方证由肝肾阴虚,虚火上炎所致,治宜滋阴降火之法。方中熟地黄、龟版滋阴潜阳,壮水制火,共为君药。黄柏、知母苦寒清热,降火保阴,同为臣药。以猪脊髓加蜂蜜为丸,取其甘润滋养,既能助君药滋补精髓,又能制黄柏之苦燥,为佐使药。

虎潜丸

【方源】《丹溪心法》。

【组成】　黄柏150 g,炙龟版120 g,炒知母、熟地黄、陈皮、白芍药各60 g,锁阳45 g,炙豹骨(原为虎骨)50 g,干姜15 g。

No. 6 Baishaoyao (*Radix Paeoniae Alba*) 60 g;

No. 7 Suoyang (*Herba Cynomorii*) 45 g;

No. 8 Zhibaogu (*Os Pardi Praeparatae*) 50 g (originally Os Tigris);

No. 9 Ganjiang (*Rhizoma Zingiberis*) 15 g.

Administration: Grind the above drugs into fine powder and make into boluses by mixing up with honey; take 9 g each time and twice daily with light salty water or with warm boiled water. Or prepare them into decoction with dosages in proportion to the original recipe.

Actions: Nourishing yin and purging fire, strengthening tendons and bones.

Clinical Application: This recipe is indicated for flaccidity syndrome, marked by soreness and weakness of the waist and knees, flaccid tendons and bones, emaciated legs and feet, weary walking, reddened tongue with little fur, thready and weak pulse. It is applicable to tuberculosis of knee joint, myodystrophy, peripheral palsy, poliomyelitis sequel and others, which manifest chiefly flaccidity of the lower limbs. The effect of reinforcing tendons and bones will be enhanced if Danggui (*Radix Angelicae Sinensis*), Niuxi (*Radix Achyranthis Bidentatae*) and mutton are added to this recipe.

Elucidation: The syndrome is caused by deficiency of essence and blood in the liver and kidney, causing interior heat and yin deficiency, and lack of nourishment in tendons and bones. It should be treated by nourishing yin and purging fire, and strengthening tendons and bones. The second ingredient is capable of nourishing kidney-yin and essence, and the first ingredient with bitter and cold nature clearing away heat and purging fire to preserve yin. Both function as monarch drugs with the effects of nourishing yin and purging away fire. Ingredient No. 4 and No. 6 bear the function of nourishing yin and blood and

【用法】 共研细末,炼蜜为丸,每次9 g,淡盐汤或温开水送下,每日 2 次。亦可作汤剂,用量按原方比例酌定。

【功用】 滋阴降火,强壮筋骨。

【临床应用】 适用于痿证。症见腰膝酸软,筋骨痿弱,腿足消瘦,步履乏力,舌红少苔,脉细弱。膝关节结核、肌营养不良症、周期性麻痹、小儿麻痹后遗症等见下肢痿软无力属肝肾阴虚有热者,可用本方治疗。若再加当归、牛膝、羊肉同用,则滋补强筋壮骨之功更为显著。

【方解】 本方证由肝肾精血不足,阴虚内热,不能濡养筋骨所致,治宜滋阴降火,强壮筋骨之法。方中龟版滋阴补肾,填精益髓;黄柏苦寒清热,降火保阴。两药配伍,滋阴降火,共为君药。熟地黄、白芍药滋阴养血,知母滋阴清热,助君药滋阴降火之力,同为臣药。豹骨强壮筋骨,锁阳温阳益精,干姜、陈皮

No. 3 nourishing yin and clearing away heat, all acting as minister drugs. Ingredient No. 8 has the effect of strengthening the tendons and bones, and No. 7 warming yang and replenishing essence; Ingredients No. 9 and No. 5, with the effect of warming the middle-energizer and regulating the stomach, can protect the stomach from impairment by the bitter and cold nature of No. 1 and No. 3, and prevent yin-nourishing tonics from inducing dampness and causing stagnation, all of these four drugs playing the role of adjuvant drug.

Cautions: This recipe is contraindicated in flaccidity of the lower limbs due to dampness or attack by exogenous pathogenic factors.

温中和胃,既可防黄柏、知母苦寒败胃,又可使阴柔之品滋而不腻,补而不滞,俱为佐药。

【注意事项】　下肢痿软因湿热浸淫或感受外邪而致者,禁用本方。

Yiguan Jian
(*Decoction for Nourishing the Liver and Kidney*)

一贯煎

Source: *Xu Mingyi Lei'an* (*Supplement to the Classified Medical Records of Celebrated Physicians*).

【方源】　《续名医类案》。

Ingredients:

No. 1 Beishashen (*Radix Glehniae*) 9 g;

No. 2 Maimendong (*Radix Ophiopogonis*) 9 g;

No. 3 Danggui (*Radix Angelicae Sinensis*) 9 g;

No. 4 Shengdihuang (*Radix Rehmanniae*) 18 - 30 g;

No. 5 Gouqizi (*Fructus Lycii*) 9 - 18 g;

No. 6 Chuanlianzi (*Fructus Mediae Toosendan*) 5 g.

【组成】　北沙参、麦门冬、当归各9 g,生地黄 18～30 g,枸杞子 9～18 g,川楝子 5 g。

Administration: Decoct the above drugs in water for oral application.

【用法】　水煎服。

Actions: Nourishing yin and dispersing stagnated liver-qi.

【功用】　滋阴疏肝。

Clinical Application: This recipe is indicated for syndrome of stagnation of liver-qi due to yin deficiency, marked by chest, epigastric and hypochondriac pain, acid regurgitation, dry throat and mouth, reddened tongue with little saliva, thready and taut pulse. It is applicable

【临床应用】　适用于阴虚肝郁证。症见胸脘胁痛,吞酸吐苦,咽干口燥,舌红少津,脉细弦。慢性肝炎、慢性胃炎、胃及十二指肠溃疡、肋间

to chronic hepatitis, chronic gastritis, gastroduodenal ulcer, intercostal neuralgia, neurosis and other diseases, which chiefly manifest pain of the chest, epigastrium, hypochondrium and costae attributable to stagnation of qi due to yin deficiency. In case of severe hypochondriac pain, add Yanhusuo (*Rhizoma Corydalis*) and Xiangfu (*Rhizoma Cyperi*) to enhance the effect of dispersing stagnated liver-qi. In case of severe epigastric pain, add Baishaoyao (*Radix Paeoniae Alba*) and Gancao (*Radix Glycyrrhizae*) to relieve pain. In case of hypochondriac and costal distention with abdominal mass, add Biejia (*Carapax Trionycis*) to moisten and remove mass. If concomitant with disorder of the stomach-qi manifesting nausea and vomiting, add Sharen (*Fructus Amomi*) and Banxia (*Rhizoma Pinelliae*) (decocted in ginger decoction) to regulate the stomach and descend the stomach-qi.

Elucidation: The syndrome is caused by yin deficiency of the liver and kidney, unsmooth flow of the liver-qi, causing qi stagnation, and invadion of the stomach by stagnant live-qi. It should be treated by nourishing yin and dispersing stagnated liver-qi. Ingredient No. 4 in larger dosage is meant to nourish yin and blood so as to invigorate the liver and kidney and used as monarch drug. Ingredients No. 1, No. 2, No. 3 and No. 5 act as minister drug to help bring about the effect of the monarch drug. The last ingredient, which serves as adjuvant drug, is aimed at dispersing stagnated liver-qi and purging heat, promoting the flow of qi and relieving pain so that liver-qi can spread out freely.

Cautions: This recipe is contraindicated for cases concomitant with phlegm-dampness manifesting greasy and whitish fur.

Baihe Gujin Tang
(*Lily Decoction for Strengthening the Lung*)
Source: *Shenzhai Yishu*

神经痛、神经官能症等以胸脘胁肋诸痛为主症,属阴虚气滞者,可用本方治疗。若胁痛较甚者,可再加延胡索、香附以加强疏肝解郁作用;若胃脘疼痛明显者,可加白芍药、甘草以缓急止痛;若胁肋胀痛并有痞块者,可加鳖甲以软坚散结;若兼胃气不和,恶心呕吐者,可加砂仁、姜半夏以和胃降逆。

【方解】　本方证由肝肾阴虚,肝失所养,以致疏泄失常,气郁而滞,进而横逆犯胃所致,治宜滋阴疏肝之法。方中重用生地黄滋阴养血,补益肝肾,为君药。北沙参、麦门冬、当归、枸杞子助君药滋阴养血柔肝,同为臣药。少加川楝子疏肝泄热,行气止痛,遂顺肝木条达之性,为佐药。

【注意事项】　若兼挟痰湿,舌苔白腻者,禁用本方。

百合固金汤

【方源】《慎斋遗书》。

Ingredients：

No. 1 Baihe (*Bulbus Lilii*) 12 g；

No. 2 Shudihuang (*Rhizoma Rehmanniae Praeparatae*) 9 g；

No. 3 Shengdihuang (*Rhizoma Rehmanniae*) 9 g；

No. 4 Danggui (*Radix Angelicae Sinensis*) 9 g；

No. 5 Baishaoyao (*Radix Paeoniae Alba*) 6 g；

No. 6 Gancao (*Radix Glycyrrhizae*) 3 g；

No. 7 Jiegeng (*Radix Platycodi*) 6 g；

No. 8 Xuanshen (*Radix Scrophulariae*) 3 g；

No. 9 Chuanbeimu (*Bulbus Fritillariae Cirhosae*) 6 g；

No. 10 Maimendong (*Radix Ophiopogonis*) 9 g.

Administration：Decoct the above drugs in water for oral application.

Actions：Reinforcing the lung and kidney, relieving cough and resolving sputum.

Clinical Application：This recipe is indicated for syndrome of yin deficiency of the lung and kidney marked by cough, dyspnea, hemoptysis, dry and painful throat, vertigo, dysphoria with feverish sensation in chest, palms and soles especially in the afternoon, reddened tongue with little fur, thready and rapid pulse. It is applicable to tuberculosis, chronic bronchitis, bronchiectasic hemoptysis, chronic laryngopharyngitis, spontaneous pneumothorax and others, which pertain to yin deficiency of the lung and kidney. In case of profuse yellowish sputum, add Danxing (*Arisaema cum Bile*), Huangqin (*Radix Scutellariae*) and Gualoupi (*Pericarpium Trichosanthis*) to clear away heat from the lung for reducing sputum. In case of severe dyspnea, add Xingren (*Semen Armeniacae Amarum*), Wuweizi (*Fructus Schisandrae*) and Kuandonghua (*Flos Farfarae*) to relieve cough and dyspnea. In case of severe hemoptysis, subtract No. 7 or add Baiji (*Rhizoma Bletillae*), Baimaogen (*Rhizoma*

【组成】 百合12 g,熟地黄、生地黄、当归各9 g,白芍药6 g,甘草3 g,桔梗6 g,玄参3 g,川贝母6 g,麦门冬9 g。

【用法】 水煎服。

【功用】 滋补肺肾,止咳化痰。

【临床应用】 适用于肺肾阴亏证。症见咳嗽气喘,咳痰带血,咽喉燥痛,头晕目眩,五心烦热,午后尤甚,舌红少苔,脉细数。肺结核、慢性支气管炎、支气管扩张咯血、慢性咽喉炎、自发性气胸等属肺肾阴虚者,可用本方治疗。若痰多而色黄者,加胆星、黄芩、瓜蒌皮以清肺化痰;若咳喘甚者,可加杏仁、五味子、款冬花以止咳平喘;若咳血重者,可去桔梗之升提,或加白及、白茅根、仙鹤草以增止血之功。

Imperatae) and Xianhecao (*Herba Agrimoniae*) to enhance the effect of arresting bleeding.

Elucidation: The syndrome is caused by yin deficiency of the lung and kidney, the flaring up of deficiency fire, impairment of the lung collateral and failure of the lung to disperse and descend. It should be treated by invigorating the lung and kidney to relieve cough and reduce sputum. The first ingredient is capable of nourishing the lung-yin and promoting production of body fluid so as to relieve cough; Ingredients No. 2 and No. 3 can nourish the kidney-yin and remove heat from the blood. These three ingredients are monarch drugs in the recipe. The last ingredient helps the first one in nourishing the lung-yin and clearing away heat, and No. 8 assists No. 2 and No. 3 in nourishing kidney yin and cooling blood to stop bleeding. Both act as minister drugs. Functioning as adjuvant drugs, ingredients No. 4 and No. 5 can nourish yin and blood, No. 9 moisten the lung and resolve phlegm, and No. 7 is good for throat and can guide other drugs upward. Ingredient No. 6 purges fire and mediates the properties of other drugs and serves as guiding drug.

【方解】 本方证由肺肾阴亏,虚火上炎,灼伤肺络,肺失清肃所致,治宜滋补肺肾,止咳化痰之法。方中百合养阴润肺,生津止咳;生地黄、熟地黄滋阴补肾,清热凉血,共为君药。麦门冬协百合以滋阴清热,润肺止咳;玄参助二地滋阴壮水,凉血止血,同为臣药。当归、白芍药滋阴养血和血,贝母润肺化痰止咳,桔梗利咽化痰,载药上行,俱为佐药。生甘草清热泻火,调和药性,为使药。

2.6.5 Prescriptions for Nourishing Yang

Shenqi Wan
(*Pill for Invigorating Kidney Qi*)

Source: *Jingui Yaolue (Synopsis of Prescriptions of the Golden Cabinet)*.

Ingredients:

No. 1 Shengdihuang (*Radix Rehmanniae*) 240 g;

No. 2 Shanyao (*Rhizoma Dioscoreae*) 120 g;

No. 3 Shanzhuyu (*Fructus Corni*) 120 g;

No. 4 Zexie (*Rhizoma Alismatis*) 90 g;

No. 5 Fuling (*Poria*) 90 g;

第五节　补阳剂

肾气丸

【方源】 《金匮要略》。

【组成】 生地黄240 g,山药、山茱萸各120 g,泽泻、茯苓、牡丹皮各90 g,桂枝、附子各30 g。

No. 6 Mudanpi (*Cortex Moutan Radicis*) 90 g;

No. 7 Guizhi (*Ramulus Cinnamomi*) 30 g;

No. 8 Fuzi (*Radix Aconiti*) 30 g.

Administration: Grind the above drugs into fine powder and mix up with honey to make pills; take 6 g each time and twice daily with warm boiled water or light salty water. Or prepare them into decoction with dosages in proportion to the original recipe.

Actions: Warming and invigorating kidney-yang.

Clinical Application: This recipe is indicated for syndrome of deficiency of kidney-yang marked by soreness and weakness of the waist and knees, cold feeling in the lower body, contracture of the lower abdomen, dysuria or polyuria, pale and large tongue, feeble pulse with deep and faint chi pulse, as well as phlegm-retention, edema, diabetes, beriberi and dysuria with lower abdominal colic. It is applicable to chronic nephritis, nephrogenic edema, diabetes, hypothyroidism, neurosis, hypoadrenocorticism, recurrence of bronchial asthma, menopausal syndrome and others, which pertain to deficiency of kidney-yang. Presently the prepared form of the first ingredient is often used clinically. Ingredient No. 7 may be replaced with Rougui (*Cortex Cinnamomi*), aiming to enhance the effect of warming yang. In case of severe edema, add Cheqianzi (*Semen Plantaginis*) and Niuxi (*Radix Achyranthis Bidentatae*) to promote diuresis and relieve edema, forming another recipe entitled Jiawei Shenqi Wan. If concomitant with sexual impotence, add Yinyanghuo (*Herba Epimedii*), Buguzhi (*Furctus Psoraleae*) and Bajitian (*Radix Morindae Officinalis*) to strengthen kidney-yang.

Elucidation: The syndrome is caused by deficiency of kidney-yang, which fails to activate qi to promote diuresis. It should be treated by warming and invigorating

【用法】 共研细末,炼蜜为丸,每次6 g,温开水或淡盐汤送下,每日2次。亦可作汤剂,用量按原方比例酌定。

【功用】 温补肾阳。

【临床应用】 适用于肾阳不足证。症见腰膝酸软,下半身常有冷感,少腹拘急,小便不利,或小便反多,舌淡而胖,脉虚弱,尺部沉细,以及痰饮、水肿、消渴、脚气、转胞等。慢性肾炎、肾性水肿、糖尿病、甲状腺功能低下、神经衰弱、肾上腺皮质功能减退、支气管哮喘反复发作、更年期综合征等属肾阳不足者,可用本方治疗。方中干地黄,现临床多改用熟地黄。若欲增强温阳之力,可将桂枝改为肉桂;若水肿明显者,可加车前子、牛膝以助利水消肿之效,即加味肾气丸;若兼阳痿者,可加淫羊藿、补骨脂、巴戟天以增壮阳起痿之功。

【方解】 本方证由肾阳不足,不能化气行水所致,治宜温补肾阳之法。方中附子、

kidney-yang. Ingredients No. 8 and No. 7 are monarch drugs with the effects of warming and invigorating kidney-yang. The first three ingredients function as minister drugs to nourish kidney-yin. The combination of monarch and minister drugs is meant to warm kidney-yang while nourishing kidney-yin so as to enhance the former's effect. Since the recipe consists of less ingredients for invigorating yang than those for nourishing yin, it can slightly generate fire so as to activate kidney-qi. Used as adjuvant drugs, ingredients No. 4, No. 5 and No. 6 can promote diuresis and blood circulation on the one hand, and prevent tonics from generating dampness on the other. The combined application of all ingredients, which are warm but not dry and tonic but not induce dampness, activates kidney-yang and healthy qi so that all symptoms are relieved.

Cautions: This recipe is contraindicated for patients with dry throat and mouth, reddened tongue and little fur.

Yougui Wan
(Pill for Reinforcing Kidney-yang)

Source: *Jingyue Quanshu* (*Complete Works of Zhang Jingyue*).

Ingredients:

No. 1 Shudihuang (*Rhizoma Rehmanniae Praeparatae*) 240 g;

No. 2 Chaoshanyao (*Rhizoma Dioscoreae Praeparatae*) 120 g;

No. 3 Shanzhuyu (*Fructus Corni*) 90 g;

No. 4 Gouqizi (*Fructus Lycii*) 120 g;

No. 5 Tusizi (*Semen Cuscutae*) 120 g;

No. 6 Lujiaojiao (*Colla Cornus Cervi*) (parched into pearls) 120 g;

No. 7 Duzhong (*Cortex Eucommiae*) 120 g;

桂枝温补肾阳,共为君药。生地黄、山茱萸、山药滋补肾阴,同为臣药。君臣相合,意在阴中求阳,以加强补阳之效,且补阳药少而滋阴药多,具有微微生火,以鼓舞肾气之功。泽泻、茯苓、牡丹皮渗湿利水活血,并防补药之滋腻,俱为佐药。诸药合用,温而不燥,滋而不腻,使肾阳振奋,气化复常,诸症自除。

【注意事项】 咽干口燥,舌红少苔者,禁用本方。

右归丸

【方源】《景岳全书》。

【组成】 熟地黄240 g,炒山药120 g,山茱萸90 g,枸杞子、菟丝子、鹿角胶(炒珠)、杜仲各120 g, 当归90 g,肉桂60 g,制附子60 g。

No. 8 Danggui（*Radix Angelicae Sinensis*）90 g;

No. 9 Rougui（*Cortex Cinnamomi*）60 g;

No. 10 Zhifuzi（*Radix Aconiti Praeparatae*）60 g.

Administration：Make the first ingredient into paste after steamed and grind the rest into fine powder; then make the powder into boluses by mixing it with honey; take 9 g each time and twice daily with warm boiled water or with light salty water. Or make into decoction with dosages in proportion to the original recipe.

Actions：Warming and enriching kidney-yang, and replenishing essence and marrow.

Clinical Application：This recipe is indicated for syndrome of insufficient kidney-yang and decline of fire in mingmen, marked by qi deficiency and mental fatigue from senility or protracted diseases, aversion to cold and cold limbs, soreness and weakness of the waist and knees, or infertility due to yang deficiency, pale tongue with whitish fur, deep and slow pulse. It is applicable to nephrotic syndrome, senile osteoporosis, infertility from spermacrasia, anemia, leukopenia and others, which belong to kidney-yang deficiency. If concomitant with seminal emission, add Buguzhi（*Fructus Psoraleae*）and Yizhiren（*Fructus Alpiniae Oxyphyllae*）to consolidate the kidney and prevent emission. In case of sexual impotence, add Bajitian（*Radix Morindae Officinalis*）and Yinyanghuo（*Herba Epimedii*）to activate kidney-yang. In case of mental fatigue due to qi deficiency, add Renshen（*Radix Ginseng*）to reinforce the primordial qi. If concomitant with poor appetite and loose stool due to deficiency of the spleen and stomach, add Ganjiang（*Rhizoma Zingiberis*）and Baizhu（*Rhizoma Atractylodis Macrocephalae*）to warm the middle-energizer and improve the function of the spleen.

Elucidation：The syndrome is caused by kidney-

【用法】　将熟地黄蒸烂杵膏，余研细末，炼蜜为丸，每次9 g，温开水或淡盐汤送服，每日 2 次。亦可作汤剂，用量按原方比例酌定。

【功用】　温补肾阳，填精益髓。

【临床应用】　适用于肾阳不足，命门火衰证。症见年老或久病气衰神疲，畏寒肢冷，腰膝酸软，或阳衰无子，舌淡苔白，脉沉而迟。肾病综合征、老年骨质疏松症、精少不育症、贫血、白细胞减少症等属肾阳不足者，可用本方治疗。若兼肾虚遗精者，可加补骨脂、益智仁以固肾涩精止遗；若兼阳痿者，可加巴戟天、淫羊藿以补肾壮阳起痿；若气虚神疲明显者，可加人参以大补元气；若兼脾胃虚弱，食少便溏者，可加干姜、白术以温中健脾助运。

【方解】　本方证由肾阳

yang deficiency and decline of fire in mingmen, and should be treated by warming and activating kidney-yang and replenishing kidney essence. Ingredients No. 10, No. 9 and No. 6 can greatly invigorate kidney-yang and function as monarch drugs. Ingredients No. 1, No. 3, No. 4 and No. 2 act as minister drugs, which nourish kidney-yin, reinforce the liver and spleen, and replenish kidney essence. Used as adjuvant drugs, ingredients No. 5 and No. 7 bear the effects of invigorating kidney-yang and strengthening waist and knees, while No. 8 has the function of nourishing and regulating blood. All in compatibility achieves tonic effect without any purgative effect, and activates kidney-yang while nourishing kidney-yin. This recipe possesses a drastic effect of activating kidney-yang and replenishing kidney essence.

Cautions: This recipe is very likely to generate dampness, and therefore should not be used by patients with kidney deficiency and dampness.

不足,命门火衰所致,治宜温补肾阳,填精益髓之法。方中附子、肉桂、鹿角胶大补肾中元阳,共为君药。熟地黄、山茱萸、枸杞子、山药滋阴益肾,养肝补脾,填精补髓,同为臣药。菟丝子、杜仲补肾阳,强腰膝,当归养血和血,均为佐药。诸药配伍,纯补无泻,阴中求阳,为峻补元阳,温煦命火,填精补髓之剂。

【注意事项】 本方药性颇为滋腻,肾虚而兼有湿浊者禁用。

2.7 Prescriptions with Astringent Effects

第七章
固涩剂

Prescriptions with astringent effects refer to those mainly composed of astringents with restraining and consolidating functions, which are applied for treating syndrome of consumption or excessive loss of qi, blood, essence and body fluid.

This syndrome may have varied causes, different affected parts of the body and manifest respective characteristics. Thus, prescriptions with astringent effects may be accordingly classified as follows. They are prescriptions for consolidating superficies to arrest perspiration, those for consolidating the intestine to stop diarrhea, those for restraining emission or enuresis and those for relieving metrorrhagia and leukorrhagia.

Prescriptions for consolidating superficies to arrest perspiration mainly consist of drugs of astringing and arresting sweating and are suitable for spontaneous perspiration and night sweating due to superficial weakness and discharge of yin-fluid. Prescriptions for consolidating the intestine to stop diarrhea chiefly comprise astringents and antidiarrheals, and are fit for protracted diarrhea and dysentery due to yang deficiency of the spleen and kidney as well as failure of the large intestine to control defecation. Prescriptions for restraining emission or enuresis are chiefly made up of drugs with the effects of storing essence and controlling urination and indicated in spermatorrhea and enuresis due to deficiency of the kidney and failing to control essence or dysfunction of the urinary

凡以收涩药为主组成,具有收敛固涩作用,用于治疗气、血、精、津液耗散滑脱证候的方剂,统称固涩剂。

由于气、血、精、津滑脱证候的病因及发病部位不同,其临床表现亦各有特点,因而固涩剂相应地分为固表止汗剂、涩肠固脱剂、涩精止遗剂以及固崩止带剂四类。

固表止汗剂由收涩止汗药为主组成,具有敛汗固表作用,适用于表虚不固,阴液外泄的自汗、盗汗。涩肠固脱剂由收涩止泻药为主组成,具有固肠止泻作用,适用于脾肾阳虚,大肠滑脱不禁的久泻、久痢。涩精止遗剂由收涩固精药为主组成,具有涩精缩尿作用,适用于肾虚精关不固或膀胱失约的遗精、遗尿。固崩止带剂由收涩止血或止带药为主组成,具有固冲止带作用,适用于冲任虚损或带脉失约

bladder. Prescriptions for relieving metrorrhagia and leukorrhagia are composed of drugs for relieving metrorrhagia and leukorrhagia and fit for metrorrhagia and leukorrhagia due to deficiency of the thoroughfare vessel and conception vessel and disorder of belt vessel.

In the clinical application of this group of prescriptions, attention should be paid to preventing accumulation of pathogenic factors. They are contraindicated for perspiration due to febrile diseases, diarrhea or dysentery due to improper diet, nocturnal emission due to pathogenic fire or metrorrhagia due to blood heat. In case of deficiency complicated with excess, pure astringents are strictly forbidden. If necessary, drugs of eliminating pathogenic factor may be used simultaneously.

2.7.1 Prescriptions for Consolidating Superficies to Arrest Perspiration

Muli San
(*Oyster Shell Powder*)

Source: *Taiping Huimin Hejiju Fang* (*Benevolent Prescriptions from Taiping Pharmaceutical Bureau*).

Ingredients:

No. 1 Huangqi (*Radix Astragali seu Hedysari*) 30 g;

No. 2 Mahuanggen (*Radix Ephedrae*) 30 g;

No. 3 Duanmuli (*Concha Ostreae*) (calcined) 30 g.

Administration: Grind the above drugs into powder; decoct 9 g with 30 g of Xiaomai (*Fructus Tritici Aestivi*) each time and twice daily for oral administration after the residue is removed.

Actions: Replenishing qi and consolidating superficial resistance, preserving yin and arresting sweat.

Clinical Application: This recipe is indicated for spontaneous perspiration and night sweat, marked by

的崩漏、带下。

临床使用固涩剂应注意防止收涩敛邪。凡属热病汗出、伤食泄痢、火扰精泄或血热崩漏等因实邪而致者禁用固涩剂；若证候虚中挟实者，切忌纯用收涩，必要时配伍祛邪药同用。

第一节　固表止汗剂

牡蛎散

【方源】《太平惠民和剂局方》。

【组成】 黄芪、麻黄根、煅牡蛎各30 g。

【用法】 共研粗末，每次9 g，加小麦30 g，同煎，去滓热服，每日2次。

【功用】 益气固表，敛阴止汗。

【临床应用】 适用于自汗、盗汗。症见身常汗出，夜

constant perspiration, especially while asleep at night, palpitation, susceptibility to fright, shortness of breath, vexation, lassitude, reddish tongue, thready and feeble pulse. It is applicable to spontaneous perspiration and night sweat due to weakened constitution after illness or operation or delivery, and others, which belong to failure of healthy qi to consolidate superficies. In case of cold limbs after perspiration with aversion to cold and preference for warmth, add Fuzi (*Radix Aconiti Praeparatae*) to dispel cold. In case of perspiration with shortness of breath, which gets aggravated with slight exertion, increase the dosage of the first ingredient and add Renshen (*Radix Ginseng*) and Baizhu (*Rhizoma Atractylodis Macrocephalae*) to replenish qi and restore body resistance. In case of night sweat with dry mouth, reddened tongue and little fur, add Shanzhuyu (*Fructus Corni*) and Baishaoyao (*Radix Paeoniae Alba*) to nourish and preserve yin.

Elucidation: The syndrome is caused by superficial weakness and discharge of yin fluid, leading to impairment of heart-yin and failing to store yang. It should be treated by supplementing qi and consolidating superficies as well as preserving yin and arresting sweat. The last ingredient is used as monarch drug, capable of arresting sweat, preserving yin and suppressing the hyperactive yang. The first ingredient can strengthen body resistance and replenish qi for arresting perspiration, and acts as minister drug. Ingredient No. 2 is specialized in arresting sweating and Xiaomai (*Fructus Tritici Aestivi*) in invigorating the heart and relieving vexation, both serving as adjuvant drugs.

Yupingfeng San and this recipe both bear the action of consolidating superficies and arresting perspiration in the treatment of polyhidrosis of the weak. But this recipe is very good at its astringent and anhidrotic effect and widely used for spontaneous perspiration or night sweat, which

卧尤甚,心悸怵惕,短气烦倦,舌淡红,脉细弱。病后、术后或产后体虚自汗、盗汗属正虚不固者,可用本方治疗。若汗出肢冷,畏寒喜温者,可加附子以助阳祛寒;若汗出气短,动则尤甚者,可重用黄芪,再加人参、白术以益气补虚;若盗汗口干,舌红少苔者,可加山茱萸、白芍药以滋阴涩津。

【方解】　本方证由表虚不固,阴液外泄,心阴受损,阳不潜藏所致,治宜益气固表,敛阴止汗之法。方中煅牡蛎收涩止汗,敛阴潜阳,为君药。黄芪益气实卫,固表止汗,为臣药。麻黄根功专止汗,小麦养心除烦,均为佐药。

本方与玉屏风散均具有固表止汗作用,用于虚人汗出过多。但本方长于收敛止汗,不论自汗或盗汗,凡属体虚而腠理失固者均可用之;玉屏风

are ascribed to weak body and striae of the skin and muscles being not strong. However, the former is effective in supplementing qi and consolidating the superficies and has dispersing action, thus is fit for spontaneous perspiration due to weakened superficies or for general debility likely to be attacked by pathogenic wind.

　　Danggui Liuhuang Tang and this recipe are both used in the treatment of night sweat. But the latter has a mild efficacy with astringent and anhidrotic effect and belongs to prescriptions for treating the secondary aspect of a disease. It can be modified to treat spontaneous perspiration or night sweat due to general debility, which are ascribed to weakened superficial resistance or failure of yin-fluid in staying in the interior due to qi deficiency. The former, however, is cold in nature and functions mainly to nourish yin and purge away fire, which belongs to prescriptions for clearing away heat and dealing with the primary cause of a disease. It, thus, is only indicated in hyperactivity of fire due to yin deficiency with manifestations as fever and night sweat. In case of severe night sweat from hyperactivity of fire due to yin deficiency, it is advisable to combine both for application.

　　Cautions：Drastic as this recipe is in its astringent and anhidrotic effect, it should be used with great caution for the case of excessive interior heat or that complicated with phlegm-dampness, manifesting dry mouth and throat, dry yellowish or greasy fur.

散则长于益气固表,同时兼有疏散之功,适宜于表虚自汗,或虚人易感风邪之证。

　　本方与当归六黄汤均可治疗盗汗证,但本方药性平和,以收敛止汗为主,属固涩治标之剂,凡虚人自汗或盗汗属气虚腠理失固或阴液不能内守者均可加减治疗;当归六黄汤则药性寒凉,以滋阴降火为主,属清热治本之剂,仅适宜于阴虚火扰,发热盗汗之证。若阴虚火旺,盗汗较著,可将两方结合使用。

　　【注意事项】 本方收敛止汗作用较强,若内热较重或兼挟痰湿,口干咽燥,舌苔黄燥或腻者慎用。

2.7.2　Prescriptions for Consolidating the Intestines to Stop Diarrhea

Zhenren Yangzang Tang
（**Zhenren Decoction for Nourishing the Zang Organs**）

Source：*Taiping Huimin Hejiju Fang*（*Benevo-*

第二节　涩肠固脱剂

真人养脏汤

【方源】《太平惠民和剂

lent Prescriptions from Taiping Pharmaceutical Bureau).

Ingredients：

No. 1 Renshen（*Radix Ginseng*）18 g；

No. 2 Danggui（*Radix Angelicae Sinensis*）18 g；

No. 3 Chaobaizhu（*Rhizoma Atractylodis Macrocephalae Praeparatae*）18 g；

No. 4 Roudoukou（*Semen Myristicae*）15 g；

No. 5 Rougui（*Cortex Cinnamomi*）24 g；

No. 6 Zhigancao（*Radix Glycyrrhizae Praeparatae*）24 g；

No. 7 Baishaoyao（*Radix Paeoniae Alba*）48 g；

No. 8 Muxiang（*Radix Aucklandiae*）42 g；

No. 9 Hezi（*Fructus Chebulae*）36 g；

No. 10 Yingsuke（*Pericarpium Papaveris*）108 g.

Administration：Grind the above drugs into powder and decoct 6 -12 g each time in water for oral application.

Actions：Astringing the intestines to stop diarrhea and warming the middle-energizer and reinforcing the spleen.

Clinical Application：This recipe is indicated for syndrome due to deficiency cold of the spleen and stomach and failure of the intestine to astringe, marked by protracted diarrhea or dysentery occurring irregularly day and night, abdominal pain with preference for warmth and pressure, lassitude, poor appetite, pale tongue with whitish fur, thready and slow pulse. It is applicable to longstanding cases of chronic or allergic colitis and others, which belong to weakness of the middle energizer. In case of severe aversion to cold with cold limbs, add Fuzi（*Radix Aconiti Praeparatae*）and Ganjiang（*Rhizoma Zingiberis*）to strengthen the effect of warming the spleenyang. In case of marked tenesmic sensation in rectum or prolapse of rectum, add Huangqi（*Radix Astragali seu Hedysari*）and Shengma（*Rhizoma Cimicifugae*）to sup-

局方》。

【组成】　人参、当归、炒白术各18 g，肉豆蔻15 g，肉桂、炙甘草各24 g，白芍药48 g，木香42 g，诃子36 g，罂粟壳108 g。

【用法】　共研粗末，每次6～12 g，水煎服。

【功用】　涩肠止泻，温中补脾。

【临床应用】　适用于脾胃虚寒，肠失固摄证。症见久泻久痢，日夜无度，腹痛喜温喜按，倦怠食少，舌淡苔白，脉细而迟。慢性结肠炎、过敏性结肠炎日久不愈，属中虚失固者，可用本方治疗。若畏寒怕冷较著，手足不温者，可加附子、干姜以助温阳暖脾之力；若肛门下坠感明显或脱肛者，可加黄芪、升麻以益气升阳举陷。

plement qi and lift up the spleen-yang.

Elucidation: The syndrome is caused by impairment of the spleen-yang and failure of the intestine in astringent effect as the result of protracted diarrhea or dysentery. It should be treated by consolidating the intestines to relieve diarrhea and warming the middle energizer and invigorating the spleen. The last ingredient is monarch drug, in larger dosage and with the effect of consolidating the intestines and relieving diarrhea. Ingredients No. 9 and No. 4, help bring about the effect of the monarch drug on the one hand, and warm the middle-energizer on the other, acting as minister drugs. Ingredients No. 1 and No. 3 can invigorate qi and the spleen, No. 2 and No. 7 can nourish and regulate the flow of blood as well as relieve pain; No. 5 can warm the kidney and spleen, and No. 8 can regulate the flow of qi and activate the spleen, preventing qi stagnation possibly induced by tonic and astringent drugs. These six ingredients together play the role of adjuvant drug. Combined with No. 1 and No. 3, ingredient No. 6 can achieve the effects of invigorating the middle-energizer and supplementing qi, and relieving spasm in combination with No. 7. Besides it also mediates the efficacy of other ingredients and serves as guiding drug.

Cautions: It is contraindicated for the early stage of diarrhea or dysentery, when the accumulation of damp heat is not yet removed.

Sishen Wan
(*Pill of Four Miraculous Drugs*)

Source: *Neike Zhaiyao* (*Summary from Internal Medicine*).

Ingredients:

No. 1 Roudoukou (*Semen Myristicae*) 60 g;

No. 2 Buguzhi (*Fructus Psoraleae*) 120 g;

No. 3 Wuweizi (*Fructus Schisandrae*) 60 g;

【方解】 本方证由泻痢日久,伤及脾阳,肠失固摄所致,治宜涩肠止泻,温中补脾之法。方中重用罂粟壳涩肠止泻,为君药。诃子、肉豆蔻助君药涩肠止泻,又可暖脾温中,同为臣药。人参、白术益气健脾,当归、白芍药养血和血,缓急止痛,肉桂温肾暖脾,木香理气醒脾,使诸补涩之品不致壅滞气机,均为佐药。炙甘草合人参、白术补中益气,合白芍药缓急止痛,又能调和药性,为佐使药。

【注意事项】 泻痢初起,湿热积滞未去者,禁用本方。

四神丸

【方源】《内科摘要》。

【组成】 肉豆蔻60 g,补骨脂120 g,五味子60 g,吴茱萸30 g。

No. 4 Wuzhuyu (*Fructus Evodiae*) 30 g.

Administration：Grind the above drugs into powder, which is then mixed with 240 g of Shengjiang (*Rhizoma Zingiberis Recens*) and 50 pieces of Dazao (*Fructus Ziziphi Jujubae*) after they are boiled and the cores removed; make the mixture into pills and take 6 - 9 g each time and twice daily. Or otherwise make into decoction with dosages in proportion to the original recipe.

Actions：Warming and invigorating the spleen and kidney and astringing the intestine to stop diarrhea.

Clinical Application：This recipe is indicated for syndrome of diarrhea before dawn, marked by diarrhea at dawn, anorexia, or protracted diarrhea, abdominal pain relieved with warmth, soreness of waist and cold limbs, mental fatigue and lassitude, pale and large tongue with thin whitish fur, deep slow and feeble pulse. It is applicable to chronic or allergic colitis with morning diarrhea, which belong to yang deficiency of the spleen and kidney. In case of severe soreness of waist and cold limbs, add Fuzi (*Radix Aconiti Praeparatae*) and Rougui (*Cortex Cinnamomi*) to enhance the effect of warming and activating kidney-yang. If concomitant with prolapse of rectum, add Huangqi (*Radix Astragali seu Hedysari*) and Shengma (*Rhizoma Cimicifugae*) to replenish qi and lifting up yang.

Elucidation：The syndrome is caused by deficiency of kidney-yang, leading to failure of fire in warming earth. It should be treated by warming and invigorating the spleen and kidney to relieve diarrhea. As monarch drug, Ingredient No. 2 is capable of activating kidney-yang and warming the spleen to relieve diarrhea. The first ingredient acts as minister drug to warm the kidney and spleen. Ingredient No. 3 has an astringent and antidiarrheal action, and No. 4 bears the effect of warming the interior and dispelling cold. Shengjiang (*Rhizoma Zingiberis*

【用法】　共研粗末，用生姜240 g，红枣 50 枚，煮熟取枣肉，和药末为丸，每次 6～9 g，每日 2 次。亦可作汤剂，用量按原方比例酌定。

【功用】　温补脾肾，涩肠止泻。

【临床应用】　适用于五更泄泻。症见黎明前腹泻，不思饮食，或久泻不愈，腹痛喜温，腰酸肢冷，神疲乏力，舌淡胖，苔薄白，脉沉迟无力。慢性结肠炎、过敏性结肠炎出现五更泄泻属脾肾阳虚者，可用本方治疗。若腰酸肢冷较甚者，可加附子、肉桂以增强温阳补肾之力；若兼脱肛者，可加黄芪、升麻以益气升阳举陷。

【方解】　本方证由肾阳虚衰，火不暖土所致，治宜温补脾肾，涩肠止泻之法。方中补骨脂补肾助阳，温脾止泻，为君药。肉豆蔻温肾暖脾，涩肠止泻，为臣药。五味子收敛止泻，吴茱萸温里祛寒，生姜、大枣补脾和胃，助君臣药补虚收涩之力，俱为佐药。

Recens) and Dazao (*Fructus Ziziphi Jujubae*) are effective in invigorating the spleen and regulating the stomach, and strengthen the effects of the monarch and minister drugs, serving as adjuvant drugs together with No. 3 and No. 4.

Both this recipe and Zhenren Yangzang Tang possess the action of consolidating the intestines and relieving diarrhea and are both used for treating protracted diarrhea and prolapse of rectum. But the former is good at warming the kidney and spleen, and a typical recipe for morning diarrhea caused by deficiency of the kidney-yang and failure of fire to warm earth. While the latter focuses on warming the spleen-yang and is fit for protracted diarrhea due to impairment of the spleen and failure of the intestine in astringent action.

Cautions: It is contraindicated for cases concomitant with damp heat manifesting yellowish and greasy fur.

本方与真人养脏汤均有涩肠固脱作用,适宜治疗泻痢日久,滑脱不禁。但本方长于温肾暖脾,为治疗肾阳虚衰,火不暖土而致五更泄泻的代表方;真人养脏汤则偏重于温补脾阳,涩肠止泻,宜于久痢伤脾,肠失固摄而致的泻痢不止。

【注意事项】 若兼挟湿热,舌苔黄腻者,禁用本方。

2.7.3 Prescriptions for Restraining Emission or Enuresis

Jinsuo Gujing Wan
(*Golden Lock Pill for Preserving Kidney Essence*)

Source: *Yifang jijie* (*Variorum of Prescriptions*).

Ingredients:

No. 1 Shayuanjili (*Semen Astragali Complanti*) 60 g;

No. 2 Qianshi (*Semen Euryales*) 60 g;

No. 3 Lianxu (*Stamen Nelumbinis*) 60 g;

No. 4 Duanlonggu (*Os Draconis*) (calcined) 30 g;

No. 5 Duanmuli (*Concha Ostreae*) (calcined) 30 g.

Administration: Grind the above drugs into fine powder, which is then mixed with the paste of Lianzi (*Semen Nelumbinis*) and made into pills; take 9 g each time and twice daily with light salty water when stomach

第三节 涩精止遗剂

金锁固精丸

【方源】《医方集解》。

【组成】 沙苑蒺藜、芡实、莲须各60 g,煅龙骨、煅牡蛎各30 g。

【用法】 共研细末,以莲子粉糊丸,每次9 g,空腹淡盐汤送下,每日2次。亦可作汤剂,用量按原方比例酌定,并

is empty. Or add proper amount of Lianzi (*Semen Nelumbinis*) to the above to make decoction for oral application with dosages in proportion to the original recipe.

Actions : Nourishing the kidney and astringing emission.

Clinical Application : This recipe is indicated for syndrome of seminal emission due to deficiency of the kidney, marked by spermatorrhea, frequent diarrhea, soreness of waist, tinnitus, mental fatigue, lassitude, pale tongue with whitish fur, thready feeble pulse. It is applicable to spermatorrhea, prospermia, enuresis, chyluria and others, which belong to instability of kidney-qi due to kidney-deficiency. In case of severe soreness of waist and knees, add Duzhong (*Cortex Eucommiae*) and Xuduan (*Radix Dipsaci*) to invigorate the kidney and strengthen waist and knees. In case of fire failing to warm earth with loose stool, add Buguzhi (*Fructus Psoraleae*) and Wuweizi (*Fructus Schisandrae*) to warm kidney-yang and relieve diarrhea. In case of scanty essence due to deficiency of the kidney and constipation due to dryness of intestines, add Shudihuang (*Rhizoma Rehmanniae Praeparatae*) and Roucongrong (*Herba Listanchis*) to reinforce the kidney and supplement essence as well as nourish blood and moisten the intestines.

Elucidation : The syndrome is caused by failure of the kidney in storing essence due to kidney deficiency and spontaneous discharge of sperms. It should be treated by reinforcing the kidney and arresting emission. The first ingredient can not only reinforce the kidney, but also restrain emission, acting as monarch drug. As minister drugs, ingredient No. 2 and Lianzi (*Semen Nelumbinis*) enhance the effect of the monarch drug. The rest three ingredients are all major astringent drugs for restraining sperms, and function as adjuvant drugs, the combination

加莲子适量,水煎服。

【功用】　补肾涩精。

【临床应用】　适用于肾虚遗精证。症见遗精滑泄,腰酸耳鸣,神疲乏力,舌淡苔白,脉细弱。遗精、早泄、遗尿、乳糜尿等属肾虚下元不固者,可用本方治疗。若腰膝酸痛明显者,可加杜仲、续断以补肾而壮腰膝;若火不暖土,大便溏泄者,可加补骨脂、五味子以温肾助阳,涩肠止泻;若肾虚精亏,肠燥便秘者,可加熟地黄、肉苁蓉以补肾益精,养血润肠。

【方解】　本方证由肾虚封藏失职,精关不固所致,治宜补肾涩精之法。方中沙苑蒺藜既可益肾补虚,又能固精止遗,为君药。芡实、莲子益肾补脾,固精止遗,可加强君药补肾固精的作用,同为臣药。煅龙骨、煅牡蛎、莲须均为收敛涩精的要药,与君臣诸药相合,收敛固涩之功更为显

with the monarch and minister drugs of which achieves an even better result. The combined application of all ingredients can arrest spontaneous discharge of sperms on the one hand, and invigorate kidney-yang on the other hand, giving consideration to both the primary and secondary aspects of the disease with stress laid on astringing nocturnal seminal emission, so this recipe is named the Gold Lock.

Cautions: This recipe is contraindicated for spermatorrhea due to hyperactivity of the ministerial fire (kidney-fire) or due to downward flow of damp heat.

Sangpiaoxiao San
(*Manthis Egg-case Powder*)

Source: *Bencao Yanyi* (*Amplified Materia Medica*).

Ingredients:

No. 1 Sangpiaoxiao (*Ootheca Mantidis*) 30 g;

No. 2 Yuanzhi (*Radix Polygalae*) 30 g;

No. 3 Shichangpu (*Rhizoma Acori Graminei*) 30 g;

No. 4 Longgu (*Os Draconis*) 30 g;

No. 5 Renshen (*Radix Ginseng*) 30 g;

No. 6 Fushen (*Sclerotium Poriae Circum Radicem Pini*) 30 g;

No. 7 Danggui (*Radix Angelicae Sinensis*) 30 g;

No. 8 Zhiguiban (*Plastrum Testudinis Praeparatae*) 30 g.

Administration: Grind the above except No. 5 into fine powder, take 6 g each time with the decoction of No. 5 before going to bed. Or decoct them for oral application with dosages in proportion to the original recipe.

Actions: Regulating and invigorating the heart and kidney to arrest emission and enuresis.

Clinical Application: This recipe is indicated for seminal emission or enuresis due to deficiency of the heart and kidney, marked by spermatorrhea or enuresis, or frequent micturition, turbid urine like rice-washing water,

著,均为佐药。诸药配伍,既可固外泄之精液,又能补亏损之肾元,标本兼顾,侧重于固涩精关,故方以"金锁"名之。

【注意事项】 遗精因相火妄动或湿热下注所致者,禁用本方。

桑螵蛸散

【方源】 《本草衍义》。

【组成】 桑螵蛸、远志、石菖蒲、龙骨、人参、茯神、当归、炙龟版各30 g。

【用法】 除人参外,共研细末,每次6 g,睡前以人参汤调下。亦可作汤剂,用量按原方比例酌定。

【功用】 调补心肾,涩精止遗。

【临床应用】 适用于心肾两虚之遗尿遗精。症见遗尿或遗精,或小便频数,尿如米泔,或心神恍惚,健忘,舌淡

or absentmindedness, amnesia, pale tongue with whitish fur, thready feeble pulse. It is applicable to infantile enuresis, spermatorrhea, diabetes, neurosis and others, which pertain to deficiency of the heart and spleen, and are characterized by enuresis or spermatorrhea with absentmindedness. In case of failure of the kidney in arresting sperms with excessive emission, add Shayuanjili (*Semen Astragali Complanti*) and Shanzhuyu (*Fructus Corni*) to strengthen the effect of reinforcing the kidney to restrain sperms. In case of marked yang deficiency with soreness of waist and cold limbs, add Buguzhi (*Fructus Psoraleae*) and Tusizi (*Semen Cuscutae*) to enhance the effect of warming kidney-yang.

Elucidation: The syndrome is caused by deficiency of both the heart and kidney, discordance between water and fire, kidney's failing to astringe essence and uncontrolled urination of urinary bladder. It should be treated by regulating and reinforcing the heart and kidney to restrain emission or enuresis. The first ingredient is monarch drug with the effects of reinforcing the kidney, restraining sperms and relieving enuresis. Ingredient No. 4 bears the action of tranquilizing mind and helps the monarch drug with the astringent effect. The last ingredient is capable of nourishing kidney-yin and reinforcing the kidney, and can nourish yin and suppress yang when combined with No. 4. Both function as minister drugs. Ingredient No. 5 can replenish the primordial qi and No. 7 nourish the heart-blood to ease mind. No. 6, No. 2 and No. 3 possess the effects of tranquilizing mind, inducing resuscitation and disolving phlegm, which are helpful in restoring coordination between the heart and kidney when in compatibility with other tonic ingredients. These five ingredients together serve as adjuvant drugs.

Cautions: This recipe is contraindicated for

苔白,脉细弱。小儿遗尿、遗精、糖尿病、神经衰弱等属心肾两虚,以遗尿或遗精而伴心神恍惚为特征者,可用本方治疗。若精关不固,遗精较甚者,可加沙苑蒺藜、山茱萸以助补肾涩精之力;若阳虚明显,腰酸肢冷者,可加补骨脂、菟丝子以增温肾助阳之功。

【方解】　本方证由心肾两虚,水火不交,肾虚不固,膀胱失约所致,治宜调补心肾,涩精止遗之法。方中桑螵蛸补肾固精缩尿,为君药。龙骨宁心安神,涩精止遗,助君药固涩止遗;龟版滋肾养阴,培补下元,合龙骨滋阴潜阳,同为臣药。人参补元气以益智,当归养心血以宁神,两药双补气血;茯神、远志、石菖蒲安神定志,开窍化痰,与诸补益药相伍,有助于心肾之交通,俱为佐药。

【注意事项】　湿热下注

frequent micturition and enuresis due to downward flow of damp heat or yang deficiency of the spleen and kidney.

Suoquan Wan
(*Pill for Reducing Urination*)

Source: *Weishi Jiacang Fang* (*Secret Prescriptions of Wei's Family*).

Ingredients:

No. 1 Wuyao (*Radix Linderae*);

No. 2 Yizhiren (*Fructus Alpiniae Oxyphyllae*);

Equal in dosage.

Administration: Grind the above into fine powder and make the powder into small pills by means of the paste of wine-parched Shanyao (*Rhizoma Dioscoreae*); take 9 g each time and twice daily with light salty water or rice gruel. Or decoct the above in water for oral application with dosages in proportion to the original recipe.

Actions: Warming the kidney to reduce urination.

Clinical Application: This recipe is indicated for enuresis due to kidney deficiency, marked by frequent micturition or enuresis, pale tongue, thready feeble pulse. It is applicable to infantile enuresis, nervous frequent micturition, diabetes insipidus as well as hypersalivation and excessive nasal discharge and others, which pertain to instability of kidney-qi. Since this recipe is simple in composition and mild in efficacy, it is necessary to add Buguzhi (*Fructus Psoraleae*), Tusizi (*Semen Cuscutae*), Sangpiaoxiao (*Ootheca Mantidis*) and Fupenzi (*Fructus Rubi*) in severe case to enhance the effect of warming and consolidating the kidney.

Elucidation: The syndrome is caused by deficiency of kidney-qi, leading to deficiency cold syndrome of the urinary bladder and its failure in restraining fluid. It should be treated by warming the kidney. The second ingredient acts as monarch drug to invigorate kidney-yang

或脾肾阳虚之尿频、遗尿者，禁用本方。

缩泉丸

【方源】 《魏氏家藏方》。

【组成】 乌药、益智仁各等分。

【用法】 共研细末，以酒煎山药末为糊制成小丸，每次9 g，淡盐汤或米汤送服，每日2次。亦可作汤剂，用量按原方比例酌定。

【功用】 温肾缩尿。

【临床应用】 适用于肾虚遗尿证。症见小便频数或遗尿，舌淡，脉细弱。小儿遗尿、神经性尿频、尿崩症，以及多唾、多涕症等属肾气不固者，可用本方治疗。本方药简力薄，若病情较重者，宜酌加补骨脂、菟丝子、桑螵蛸、覆盆子等以加强温肾固摄的作用。

【方解】 本方证由肾气不足，膀胱虚寒，不能约束水液所致，治宜温肾缩尿之法。方中益智仁补肾助阳，固精缩尿，为君药。乌药温肾散寒，

and preserve essence to relieve enuresis. The first ingredient is capable of warming the kidney and dispelling cold
and helps bring about the effect of the monarch drug,
functioning as minister drug. Shanyao (*Rhizoma Dioscoreae*) is used as adjuvant drug with the effect of reinforcing the spleen and kidney and preserving essential qi.
All drugs together, warm but not dry, with astringent
effect but not leading to stagnation of pathogenic factors,
restore the function of the kidney and urinary bladder,
thus relieving frequent micturition and enuresis.

缩尿止遗,助君药温暖下元,
固肾缩尿,为臣药。山药补脾
肾而涩精气,为佐药。诸药合
用,温而不燥,涩而不滞,使肾
气复而膀胱约束有权,则尿
频、遗尿可愈。

2.7.4　Prescriptions for Relieving Metrorrhagia and Leukorrhagia

第四节　固崩止带剂

Guchong Tang
(*Decoction for Strengthening the Thoroughfare Vessel*)

固冲汤

Source：*Yixue Zhongzhong Canxilu* (*Discourse on Medical Problems by Integrated Traditional Chinese and Western Medicine*).

【方源】《医学衷中参西录》。

Ingredients：

No. 1 Chaobaizhu (*Rhizoma Atractylodis Macro-cephalae Praeparatae*) 30 g;

No. 2 Huangqi (*Radix Astragali seu Hedysari*) 18 g;

No. 3 Duanlonggu (calcined *Os Draconis*) 24 g;

No. 4 Duanmuli (calcined *Concha Ostreae*) 24 g;

No. 5 Shanzhuyu (*Fructus Corni*) 24 g;

No. 6 Baishaoyao (*Radix Paeoniae Alba*) 12 g;

No. 7 Haipiaoxiao (*Os Sepiiellae seu Sepiae*) 12 g;

No. 8 Qiancao (*Radix Rubiae*) 9 g;

No. 9 Zonglütan (*Trachycarpi Carbonisa tus*) 6 g;

No. 10 Wubeizi (*Galla Chinensis*) 1.5 g.

【组成】　炒白术30 g,黄
芪18 g,煅龙骨24 g,煅牡蛎
24 g,山茱萸24 g,白芍药12 g,
海螵蛸12 g,茜草9 g,棕榈炭
6 g,五倍子1.5 g。

Administration：Decoct the above drugs in water for oral application.

【用法】　水煎服。

Actions: Replenishing qi and invigorating the spleen, consolidating thoroughfare vessel and controlling blood.

Clinical Application: This recipe is indicated for debility of thoroughfare vessel due to deficiency of spleen-qi, marked by metrorrhagia or profuse but thin light-color or menstruation, palpitation, shortness of breath, soreness and weakness of waist and knees, pale tongue, thready and feeble pulse. It is applicable to dysfunctional uterine bleeding, which belong to debility of the chong meridian due to spleen deficiency. If concomitant with cold limbs and perspiration, thready and feeble pulse, which are indicative of yang exhaustion, increase the dosage of ingredient No. 2 and use Shenfu Tang 〔Renshen (*Radix Ginseng*) and Fuzi (*Radix Aconiti Praeparatae*)〕 simultaneously so as to supplement qi and restore yang.

Elucidation: The syndrome is caused by failure of the spleen in controlling blood and debility of thoroughfare vessel. It should be treated by replenishing qi and invigorating the spleen, reinforcing the thoroughfare vessel to arrest bleeding. In larger dosages, the first two ingredients are meant to supplement qi and reinforce the spleen to control blood and used as monarch drugs. Ingredients No. 5 and No. 6 function as minister drugs with the effects of invigorating the liver and kidney, nourishing blood and preserving yin. Ingredients No. 3, No. 4, No. 9 and No. 10 astringe and enrich blood, while No. 7 and No. 8 can resolve blood stasis to stop bleeding. Therefore, their combination can result in the effect of stopping bleeding without retaining blood stasis. These six ingredients play the role of adjuvant drug.

Cautions: This recipe is contraindicated for patients with metrorrhagia due to heat in the blood.

【功用】 益气健脾,固冲摄血。

【临床应用】 适用于脾气虚弱,冲脉不固证。症见血崩或月经过多,色淡质稀,心悸气短,腰膝酸软,舌质淡,脉细弱。功能性子宫出血属脾虚冲脉不固者,可用本方治疗。若兼肢冷汗出,脉细微者,为阳脱之象,需加重黄芪用量,并合参附汤(人参、附子)以益气回阳。

【方解】 本方证由脾气虚弱,失其统摄,冲脉不固所致,治宜益气健脾,固冲摄血之法。方中重用白术、黄芪补气健脾以摄血,共为君药。山茱萸、白芍药补益肝肾,养血敛阴,同为臣药。煅龙骨、煅牡蛎、棕榈炭、五倍子收涩止血,海螵蛸、茜草化瘀止血,使血止而无留瘀之弊,俱为佐药。

【注意事项】 血热妄行而致崩中漏下者,禁用本方。

Wandai Tang

(*Decoction for Treating Leukorrhagia*)

Source：*Fu Qingzhu Nüke* (*Fu Qingzhu's Obsterics and Gynecology*).

Ingredients：

No.1 Chaobaizhu (*Rhizoma Atractyodis Praeparatae*) 30 g;

No.2 Chaoshanyao (*Rhizoma Dioscoreae Praeparatae*) 30 g;

No.3 Renshen (*Radix Ginseng*) 6 g;

No.4 Chaobaishaoyao (*Radix Paeoniae Praeparatae*) 15 g;

No.5 Chaocheqianzi (*Semen Plantaginis Praeparatae*) 9 g;

No.6 Cangzhu (*Rhizoma Atractylodis*) 9 g;

No.7 Gancao (*Radix Glycyrrhizae*) 3 g;

No.8 Chenpi (*Pericarpium Citri Reticulatae*) 1.5 g;

No.9 Chaojingjiesui (*Spica Schizonepetae*) 1.5 g;

No.10 Chaihu (*Radix Bupleuri*) 1.8 g.

Administration：Decoct the above drugs in water for oral application.

Actions：Invigorating the middle-energizer and reinforcing the spleen, eliminating dampness and relieving leukorrhagia.

Clinical Application：This recipe is indicated for leukorrhagia due to deficiency of the spleen, marked by thin whitish or yellowish leukorrhea without foul smell, pale complexion, lassitude, loose stool, pale tongue with whitish fur, soft and feeble pulse. It is applicable to cervicitis, vaginitis, and chronic pelvic inflammation, which are marked by lingering thin whitish leukorrhagia due to deficiency of spleen-qi. In case of lower abdominal pain with localized cold sensation, add Paojiang (*Rhizoma Zingiberis Praeparatae*) and Xiaohuixiang (*Fructus Foeniculi*) to warm yang and dispel cold. If concomitant

完带汤

【方源】　《傅青主女科》。

【组成】　炒白术30 g,炒山药30 g,人参6 g,炒白芍药15 g,炒车前子9 g,苍术9 g,甘草3 g,陈皮1.5 g,炒荆芥穗1.5 g,柴胡1.8 g。

【用法】　水煎服。

【功用】　补中健脾,化湿止带。

【临床应用】　适用于脾虚带下证。症见带下色白或淡黄,清稀无臭,面色㿠白,倦怠便溏,舌淡苔白,脉濡弱。宫颈炎、阴道炎、慢性盆腔炎而见带下绵绵,清稀色白属脾气虚弱者,可用本方治疗。若兼小腹冷痛者,可加炮姜、小茴香以温阳祛寒;若兼腰膝酸软者,可加杜仲、续断以补肝肾,强腰膝;若带下量多不止

with soreness and weakness of waist and knees，add Duzhong (*Cortex Eucommiae*) and Xuduan (*Radix Dipsaci*) to reinforce the liver and kidney and strengthen waist and knees. In case of incessant leukorrhea in larege amount，add Duanlonggu (*calcined Os Draconis*) and Duanmuli (*calcined Concha Ostreae*) to stop leukorrhagia. In case of yellowish leukorrhea，add Huangbai (*Cortex Phellodendri*) and Cheqianzi (*Semen Plantaginis*) to eliminate damp heat.

Elucidation：The syndrome is caused by stagnation of the liver subjugating the spleen and dysfunction of the spleen in transportation due to deficiency，leading to accumulation and downward attack of damp turbidity. It should be treated by reinforcing the spleen and eliminating dampness. The first two ingredients in larger dosages are meant to invigorate qi of the middle-energizer and reinforce the spleen to remove dampness，acting as monarch drugs. Ingredients No. 3 and No. 6 bear the respective function of restoring qi and drying dampness，helping bring about the effect of the monarch drug. Ingredients No. 4 and No. 10 possess the respective function of nourishing the liver and regulating the stagnated liver-qi，relieving the accompanying symptoms as stagnation of the liver-qi. These four together serve as minister drugs. Ingredient No. 5 possesses the effect of promoting diuresis，No. 8 promoting the flow of qi to eliminate dampness and No. 9 dispersing the stagnated liver-qi and lifting yang，which all play the role of adjuvant drug. Used as guiding drug，No. 7 can supplement qi and mediate the properties of other drugs.

Cautions：This recipe is contraindicated for stenchy yellowish leukorrhea with greasy yellowish fur.

者,可加煅龙骨、煅牡蛎以固涩止带；若带下兼黄色者,可加黄柏、车前子以清利湿热。

【方解】 本方证由肝郁乘脾,脾虚不运,以致湿浊内停,下注成带,治宜补中健脾、化湿止带之法。方中重用白术、山药益气补中,健脾燥湿,共为君药。人参补气,苍术燥湿,共助君药以补中祛湿；白芍药柔肝,柴胡疏郁,同解兼证之肝气郁滞,均为臣药。车前子渗利湿浊,陈皮行气化湿,荆芥穗疏肝升阳,俱为佐药。炙甘草益气补中,调和药性,为使药。

【注意事项】 带下色黄,其气腥秽,舌苔黄腻者,禁用本方。

2.8 Sedative Prescriptions

第八章

安神剂

Sedative prescriptions refer to those mainly composed of sedatives with the effect of tranquilizing mind for the treatment of mental disorders.

By mental disorders is meant mental derangement with chief clinical manifestations as palpitation, insomnia, dysphoria and mania, the basic pathology of which may either be disturbed mentality by pathogenic heat or failure of blood to nourish the heart. Therefore, these prescriptions are accordingly subdivided into prescriptions with heavy sedatives and those with tonic sedatives.

Prescriptions with heavy sedatives are chiefly made up of tranquilizers of great weight, which bear the properties of tranquilizing mind, suppressing yang and purging away fire. They are indicated for restlessness of mind with chief pathologic changes as yang hyperactivity of the heart and liver as well as mental disturbance due to heat and fire. Prescriptions with tonic sedatives possess the effect of tranquilizing mind and nourishing yin and blood. They are suitable for irritability as a result of failure of blood to nourish the heart and liver due to deficiency.

Minerals, metals or shells in prescriptions with heavy sedatives are apt to impair stomach-qi. Prolonged administration is therefore inadvisable. Patients with usual weakness of the spleen and stomach should use some drugs which can regulate the spleen and stomach. Though in this group of prescriptions, Zhusha (*Cinnabaris*) is very

凡以安神药为主组成,具有安神定志作用,用于治疗神志不安疾患的方剂,统称安神剂。

所谓神志不安疾患,是指以心悸、失眠、烦躁、惊狂等心神失宁症状为主要临床表现的一类疾病,其基本病理或为热扰心神,或为血不养心,因而安神剂相应地分为重镇安神剂与滋养安神剂两类。

重镇安神剂由重镇安神药为主组成,具有镇心安神,潜阳泻火作用,适用于以心肝阳亢或火热扰心为主要病理变化的心神失宁。滋养安神剂由补养安神药为主组成,具有养心安神,滋阴补血作用,适用于以阴血不足、心肝失养为主要病理变化的心神失宁。

重镇安神剂中的金石类药物易伤胃气,不宜久服,对于素体脾胃虚弱的患者,应配合服用健脾和胃之品。本类方剂中的朱砂虽为安神良药,但因其主要成分为硫化汞,因

effective in tranquilizing mind, it should not be taken in large dosage or for a long time to prevent mercurialism because its chief ingredient is mercuric sulfide.

而不宜多服或久服,以防引起汞中毒。

2.8.1 Prescriptions with Heavy Sedatives

第一节　重镇安神剂

Zhusha Anshen Wan
(*Cinnabar Sedative Pill*)

朱砂安神丸

Source：*Yixue Faming* (*Medical Inventions*).

Ingredients：

No. 1 Zhusha (*Cinnabaris*) 15 g;

No. 2 Huanglian (*Rhizoma Coptidis*) 18 g;

No. 3 Zhigancao (*Radix Glycyrrhizae Praeparatae*) 16 g;

No. 4 Shengdihuang (*Radix Rehmanniae*) 8 g;

No. 5 Danggui (*Radix Angelicae Sinensis*) 8 g.

【方源】《医学发明》。

【组成】　朱砂15 g,黄连18 g,炙甘草16 g,生地黄、当归各8 g。

Administration：Grind the first ingredient in water or grind it into extremely fine powder; then mix it well with the fine powder of the rest; make the mixture into pills with honey and take 6 - 9 g each time with warm boiled water before going to bed. Or decoct the above except No. 1 in water with dosages modified proportionally on the basis of the original recipe, take with this decoction the first ingredient after it is ground in water.

【用法】　朱砂水飞或粉碎成极细粉,其余四味研成细末,和匀,炼蜜为丸,每次 6～9 g,睡前温开水送下。亦可作汤剂,用量按原方比例酌情增减,朱砂水飞,以药汤送服。

Actions：Tranquilizing mind and purging away fire from the heart.

【功用】　重镇安神,清心泻火。

Clinical Application：This recipe is indicated for mental derangement due to hyperactivity of heart-fire and deficiency of yin and blood, marked by insomnia, dreaminess, severe palpitation with fright, vexation, irritability, reddened tongue, thready and rapid pulse. It is applicable to palpitation, amnesia, and insomnia induced by neurosis, or to vague mind induced by mental depression

【临床应用】　适用于心火亢盛,阴血不足,神志不安证。症见失眠多梦,惊悸怔忡,心烦神乱,舌红,脉细数。神经衰弱所致的心悸、健忘、失眠,或精神抑郁症引起的神志恍惚等属心火上炎,阴血不

and others, which belong to the flaring up of heart fire and deficiency of yin and blood. If complicated with phlegm-heat manifesting chest distress and greasy fur, add Quangualou (*Fructus Trichosanthis*) and Zhuru (*Caulis Bambusae in Taeniam*) to clear away heat and eliminate phlegm. In case of severe palpitation and insomnia, add Longgu (*Os Draconis*), Muli (*Concha Ostreae*) and Cishi (*Magnetitum*) to enhance the effect.

Elucidation: The syndrome results from hyperactivity of the heart-fire, causing impairment of yin blood and lack of nourishment in the heart. It should be treated with heavy sedatives and by purgating heart fire. The first ingredient is heavy and cold in nature and takes effect directly in the heart meridian. It acts as monarch drug with the effect of easing mind and purging fire from the heart. The second ingredient functions as minister drug to help bring about the effect of the monarch drug. The combination of both achieves a remarkable effect of clearing away heat from the heart and relieving vexation. Ingredients No. 5 and No. 4 have the respective effect of nourishing blood and yin and are used as adjuvant drugs. Serving as guiding drug, Ingredient No. 3 can supplement qi and regulate the middle-energizer, prevent No. 1 from impairing the stomach, and mediate the properties of other drugs.

Cautions: This recipe is contraindicated for those with general debility or weakness of the spleen and stomach.

Cizhu Wan
(*Medicated Leaven Pill*)

Source: *Beiji Qianjin Yaofang (Valuable Prescriptions for Emergency)*.

Ingredients:

No. 1 Cishi (*Magnetitum*) 60 g;

No. 2 Zhusha (*Cinnabaris*) 30 g;

No. 3 Shenqu (*Massa Dermentata Medicinalis*) 120 g.

足者,可用本方治疗。若兼挟痰热,见胸闷苔腻者,可酌加全瓜蒌、竹茹以清热化痰;若心悸、怔忡、失眠较重者,宜加龙骨、牡蛎、磁石以加强重镇安神之力。

【方解】 本方证由心火亢盛,灼伤阴血,心失所养所致,治宜重镇安神,清心泻火之法。方中朱砂质重性寒,专入心经,重镇安神,清心泻火,为君药。黄连清心泻火,助君药清心安神,为臣药。两药相伍,重镇安神,清心除烦之功颇著。当归养血,生地黄滋阴,两药同用以补充为心火所灼之阴血,为佐药。炙甘草益气和中,可防朱砂质重碍胃,又能调和药性,为佐使药。

【注意事项】 素体阴虚或脾胃虚弱者,禁用本方。

磁朱丸

【方源】 《备急千金要方》。

【组成】 磁石60 g,朱砂30 g,神曲120 g。

Administration: Grind the above drugs separately into extremely fine powder, then mix them with honey after being sieved to make boluses; take 6 g each time and once daily with warm boiled water.

Actions: Tranquilizing mind, suppressing yang and improving eyesight.

Clinical Application: This recipe is applicable to restlessness due to disharmony between the heart and kidney, marked by palpitation, insomnia, tinnitus, deafness, and blurred vision. It is also applicable to neurosis, epilepsy, hypertension, and pathologic changes of retina, optic nerve, vitreous body and lens as well as disturbance of aqueous humor circulation. If concomitant with dizziness, xenophthalmia and photophobia that are indicative of deficiency of liver and kidney yin, Liuwei Dihuang Wan may be taken simultaneously, or Liuwei Dihuang Tang for oral administration of the boluses. In case of epilepsy with excessive phlegm, Daotan Tang 〔composed of Erchen Tang plus Tiannanxing (*Rhizoma Arisaematis*) and Zhishi (*Fructus Aurantii Immaturus*)〕 can be used for oral administration of the boluses.

Elucidation: The syndrome is caused by deficiency of the kidney-yin, hyperactive heart-yang and incoordination between the heart and kidney. It should be treated by nourishing yin and suppressing yang, restoring coordination between the heart and kidney and tranquilizing mind. The first ingredient, which is pungent and cold in nature and takes effect in the kidney, is the monarch drug with the effect of supplementing yin, suppressing hyperactive yang and easing mind. Used as minister drug, the second ingredient is sweet and cold in nature and takes effect in the heart, purging away fire from the heart and tranquilizing mind. Both in compatibility can supplement yin and suppress the hyperactive yang so that the normal physiological

【用法】 上药分别研为极细末,过筛混匀,炼蜜为丸,每次6g,温开水送服,每日1次。

【功用】 重镇安神,益阴明目。

【临床应用】 适用于心肾不交,神志不安证。症见心悸失眠,耳鸣耳聋,视物昏花。神经衰弱、癫痫、高血压病,视网膜、视神经、玻璃体、晶状体的病变,以及房水循环障碍等属心肾不交证者,可用本方治疗。若兼头晕目眩,目涩羞明等肝肾阴虚表现者,宜配伍六味地黄丸同用,或以六味地黄汤送服;若癫痫痰多者,可以导痰汤(二陈汤加天南星、枳实)送服。

【方解】 本方证由肾阴不足,心阳偏亢,心肾不交所致,治宜益阴潜阳,交通心肾,重镇安神之法。方中磁石辛寒入肾,益阴潜阳,重镇安神,为君药。朱砂甘寒入心,清心降火,重镇安神,为臣药。两药相伍,可益阴潜阳,使水火既济,精气得以上荣,心火不致上扰,心肾交泰,则目昏耳聋,心悸失眠等症自除。两药又能潜阳熄风,癫痫因阳亢风动而致者服之可平。神曲健

coordination between the heart and kidney is restored and the vital-qi can ascend to nourish head and prevent the head from being disturbed by the upward invasion of the hyperactive heart-fire. Consequently such symptoms as blurring of vision, deafness, palpitation and insomnia will be relieved. Besides these two ingredients can also suppress the hyperactive yang and stop endogenous wind. Thus, epilepsy, which is brought about by liver-wind stirring due to the hyperactive yang, is relieved with this recipe. The last ingredient functions as adjuvant drug, which regulates the spleen and stomach to promote the transportation and transformation of mineral drugs and to prevent them from impairing the stomach as well. Honey is meant to reinforce the middle-energizer and replenish qi, reduce the efficacy of other drugs and promote the transportation, transformation and distribution of the drugs.

Cautions: The first two ingredients, heavy in nature, should not be used in large dosage or for long time.

脾和胃,以助金石药之运化,并可防其重镇伤胃,为佐药。炼蜜为丸,取其补中益气,且可缓和药力,并有利于药物的运化输布。

【注意事项】　方中磁石、朱砂均为重坠之品,不宜用量过多,亦不宜久服。

2.8.2　Sedative Prescriptions with Tonic Effects

Suanzaoren Tang
(*Wild Jujube Seed Decoction*)

第二节　滋养安神剂

酸枣仁汤

Source: *Jingui Yaolue* (*Synopsis of Prescriptions of the Golden Cabinet*).

Ingredients:

No.1 Suanzaoren (*Semen Ziziphi Spinosae*) (baked after broken) 15 - 18 g;

No.2 Fuling (*Poria*) 6 g;

No.3 Zhimu (*Rhizoma Anemarrhenae*) 6 g;

No.4 Chuanxiong (*Rhizoma Ligustici Chuanxiong*) 6 g;

No.5 Gancao (*Radix Glycyrrhizae*) 3 g.

【方源】　《金匮要略》。

【组成】　酸枣仁(打碎,炒)15～18 g,茯苓6 g,知母6 g,川芎6 g,甘草3 g。

Administration：Decoct the above drugs in water for oral application.

Actions：Nourishing the blood and tranquilizing mind, clearing away heat and relieving restlessness.

Clinical Application：This recipe is indicated for syndrome of restlessness and insomnia due to deficiency, marked by insomnia, palpitation, vexation, vertigo, dry throat and mouth, reddened tongue, taut and thready pulse. It is applicable to neurosis, cardiac neurosis and menopausal syndrome with the above symptoms. The second ingredient is now often replaced with Fushen (*Sclerotium Poriae Circum Radicem Pini*). In case of excessive fire of deficiency type manifested as dysphoria with smothery sensation, insomnia and dreaminess, subtract ingredient No. 4 and add Shengdihuang (*Radix Rehmanniae*), Baishaoyao (*Radix Paeoniae Alba*) and Huanglian (*Rhizoma Coptidis*) instead to nourish yin and clear away heat for relieving dysphoria. In case of severe night sweat, add Muli (*Concha Ostreae*) and Fuxiaomai (*Fructus Tritici Levis*) to arrest sweating and restore peaceful mind. In case of frequent waking-up with a start, palpitation and dreaminess, pale tongue, taut and thready pulse, which are indicative of qi deficiency of the heart and gall bladder, add Dangshen (*Radix Codonopsis Pilosulae*) and Longchi (*Dens Draconis*) to supplement qi and relieve fright.

Elucidation：The syndrome is caused by deficiency of liver-blood, disturbance of deficiency-heat in the interior and mental irritability. It should be treated by nourishing blood and clearing away heat to restore peaceful mind and relieve dysphoria. With a larger dosage, the first ingredient acts as monarch drug with the action of nourishing blood and reinforcing the liver to tranquilize mind. Used as minister drugs, Ingredient No. 2 bears the effect

【用法】 水煎服。

【功用】 养血安神,清热除烦。

【临床应用】 适用于虚烦不眠证。症见失眠心悸,心烦不安,头目眩晕,咽干口燥,舌红,脉弦细。神经衰弱、心脏神经官能症、更年期综合征等见有上述症状者,可用本方治疗。方中茯苓,现临床多用茯神。若虚火较甚,烦热失眠多梦者,可去川芎,加生地黄、白芍药、黄连以养阴清热除烦;若盗汗较重者,可加牡蛎、浮小麦以敛汗宁心;若时有惊醒,心悸多梦,舌淡,脉弦细,属心胆气虚者,可加党参、龙齿以益气镇惊。

【方解】 本方证由肝血不足,虚热内扰,心神失宁所致,治宜养血安神,清热除烦之法。方中重用酸枣仁养血补肝,宁心安神,为君药。茯苓宁心安神,知母滋阴清热,合用以助君药除烦安神之功,同为臣药。川芎调畅气机,疏

of easing mind and No. 3 nourishing yin and clearing away heat, the combination of which promotes the function of the monarch drug in relieving dysphoria and tranquilizing mind. Ingredient No. 4 can regulate qi function and release the stagnated liver-qi. No. 1 and No. 4 are opposite and supplementary to each other, one being sour with astringent action and the other pungent with diaphoretic effect. Both play the role of adjuvant drugs, nourishing liver blood to invigorate the liver and dispersing stagnanted liver-qi to activate the liver. The last ingredient serves as guiding drug, which can clear away heat, regulate the middle-energizer and mediate the efficacy of other drugs.

Cautions: This recipe should not be used for excessive liver-fire manifesting dysphoria, insomnia, headache, flushed face, bitter mouth and dry throat, taut rapid and forceful pulse.

Tianwang Buxin Dan
(*Heavenly King Cardiotonic Pellet*)

Source: *Shesheng Mipou* (*Exposition on Health Conservation*).

Ingredients:

No. 1 Suanzaoren (*Semen Ziziphi Spinosae*) 60 g;

No. 2 Baiziren (*Semen Platycladi*) 60 g;

No. 3 Dangguishen (*Radix Angelicae Sinensis*) 60 g;

No. 4 Tianmendong (*Radix Asparagi*) 60 g;

No. 5 Maimendong (*Radix Ophiopogonis*) 60 g;

No. 6 Shengdihuang (*Radix Rehmanniae*) 120 g;

No. 7 Renshen (*Radix Ginseng*) 15 g;

No. 8 Danshen (*Radix Salviae Miltiorrhizae*) 15 g;

No. 9 Xuanshen (*Radix Scrophulariae*) 15 g;

No. 10 Baifuling (*Poria*) 15 g;

No. 11 Wuweizi (*Fructus Schisandrae*) 15 g;

No. 12 Yuanzhi (*Radix Polygalae*) 15 g;

达肝气,与酸枣仁相配,酸收与辛散同用,养肝血以补肝体,疏肝气以遂肝用,相反而相成,为佐药。甘草生用,清热和中,调和药性,为使药。

【注意事项】 肝火较甚,心烦失眠而头痛面赤,口苦咽干,脉弦数有力者,不宜使用本方。

天王补心丹

【方源】 《摄生秘剖》。

【组成】 酸枣仁、柏子仁、当归身、天门冬、麦门冬各60 g,生地黄120 g,人参、丹参、玄参、白茯苓、五味子、远志、桔梗各15 g。

No. 13 Jiegeng (*Radix Platycodi*) 15 g.

Administration: Grind the above into fine powder, which is then mixed with honey and made into pellets; coat the pellets with 9 - 15 g of Zhusha (*Cinnabaris*) after ground in water; take 6 - 9 g each time and twice daily with warm boiled water or with the decoction of longyanrou (*Arillus Longan*). Or decoct the above ingredients in water for oral application with dosages in proportion to the original recipe.

Actions: Invigorating the heart to tranquilize mind, nourishing yin and clearing away heat.

Clinical Application: This recipe is indicated for mental derangement due to yin deficiency and interior heat, marked by palpitation, insomnia, restlessness due to deficiency, mental fatigue, nocturnal emission, amnesia, feverish sensation in heart, palms and sores, orolingual boil, reddened tongue with little fur, thready and rapid pulse. It is applicable to neurosis, schizophrenia, heart disease, hyperthyroidism and others, the chief symptoms of which are mental derangement with feverish sensation in heart, palms and sores, reddened tongue with little fur, thready and rapid pulse. In case of severe insomnia, add Longchi (*Dens Draconis*) and Cishi (*Magnetitum*) to enhance the sedative effect of this recipe.

Elucidation: The syndrome is caused by deficiency of the heart and kidney, yin and blood deficiency, failure of yin to restrict yang and stirring up of deficiency fire in the interior. It should be treated by supplementing heart-qi to ease mind, nourishing yin to clear away heat. Moist in nature and with tonic action, ingredients No. 1, No. 2, No. 11 and No. 12 all possess the function of nourishing the heart and tranquilizing mind. Besides, No. 1 and No. 11, sour in flavor with astringent action, are the main components of this recipe, capable of restraining the loss

【用法】 共研细末,炼蜜为丸,用朱砂水飞 9~15 g,为衣,每次 6~9 g,温开水送下,或用龙眼肉煎汤送服,每日 2 次。亦可作汤剂,用量按原方比例酌定。

【功用】 补心安神,滋阴清热。

【临床应用】 适用于阴虚内热,神志不安证。症见心悸失眠,虚烦神疲,梦遗健忘,手足心热,口舌生疮,舌红少苔,脉细而数。神经衰弱、精神分裂症、心脏病、甲状腺功能亢进等以神志不安为主症,并伴手足心热,舌红少苔,脉细数者,可用本方治疗。若失眠较重者,可加龙齿、磁石以增强本方安神之功。

【方解】 本方证由心肾两虚,阴亏血少,阴不制阳,虚火内动所致,治宜补心安神,滋阴清热之法。方中酸枣仁、柏子仁、五味子、远志均质润性补,具养心安神之功,且酸枣仁、五味子味酸收敛,又可敛心气之耗散,为本方的主要组成部分。丹参清热凉血,除烦安神,可加强安神之功。生

and consumption of the heart-qi. Ingredient No. 8 can clear away heat from blood to cool blood, relieve dysphoria and restlessness and enhance the effect of restoring peaceful mind. No. 6, No. 9, No. 4 and No. 5 bear the action of nourishing yin and clearing away heat so as to restrain yang and relieve dysphoria. Ingredients No. 7 and No. 10 can replenish heart-qi, and No. 3 nourish the heart-blood to promote the tonic action of other sedative drugs. The last ingredient has the properties of guiding other drugs to exert their effects in the heart meridian and retain in the upper-energizer. Zhusha (*Cinnabaris*) is meant to further strengthen the effect of tranquilizing mind.

Cautions: Most ingredients in this recipe are apt to generate dampness, therefore it should not be taken for a long time by patients with deficiency cold syndrome of the spleen and stomach manifesting poor digestion, and retention of dampness and phlegm marked by greasy whitish fur.

地黄、玄参、天门冬、麦门冬滋阴清热,壮水制火而除烦热。人参、茯苓益心气;当归养心血,以助诸安神药补心之力。桔梗载药上浮,俾药力上入心经,留于上焦。丸以朱砂为衣,可进一步加强安神治标之效。

【注意事项】　本方滋腻之品较多,对于脾胃虚寒,胃纳欠佳,湿痰留滞,舌苔白腻者,均不宜长期服用。

Ganmai Dazao Tang
(*Decoction of Licorice,*
Blighted Wheat and Chinese Dates)

Source: *Jingui Yaolue* (*Synopsis of Prescriptions of the Golden Cabinet*).

Ingredients:

No. 1 Gancao (*Radix Glycyrrhizae*) 9 g;

No. 2 Xiaomai (*Fructus Tritici Aestivi*) 15 - 30 g;

No. 3 Dazao (*Fructus Ziziphi Jujubae*) 10 pcs.

Administration: Decoct the above drugs in water for oral application.

Actions: Invigorating the heart to tranquilize mind and regulating the middle-energizer to relieve pain.

Clinical Application: This recipe is indicated for intestinal dryness marked by absentmindedness, feeling like crying with grief, loss of self-control, dysphoria,

甘麦大枣汤

【方源】　《金匮要略》。

【组成】　甘草9 g,小麦15～30 g,大枣10 枚。

【用法】　水煎服。

【功用】　养心安神,和中缓急。

【临床应用】　适用于脏躁。症见精神恍惚,常悲伤欲哭,不能自主,心中烦乱,睡眠

unpeaceful sleep, even odd words and deeds, frequent yawning, reddish tongue with little fur, thready feeble and rapid pulse. It is applicable to hysteria, involuntional melancholia, neurosis and cardiac neurosis and others with the above symptoms. In case of marked yin deficiency manifesting dry mouth and throat, reddened tongue with little fur, add Shengdihuang (*Radix Rehmanniae*) and Baihe (*Bulbus Lilii*) to nourish heart-yin. If concomitant with deficiency of the liver-blood manifesting vertigo, taut and thready pulse, add Suanzaoren (*Semen Ziziphi Spinosae*) and Danggui (*Radix Angelicae Sinensis*) to nourish the liver-blood for easing mental stress.

Elucidation: The syndrome is the result of extreme anxiety or contemplation, leading to impairment of heart-yin and dysfunction of liver-qi. It should be treated by nourishing the heart and liver to relieve mental stress and pain. The second ingredient functions as monarch drug to nourish heart-yin and relieve dysphoria. The first ingredient in a big dosage is meant to invigorate heart-qi and regulate the middle-energizer and used as minister drug. The last ingredient acts as adjuvant drug with the effect of supplementing qi to regulate the middle-energizer, and moistening dryness to relieve pain. Combination of the three is a common recipe in the treatment of hysteria, which is sweet and moist in nature and mild in its tonic action.

Cautions: This recipe should be used with great caution in the case of severe phlegm-dampness with greasy whitish fur.

不安,甚则言行失常,呵欠频作,舌淡红苔少,脉细微数。癔病、更年期忧郁症、神经衰弱症、心脏神经官能症等见有上述症状者,可用本方治疗。若阴虚明显,口干咽燥,舌红少苔者,可加生地黄、百合以滋养心阴;若兼肝血不足,头目眩晕,脉弦细者,可加酸枣仁、当归以养肝补血安神。

【方解】 本方证由忧思过度,心阴受损,肝气失和所致,治宜养心安神,柔肝缓急之法。方中小麦补养心阴,除烦安神,为君药。重用甘草补养心气,和中缓急,为臣药。大枣益气和中,润燥缓急,为佐药。三药合用,味甘质润,补性平和,为养心调肝治疗脏躁之常用方剂。

【注意事项】 若痰湿较重,舌苔白腻者,慎用本方。

2.9 Prescriptions for Resuscitation

第九章
开窍剂

Those that are mainly composed of aromatic drugs with the action of inducing resuscitation and restoring consciousness in the treatment of coma are known as prescriptions for resuscitation.

Since coma may be the result of heat or cold pathogenic factors, prescriptions for resuscitation are accordingly subdivided into cold-natured prescriptions and warm-natured prescriptions for resuscitation.

The former consists mainly of drugs for restoring consciousness and those for clearing away heat and is indicated for unconsciousness due to heat, inclusive of retention of warm heat invading the pericardium and phlegm-heat blocking heart orifice. The latter is chiefly made up of drugs for inducing resuscitation and those for warming the interior and used for apoplexy, invasion by cold, qi stagnation or mental confusion due to phlegm.

Excess syndrome of stroke is characterized by coma, but it does not necessarily follow that all coma is caused by obstruction of the heart orifice. Therefore, in the application of this group of prescriptions, it is necessary to exclude coma with delirium brought about by qi prostration or by heat accumulation in the yangming meridian. Besides aromatic drugs in these prescriptions should not be decocted to prevent volatilization or reduced efficacy. That is why this group of prescriptions is often made into powder, pellets or pills, or injection. Moreover, this group

凡以芳香开窍药为主组成,具有开窍醒神作用,用于治疗神昏窍闭之证的方剂,统称开窍剂。

由于神昏窍闭证候有热闭与寒闭两种证型,因而开窍剂相应地分为凉开剂与温开剂两类。

凉开剂由开窍药配伍清热药为主组成,具有清热开窍作用,适用于温热之邪内陷心包,或痰热之邪闭阻心窍的热闭证。温开剂由开窍药配伍温里药为主组成,具有温通开窍作用,适用于中风、中寒或气郁、痰浊蒙蔽心窍的寒闭证。

窍闭证以神志昏迷为特征,但神志昏迷并非均由心窍闭阻而致,所以使用开窍剂时首先应排除因正气外脱(脱证)或热结阳明所导致的神昏谵语;其次,开窍剂中的芳香开窍药物不能加热煎煮,否则会致药性挥发,影响疗效,故一般开窍剂多制成散剂、丸剂或注射剂应用;第三,开窍剂

of prescriptions is likely to impair primordial qi and the primordial qi of fetus if taken for a long time because pungent flavor tends to disperse. Therefore they are rarely given to patients except for first aid. They should be stopped immediately when the expected result is obtained or used with great caution in pregnant women.

辛散走窜,久服易伤人元气,并有碍胎元,故临床多用于急救,且中病即止,不可久服,孕妇慎服。

2.9.1 Prescriptions for Inducing Resuscitation with Cold Drugs

第一节   凉开剂

Angong Niuhuang Wan
(*Bolus of Bezoar for Resuscitation*)

安宫牛黄丸

Source: *Wenbing Tiaobian* (*Treatise on Differentiation and Treatment of Seasonal Febrile Diseases*).

【方源】 《温病条辨》。

Ingredients:

No. 1 Niuhuang (*Calculus Bovis*) 30 g;

No. 2 Shuiniujiao (*Cornu Bubali*) (concentrated powder) 30 g [originally Xijiao (*Cornu Rhinocerotis*)];

No. 3 Huanglian (*Rhizoma Coptidis*) 30 g;

No. 4 Huangqin (*Radix Scutellariae*) 30 g;

No. 5 Zhizi (*Fructus Gardeniae*) 30 g;

No. 6 Yujin (*Radix Curcumae*) 30 g;

No. 7 Zhusha (*Cinnabaris*) 30 g;

No. 8 Xionghuang (*Realgar*) 30 g;

No. 9 Shexiang (*Moschus*) 7.5 g; (Generally use artificial one)

No. 10 Bingpian (*Borneolum*) 7.5 g;

No. 11 Zhenzhu (*Margarita*) 15 g.

【组成】 牛黄、水牛角(浓缩粉,原为犀角)、黄连、黄芩、栀子、郁金、朱砂、雄黄各30 g,麝香、冰片各7.5 g,珍珠15 g。

Administration: Grind the above ingredients into fine powder and mix the powder with honey to make boluses weighing 3 g each. Take one bolus each time and once daily, but twice or three times daily for severe case.

【用法】 共研细末,炼蜜为丸,每丸重3 g。每次 1 丸,每日 1 次,重证者,每日可服2~3 次。

Actions: Clearing away heat and inducing resuscitation, eliminating phlegm and toxin.

【功用】 清热开窍,豁痰解毒。

Clinical Application：This recipe is indicated for pathogenic heat invading the pericardium, marked by high fever, restlessness, coma with delirium, dry tongue and mouth, excessive sputum or saliva, reddened or deep-red tongue, rapid pulse. It is applicable to epidemic encephalitis B, epidemic cerebrospinal meningitis, toxic dysentery, uremia, cerebrovascular accident, hepatic coma and others, which belong to pathogenic heat invading the pericardium. In case of forceful pulse, it is advisable to take the boluses orally with the decoction of Jinyinhua (*Flos Lonicerae*) and Bohe (*Herba Menthae*) to enhance the effect of clearing away heat and inducing perspiration. In case of feeble pulse, take the boluses orally with the decoction of Renshen (*Radix Ginseng*) to promote the effect of strengthening body resistance. If concomitant with excess syndrome of the yangming fu organ manifesting coma and constipation, it is recommended to dissolve 2 boluses in water and mix it with 9 g powder of Dahuang (*Radix et Rhizoma Rhei*) for oral administration, which is known as Niuhuang Chengqi Tang.

Elucidation：The syndrome arises when warm heat invades the pericardium and phlegm-heat blocks the clear orifice. It should be treated by clearing away heat and eliminating phlegm. The first ingredient bears the action of clearing away heat from the heart, relieving convulsion, eliminating phlegm to restore consciousness. Ingredient No. 9 can remove obstruction from the twelve meridians and is good at inducing resuscitation. Both act as monarch drugs. Ingredients No. 2, No. 3, No. 4 and No. 5 possess the effect of clearing away heat and reducing fire and help the first ingredient clear away heat from the pericardium. Ingredients No. 10 and No. 6 are aromatic and can promote the effect of No. 9 in restoring mental activity. These six together serve as minister drugs. Ingredients

【临床应用】 适用于邪热内陷心包证。症见高热烦躁,神昏谵语,口干舌燥,痰涎壅盛,舌红或绛,脉数。流行性乙型脑炎、流行性脑脊髓膜炎、中毒性痢疾、尿毒症、脑血管意外、肝昏迷等属热闭心包者,可用本方治疗。若脉实有力者,可以金银花、薄荷煎汤送服,以增清热透邪之功;若脉虚无力者,可以人参煎汤送服,以助扶正祛邪之力;若兼有阳明腑实,见神昏,便秘者,可用安宫牛黄丸2粒化开,调大黄末9 g,内服,此即牛黄承气汤。

【方解】 本方证由温热之邪内陷心包,痰热蒙蔽清窍所致,治宜清热开窍,豁痰解毒之法。方中牛黄清心解毒,熄风定惊,豁痰开窍;麝香通行十二经,长于开窍醒神,两药配伍,清心开窍,共为君药。水牛角、黄连、黄芩、栀子清热泻火解毒,助牛黄以清心包之热;冰片、郁金芳香辟秽,通窍开闭,加强麝香开窍醒神之效,俱为臣药。朱砂、珍珠镇心安神,以除烦躁不安;雄黄助牛黄以豁痰解毒,均为佐

No. 7, No. 11 and No. 8 are used as adjuvant drugs, of which No. 7 and No. 11 are capable of tranquilizing mind and relieving restlessness and the last promoting No. 1 in eliminating phlegm. Honey regulates the stomach and serves as guiding drug. In the original recipe, gold foil was used as coating for the boluses, which is effective in restoring mentality. But it has presently been deleted from Chinese Pharmacopoeia.

药。以蜂蜜为丸,可和胃调中,以为使药。原方用金箔为衣,是取其重镇安神之效,现《中国药典》已将该药剔除。

Zixue Dan
(*Purple-Snow Pellet*)

Source: *Waitai Miyao* (*The Medical Secrets of an Official*).

Ingredients:

No. 1 Shigao (*Gypsum Fibrosum*) 1 500 g;

No. 2 Hanshuishi (*Calcitum*) 1 500 g;

No. 3 Huashi (*Talcum*) 1 500 g;

No. 4 Cishi (*Magnetitum*) 1 500 g;

No. 5 Shuiniujiao (*Cornu Bubali*) (concentrated powder) 5 000 g 〔originally Xijiao(*Cornu Rhinocerotis*)〕;

No. 6 Lingyangjiao (*Cornu Saigae Tattaricae*) 150 g;

No. 7 Qingmuxiang (*Radix Aristolochiae*) 150;

No. 8 Chenxiang (*Lignum Aquilariae Resinatum*) 150 g;

No. 9 Xuanshen (*Radix Scrophulariae*) 500 g;

No. 10 Shengma (*Rhizoma Cimicifugae*) 500 g;

No. 11 Zhigancao (*Radix Glycyrrhizae Praeparatae*) 250 g;

No. 12 Dingxiang (*Flos Caryophylli*) 30 g;

No. 13 Mangxiao (*Natrii Sulphas*) 1 000 g;

No. 14 Xiaoshi (*Nitrum*) 1 000 g;

No. 15 Shexiang (*Moschus*) 1.5 g; (Generally use artificial one)

No. 16 Zhusha (*Cinnabaris*) 90 g.

Administration: Grind the above into extremely

紫雪丹

【方源】《外台秘要》。

【组成】 石膏、寒水石、滑石、磁石各1 500 g,水牛角(浓缩粉,原为犀角)5 000 g,羚羊角、青木香、沉香各150 g,玄参、升麻各500 g,炙甘草250 g,丁香30 g,芒消、硝石各1 000 g,麝香1.5 g,朱砂90 g。

【用法】 共研极细末,混

fine powder and pack it in vials after mixed evenly, weighing 1.5 g each. Take orally 1.5 - 3 g each time and twice daily.

Actions: Restoring consciousness by clearing away heat, stopping wind to relieve convulsion.

Clinical Application: This recipe is indicated for syndrome of stirring of wind due to heat invading pericardium, marked by high fever, dysphoria, coma with delirium, convulsion, macular eruption, hematemesis, profuse thirst, parched lips and dryness of teeth, dark urine, constipation, reddened or deep-red tongue with dry yellowish fur, rapid and forceful or taut pulse. It is applicable to febrile and infectious diseases, such as epidemic cerebrospinal meningitis, crisis of epidemic encephalitis B, severe pneumonia, scarlet fever, and hematosepsis due to pyogenic infection. It is also indicated in high fever, coma and spasm as the result of hepatic coma, infantile hyperpyretic convulsion, and excessive heat from infantile measles.

Elucidation: The syndrome is caused by excessive heat invading the pericardium and wind stirring up due to excessive heat. It should be treated with the method of clearing away heat and calming wind to restore mentality and relieve convulsion. Ingredient No. 5 is capable of clearing away heat from the heart and blood, No. 6 calming the liver-wind to relieve convulsion, and No. 15 restoring consciousness with aromatic flavor. The three are monarch drugs in this recipe and together constitute the result of clearing away heat from the heart and liver, inducing resuscitation and relieving convulsion or spasm. Ingredients No. 1, No. 2 and No. 3 are extremely cold in nature and capable of clearing away heat, while No. 9 and No. 10 can eliminate heat and toxins, the five together playing the role of minister drugs. Ingredients No. 7, No.

匀装瓶,每瓶重1.5 g。每次1.5~3 g,每日 2 次。

【功用】　清热开窍,熄风止痉。

【临床应用】　适用于热邪内陷心包热盛动风证。症见高热烦躁,神昏谵语,痉厥,斑疹吐衄,口渴引饮,唇焦齿燥,尿赤便秘,舌红绛苔干黄,脉数有力或弦。各种发热性感染性疾病,如流行性脑脊髓膜炎、流行性乙型脑炎的极期、重症肺炎、猩红热、化脓性感染等疾患的败血症期,肝昏迷以及小儿高热惊厥、小儿麻疹热毒炽盛所致的高热神昏抽搐者,可用本方治疗。

【方解】　本方证由邪热炽盛,内陷心包,热盛动风所致,治宜清热开窍,熄风止痉之法。方中水牛角清心凉血解毒,羚羊角凉肝熄风止痉,麝香芳香开窍醒神,三药配伍,清心凉肝,开窍熄风,共为君药。石膏、寒水石、滑石大寒清热,玄参、升麻清热解毒,同为臣药。青木香、丁香、沉香行气通窍,并助麝香开窍醒神;朱砂、磁石重镇安神,兼助羚羊角平肝潜阳;芒消、硝石泄热散结,导热下行,俱为佐药。炙甘草益气安中,防寒凉

8 and No. 12 bear the action of promoting flow of qi and assisting No. 15 in restoring consciousness, while No. 16 and No. 4 are heavy in nature and can tranquilize mind and help No. 6 suppress the hyperactive liver-yang. Ingredients No. 13 and No. 14 possess the effect of purging and descending accumulated heat. These seven ingredients are used as adjuvant drugs. Ingredient No. 11 serves as guiding drug, which supplements qi and regulates the middle-energizer to prevent drugs of cold or cool nature from impairing the stomach on the one hand, and mediates the properties of other drugs on the other. Gold, which is heavy and capable of restoring consciousness, used to be included in the original recipe, but has now been deleted from *Chinese Pharmacopoeia*.

药碍胃之弊，又可调和药性，为佐使药。原方尚有黄金，乃取其重镇安神之功，现《中国药典》已将该药剔除。

Zhibao Dan
(*Bolus of Precious Drugs*)

至宝丹

Source: *Taiping Huimin Hejiju Fang* (*Benevolent Prescriptions from Taiping Pharmaceutical Bureau*).

【方源】《太平惠民和剂局方》。

Ingredients:

No. 1 Shuiniujiao (*Cornu Bubali*) (concentrated powder) 30 g 〔originally Xijiao(*Cornu Rhinocerotis*)〕;

No. 2 Zhusha (*Cinnabaris*) 30 g;

No. 3 Xionghuang (*Realgar*) 30 g;

No. 4 Daimao (*Carapax Eretmochelydis*) 30 g;

No. 5 Hupo (*Succinum*) 30 g;

No. 6 Shexiang (*Moschus*) 7.5 g; (Generally use artificial one)

No. 7 Bingpian (*Borneolum*) 7.5 g;

No. 8 Niuhuang (*Calculus Bovis*) 15 g;

No. 9 Anxixiang (*Benzoinum*) 45 g.

【组成】 水牛角（浓缩粉，原为犀角）、朱砂、雄黄、玳瑁、琥珀各30 g，麝香、冰片各7.5 g，牛黄15 g，安息香45 g。

Administration: Grind the above into fine powder and mix the powder with honey to make pills weiging 3 g each; take one pill each time and once daily with warm boiled water.

【用法】 共研细末，炼蜜为丸，每丸重3 g。每次 1 丸，温开水化服，每日 1 次。

Actions：Clearing away heat and dissolving turbid and toxic substances to induce resuscitation.

Clinical Application：This recipe is indicated for syndrome of phlegm-heat retaining in the pericardium, marked by coma, delirium, dysphoria, abundant expectoration, harsh respiration, reddened tongue with thick greasy yellowish fur, smooth and rapid pulse. It is applicable to epidemic cerebrospinal meningitis, epidemic encephalitis B, toxic dysentery, uremia, cerebrovascular accident, and hepatic coma and others which belong to phlegm-heat retaining in the pericardium. In case of deficiency of vital-qi with feeble pulse, take the pills with the decoction of Renshen (*Radix Ginseng*).

Elucidation：The syndrome is caused by retention of phlegm in the pericardium due to excessive heat. It should be treated by clearing away heat and removing phlegm. Ingredients No. 1 and No. 6 act as monarch drugs, and the combined application of both constitutes the result of clearing away heat and inducing resuscitation. Ingredients No. 7 and No. 9 are aromatic in flavor and capable of restoring consciousness, eliminating turbid substances and promoting the action of No. 6. Ingredients No. 8 and No. 4 can clear away heat and toxins, besides No. 8 can also eliminate phlegm to induce resuscitation and relive convulsion or spasm, and promote the effect of No. 1 in clearing away heat from blood. These four ingredients play the role of minister drug. Serving as adjuvant drug, No. 2 and No. 5 can relieving palpitation and tranquilize mind, and No. 3 eliminate phlegm and toxins. Gold and silver foils were used in the original recipe, which were meant to strengthen the effect of tranquilizing mind. But they have been deleted presently from Chinese Pharmacopoeia.

This recipe and Angong Niuhuang Wan, Zixue (*Pow-*

【功用】 清热开窍,化浊解毒。

【临床应用】 适用于痰热内闭心包证。症见神昏谵语,身热烦躁,痰盛气粗,舌红苔黄厚腻,脉滑数。流行性脑脊髓膜炎、流行性乙型脑炎、中毒性痢疾、尿毒症、脑血管意外、肝昏迷等属痰热内闭心包者,可用本方治疗。若正气不足,脉虚无力者,可以人参煎汤化服。

【方解】 本方证由邪热亢盛,痰浊内闭心包所致,治宜清热开窍,化浊解毒之法。方中水牛角与麝香合用,长于清热开窍,共为君药。冰片与安息香芳香开窍,辟秽化浊,助麝香芳香开窍走窜之力;牛黄、玳瑁清热解毒,牛黄又能豁痰开窍,熄风定惊,助水牛角清热凉血解毒之功,同为臣药。朱砂、琥珀镇心安神,雄黄豁痰解毒,均为佐药。原方尚用金箔、银箔,意在加强重镇安神之功,现《中国药典》已将其剔除。

本方与安宫牛黄丸、紫雪

der) are collectively named "Three Treasures", which share similar functions and chief indications and possess their respective advantages when their therapeutic effects are analyzed in detail. Angong Niuhuang Wan is good at clearing away heat and toxins and fit for cases with marked high fever and delirium as seen in unconsciousness due to heat. Zixue (*Powder*) excels in relieving convulsion and spasm and is fit for cases with convulsion and clonus. Zhibao Dan is effective in inducing resuscitation and eliminating turbid substances, thus suitable for cases with severe coma and thick greasy fur. They should be applied according to the condition of illness.

Cautions: This recipe comprises many drugs of aromatic, pungent and dry nature, which are likely to consume and impair yin and body fluid. Therefore, it should be used with great caution in patients with excessive deficiency of yin.

丹合称"三宝",其功用及主治证候相似,但细析三者功效又各有所长。其中安宫牛黄丸长于清热解毒,适宜于热闭证中高热、谵语明显者;紫雪丹长于熄风止痉,适宜于热闭证中痉厥抽搐明显者;至宝丹长于开窍化浊,适宜于热闭证中神昏较重,舌苔厚腻者。临床可根据病情有针对性地选择使用。

【注意事项】 本方芳香辛燥之品较多,有耗阴劫液之弊,阴亏较甚者慎用。

2.9.2 Warm-natured Prescriptions for Inducing Resuscitation

第二节 温开剂

Suhexiang Wan
(*Storax Pill*)

苏合香丸

Source: *Taiping Huimin Hejiju Fang* (*Benevolent Prescriptions from Taiping Pharmaceutical Bureau*).

【方源】《太平惠民和剂局方》。

Ingredients:

No.1 Suhexiang (*Resina Liquidambaris Orientalis*) 30 g;

No.2 Bingpian (*Borneolum*) 30 g;

No.3 Shexiang (*Moschus*) 60 g;(Generally use artificial one)

No.4 Anxixiang (*Benzoinum*) 60 g;

No.5 Qingmuxiang (*Radix Aristolochiae*) 60 g;

No.6 Xiangfu (*Rhizoma Cyperi*) 60 g;

No.7 Baitanxiang (*Lignum Santali*) 60 g;

【组成】 苏合香、冰片各30 g,麝香、安息香、青木香、香附、白檀香、沉香、丁香、荜茇各60 g,乳香、白术、诃子、水牛角、朱砂各60 g。

No. 8 Chenxiang (*Lignum Aquilariae Resinatum*) 60 g;

No. 9 Dingxiang (*Flos Caryophylli*) 60 g;

No. 10 Biba (*Fructus Piperis Longi*) 60 g;

No. 11 Ruxiang (*Resina Olibani*) 60 g;

No. 12 Baizhu (*Rhizoma Atractylodis Macrocephalae*) 60 g;

No. 13 Hezi (*Fructus Chebulae*) 60 g;

No. 14 Shuiniujiao (*Cornu Bubali*) 60 g [originally Xijiao (*Cornu Rhinocerotis*)];

No. 15 Zhusha (*Cinnabaris*) 60 g.

Administration: Grind the above into fine powder and mix the powder with honey to make pills weighing 3 g each; take one pill each time and once or twice daily with warm boiled water before meals.

Actions: Inducing resuscitation with aromatics, promoting the flow of qi to relieve pain.

Clinical Application: This recipe is indicated for syndrome of constipation due to pathogenic cold, marked by sudden faint, trismus, unconsciousness, whitish fur and slow pulse; also indicated in abrupt pain of the heart and abdomen and even syncope. It is applicable to unconsciousness from epidemic encephalitis B, hepatic coma, angina pectoris of coronary heart disease, myocardial infarction and others which belongs to cold stagnation in the heart orifice. It may also be used for chest or abdominal pain, which pertains to stagnation of cold and qi in the interior.

Elucidation: The syndrome results mostly from obstruction and disturbance of the mind due to cold, dampness, turbid substances, phlegm or stagnation of qi. It should be treated by inducing resuscitation and promoting flow of qi. Ingredients No. 1, No. 3, No. 2 and No. 4 are all aromatics and used as monarch drug, effective in restoring consciousness. As minister drug, No. 5, No. 7,

【用法】 共研细末,炼蜜为丸,每丸重3g。每次1丸,每日1～2次,饭前温开水送服。

【功用】 芳香开窍,行气止痛。

【临床应用】 适用于寒闭证。症见突然昏倒,牙关紧闭,不省人事,苔白,脉迟;亦治心腹卒痛,甚则昏厥。流行性乙型脑炎、肝昏迷、冠心病心绞痛、心肌梗死等神志昏迷属寒邪闭阻心窍者,或胸腹疼痛属寒凝气滞者,可用本方治疗。

【方解】 本方证多由寒邪、湿浊、痰湿或气郁闭阻,蒙蔽清窍,扰乱神明所致,治宜芳香开窍,行气止痛之法。方中苏合香、麝香、冰片、安息香等均为芳香开窍之品,合而用之,开窍醒神之功颇为显著。

No. 8, No. 11, No. 9 and No. 6 are pungent, warm and aromatic in nature and bear the properties of removing obstruction to promote flow of qi, dispelling cold to relieve pain, eliminating turbid substances to regulate blood circulation and help the monarch drugs in restoring consciousness. Ingredient No. 10 warms the middle-energizer to dispel cold and can enhance the effect of dispelling cold, relieving pain and removing obstruction when in compatibility with the above ten pungent aromatics. Ingredient No. 12 is capable of supplementing qi, invigorating the spleen, drying dampness and eliminating turbid substance, while No. 13 preserving qi by its astringent action. The use of No. 12 and No. 13 together with other aromatics can prevent the pungent aromatics from consuming vital-qi. Ingredient No. 14 has the effect of eliminating toxins from the heart, and No. 15 tranquilizing mind. The above five ingredients serve as adjuvant drugs in the recipe.

Zijin Ding (Also Named Yushu Dan)
(Knoxia and Moleplant Lozenage)

Source: *Pianyu Xinshu*.

Ingredients:

No. 1 Shancigu (*Bulbus Cremastrae*) 90 g;

No. 2 Hongdaji (*Radix Knoxiae*) 45 g;

No. 3 Qianjinzishuang (*frostlike powder of Semen Euphorbiae*) 30 g;

No. 4 Wubeizi (*Galla Chinensis*) 90 g;

No. 5 Shexiang (*Moschus*) 9 g; (Generally use artificial one)

No. 6 Xionghuang (*Realgar*) 30 g;

No. 7 Zhusha (*Cinnabaris*) 30 g.

Administration: Grind the above ingredients into fine powder and make it into pastilles with the paste of Nuomi (*Semen Oryzae Glutinosae*); then dry the pastilles

共为君药。青木香、白檀香、沉香、乳香、丁香、香附等辛温芳香,行气解郁,散寒止痛,辟秽化浊,通调血脉,并借其走窜之功以助君药开通窍闭之力,同为臣药。荜茇温中散寒,与上述十种辛香之品配伍,可增强散寒止痛开郁作用;白术补气健脾,燥湿化浊,诃子收涩敛气,与诸香药配伍,寓补气收敛于芳香走窜开窍之中,可防止辛香太过,耗散正气;水牛角清心解毒,朱砂重镇安神,俱为佐药。

紫金锭(又名玉枢丹)

【方源】《片玉心书》。

【组成】 山慈姑90 g,红大戟45 g,千金子霜30 g,五倍子90 g,麝香9 g,雄黄30 g,朱砂30 g。

【用法】 共研细末,以糯米糊制成锭,阴干。口服每次0.6~1.5 g,每日 2 次;外用醋

in the shade. Take orally 0.6 – 1.5 g each time and twice daily; or apply it externally over the affected parts after mixed with vinegar.

Actions: Eliminating phlegm for resuscitation, removing turbid and toxic substances, relieving swelling and pain.

Clinical Application: This recipe is indicated for sunstroke or seasonal pestilence, marked by epigastria and abdominal distension, fullness and pain, nausea, vomiting, diarrhea; or indicated in infantile phlegm syncope; or carbuncles, furuncles, boils; or bite wounds; or unknown swelling. This recipe can be taken orally for cases of acute gastroenteritis, food poisoning and dysentery, which are brought about by turbid substance or phlegm and manifested as thick greasy fur or grimy greasy fur. It can also be applied externally for acute pyogenic infection of the skin and soft tissues.

Elucidation: The syndrome is caused by functional disorder of the stomach and intestines in ascending and descending due to attack by turbid substances or phlegm. It should be treated by eliminating phlegm for resuscitation, removing turbid and toxic substances and relieving swelling and pain. The first ingredient is capable of clearing away heat and relieving swelling, eliminating phlegm and mass, and removing toxins. Ingredient No. 5, aromatic in flavor, can induce resuscitation and promote the circulation of qi to relieve pain. Both play the role of monarch drugs. Ingredients No. 3 and No. 2 are used as minister drugs, assisting the monarch drugs in eliminating phlegm, relieving swelling and removing mass. Ingredient No. 4 has an astringent action and can relieve diarrhea. No. 6 can eliminate turbid and toxic substances and No. 7 tranquilize mind. The above three act as adjuvant drugs. All ingredients together can restore consciousness, elimi-

磨,调敷患处。

【功用】　化痰开窍,辟秽解毒,消肿止痛。

【临床应用】　适用于中暑时疫,症见脘腹胀闷疼痛,恶心呕吐,泄泻;或小儿痰厥;或疔疮疖肿,虫咬损伤,无名肿毒。急性胃肠炎、食物中毒、痢疾等由秽恶痰浊之邪引起,舌苔厚腻或浊腻者,可以本方内服;皮肤及软组织急性化脓性感染可用本方外敷。

【方解】　本方证由感受秽恶痰浊之邪,肠胃气机闭塞,升降失常所致,治宜化痰开窍,辟秽解毒,消肿止痛之法。方中重用山慈姑清热消肿,化痰散结,并能解毒;配伍麝香芳香开窍,行气止痛,共为君药。千金子霜、红大戟助君药逐痰消肿散结,同为臣药。五倍子涩肠止泻,雄黄化痰辟秽解毒,朱砂重镇安神,俱为佐药。诸药配伍,内服可开窍化痰,辟秽解毒,外用可清热消肿,散结止痛。

nate phlegm and toxins if taken orally, and can clear away heat, relieve swelling and pain, and remove mass if applied externally.

Cautions: Ingredients No. 3 and No. 2 are drastic and poisonous in property, and therefore must not be taken with overdose or for a long time.

【注意事项】 续随子霜、红芽大戟药性峻猛而有毒,故服用本方时不可过量或久服。

2.10 Prescriptions for Regulating the Flow of Qi

第十章
理气剂

Prescriptions for regulating the flow of qi refer to those that mainly comprise drugs with the action of promoting the normal flow of qi and are applied in functional disorder of qi.

Since functional disorder of qi may manifest either qi stagnation or reversed flow of qi, this group of prescriptions is subdivided accordingly into prescriptions for promoting the flow of qi and those for descending the upward adverse flow of qi.

The former is chiefly composed of drugs, which bear the action of promoting the functional activities of qi and relieving flatulence, and fit for qi stagnation syndrome of the spleen, stomach and liver. The latter, however, consists mainly of drugs that can check the upward adverse flow of qi and is indicated for syndromes of upward flow of lung-qi and stomach-qi.

Most ingredients of this group of prescriptions are pungent, warm, aromatic and dry in nature and apt to consume qi and body fluid. Therefore, they should not be taken overdose or for long time. Besides, they should be used carefully for the aged, the weak, those with hyperactivity of fire due to yin deficiency, or pregnant women.

凡以理气药为主组成,具有调理气机作用,用于治疗气机失常病证的方剂,统称理气剂。

由于气机失常主要表现为气滞与气逆两种形式,因而理气剂相应地分为行气剂与降气剂两类。

行气剂由行气药为主组成,具有行气解郁,消痞除满作用,适用于脾胃气滞与肝郁气滞证候。降气剂由降气药为主组成,具有降逆下气,平喘止呕作用,适用于肺气上逆与胃气上逆证候。

理气剂的组成药物大多辛温香燥,易于耗气伤津,故不可过量或过久服用;年老体弱、阴虚火旺以及孕妇等慎用。

2.10.1   Prescriptions for Promoting the Flow of Qi

Yueju Wan
(**Pill for Relieving Stagnation**)

Source: *Danxi Xinfa* (*Danxi's Experience on Medicine*).

Ingredients:

No. 1 Cangzhu (*Rhizoma Atractylodis*);

No. 2 Xiangfu (*Rhizoma Cyperi*);

No. 3 Chuanxiong (*Rhizoma Ligustici Chuanxiong*);

No. 4 Shenqu (*Massa Fermentata Medicinalis*);

No. 5 Zhizi (*Fructus Gardeniae*);

All in equal dosage.

Administration: Grind the above into fine powder and make it into pills with water; take orally 6 - 9 g each time and twice daily with warm boiled water. Or decoct the above drugs in water with dosages in proportion to the original recipe.

Actions: Promoting the flow of qi to eliminate stagnation.

Clinical Applicantion: This recipe is indicated for syndromes of stagnancy of qi, blood, phlegm, fire, dampness or food, marked by chest distress and fullness, epigastric and abdominal distension and pain, acid regurgitation, vomiting, and indigestion. It is applicable to the above symptoms as seen in gastric neurosis, gastroduodenal ulcer, chronic gastritis, cholelithiasis, cholecystitis, hepatitis, intercostal neuralgia, dysmenorrhea, and irregular menstruation. In case of excessive stagnancy of qi, enlarge the dosage of No. 2, and add Muxiang (*Radix Aucklandiae*) and Zhike (*Fructus Aurantii*) to promote the circulation of qi. In case of dominant blood stasis, enlarge

第一节　行气剂

越鞠丸

【方源】《丹溪心法》。

【组成】　苍术、香附、川芎、神曲、栀子各等份。

【用法】　共研细末，水泛为丸，每次 6～9 g，温开水送下，每日 2 次。亦可作汤剂，用量按原方比例酌定。

【功用】　行气解郁。

【临床应用】　适用于气、血、痰、火、湿、食六郁证。症见胸膈痞闷，脘腹胀痛，吞酸呕吐，饮食不消。胃神经官能症、胃及十二指肠溃疡、慢性胃炎、胆石症、胆囊炎、肝炎、肋间神经痛、妇女痛经、月经不调等见有上述症状者，可用本方治疗。若气郁偏重者，可重用香附，酌加木香、枳壳以行气；若血郁偏重者，可重用川芎，酌加桃仁、红花以活血；

the dosage of No. 3 and add Taoren (*Semen Persicae*) and Honghua (*Flos Carthami*) to promote blood circulation. In case of retention of dampness, enlarge the dosage of No. 1 and add Fuling (*Poria*) and Zexie (*Rhizoma Alismatis*) for diuretic purpose. In case of indigestion, enlarge the dosage of No. 4 and add Shanzha (*Fructus Crataegi*) and Maiya (*Fructus Hordei Germinatus*) to promote digestion. In case of fire stagnancy, enlarge the dosage of No. 5 and add Huangqin (*Radix Scutellariae*) and Huanglian (*Rhizoma Coptidis*) to purge away fire. In case of phlegm retention, add Banxia (*Rhizoma Pinelliae*) and Gualou (*Fructus Trichosanthis*) to remove phlegm.

Elucidation: The syndrome is the result of qi stagnation of the liver and spleen. Prolonged stagnation of liver-qi or failure of the liver in its dispersing function leads to dysfunction of the spleen in transportation and transformation. It further causes phlegm generation from dampness, indigestion or obstructed circulation of blood or fire transformation. Of the six stagnancy syndromes, qi stagnation originates first. Therefore treatment should focus on promoting the flow of qi to relieve stagnation. No. 2 is the monarch drug, aimed at promoting the flow of qi. With the effect of removing blood stasis to promote blood flow, No. 3 can also help No. 2 carry out its action. No. 5 is meant to clear away heat and purge away fire, No. 1 to activate the spleen by removing dampness, and No. 4 to promote digestion. These four ingredients function as minister and adjuvant drugs. Retention of phlegm usually generates from dampness in the spleen and is also related to qi, fire and food. When a smooth flow of qi occurs, all the other stagnancy syndromes will be relieved. This is what is called in TCM "treatment aiming at the root cause of a disease".

Cautions: Although this recipe is used in the

【方解】　本方证是由肝脾气机郁滞而致。肝郁日久，或因疏泄失职而致脾失健运，聚湿生痰，食滞不化，或致血行不畅，或郁而化火，以致气、血、痰、火、食、湿六郁并见，因而诸郁之中是以气郁为先，治法应以行气解郁为主。方中香附行气解郁，以治气郁，为君药。川芎活血祛瘀，以治血郁，又可助香附行气解郁；栀子清热泻火，以治火郁；苍术燥湿运脾，以治湿郁；神曲消食导滞，以治食郁，共为臣佐药。痰郁多由脾湿所生，亦与气、火、食有关，气机流畅，诸郁得解，则痰郁亦随之而消，此亦治病求本之意。

【注意事项】　本方虽通

若湿郁偏重者，可重用苍术，酌加茯苓、泽泻以利湿；若食郁偏重者，可重用神曲，酌加山楂、麦芽以消食；若火郁偏重者，可重用栀子，酌加黄芩、黄连以泻火；若痰郁偏重者，可酌加半夏、瓜蒌以祛痰。

treatment of the above six stagnancy syndromes, its com-patibility is supposed chiefly to present a fundamental principle in treating such syndromes. Clinically it should be dealt with in accordance with the order of severity of various stagnancy syndromes.

治六郁,但组方配伍重在示人以治郁大法,临床应根据诸郁的轻重主次加以灵活化裁。

Chaihu Shugan San
(*Bupleurum Powder for Relieving Liver Qi*)

柴胡疏肝散

Source: *Jingyue Quanshu* (*Complete Works of Zhang Jingyue*).

【方源】《景岳全书》。

Ingredients:

No. 1 Jupi (*Pericarpium Citri Reticulatae*) 6 g;

No. 2 Chaihu (*Radix Bupleuri*) 6 g;

No. 3 Chuanxiong (*Rhizoma Ligustici Chuanxiong*) 5 g;

No. 4 Xiangfu (*Rhizoma Cyperi*) 5 g;

No. 5 Zhike (*Fructus Aurantii*) 5 g;

No. 6 Shaoyao (*Radix Paeoniae*) 5 g;

No. 7 Zhigancao (*Radix Glycyrrhizae Praeparatae*) 3 g.

【组成】 橘皮、柴胡各6 g,川芎、香附、枳壳、芍药各5 g,炙甘草3 g。

Administration: Decoct the above ingredients in water for oral application.

【用法】 水煎服。

Actions: Soothing the liver to relieve stagnation of liver-qi, and promoting the flow of qi to alleviate pain.

【功用】 疏肝解郁,行气止痛。

Clinical Applicantion: This recipe is indicated for syndrome of stagnancy of liver-qi, marked by distension and pain of the hypochondrium, epigastrium and abdo-men, belching and sighing, taut pulse. It is applicable to hepatitis, chronic gastritis, and intercostal neuralgia and others, which pertain to stagnancy of liver-qi. Clinically Baishaoyao (*Radix Paeoniae Alba*) is often used as No. 6. In case of sharp pain, add Danggui (*Radix Angelicae Sinensis*) and Yujin (*Radix Curcumae*) to enhance the action of promoting the circulation of qi and blood to re-lieve pain. In case of fire transformation from stagnated liver-qi with dry mouth and reddened tongue, add Zhizi (*Fructus Gardeniae*) and Chuanlianzi (*Fructus Meliae*

【临床应用】 适用于肝气郁滞证。症见胁肋脘腹胀痛,嗳气太息,脉弦。肝炎、慢性胃炎、肋间神经痛等属肝郁气滞者,可用本方治疗。方中芍药,现临床常用白芍药。若疼痛较甚者,可加当归、郁金以增强行气活血止痛之力;若肝郁化火,口干舌红者,可加栀子、川楝子以清肝泻火。

Toosendan) to purge away fire from the liver.

Elucidation：The syndrome is the result of dysfunction of the liver due to mental depression and qi stagnation, which should be treated by dispersing the stagnated liver-qi to relieve pain. Ingredient No. 2 is good at this respect and used as monarch drug. No. 4 is capable of regulating the flow of qi and No. 3 promoting the circulation of both qi and blood, which together function as minister drugs. No. 5 and No. 1 bear the action of regulating qi and removing stagnation, while No. 6 and No. 7 possess the effect of nourishing blood and the liver and relieving spasm and pain, the four serving as adjuvant drugs. No. 7 also plays the part of guiding drug because it can mediate the properties of other ingredients.

Banxia Houpo Tang
(*Decoction of Pinellia and Magnolia Bark*)

Source：*Jingui Yaolue* (*Synopsis of Prescriptions of the Golden Cabinet*).

Ingredients：

No. 1 Banxia (*Rhizoma Pinelliae*) 12 g;

No. 2 Houpo (*Cortex Magnoliae Officinalis*) 9 g;

No. 3 Fuling (*Poria*) 12 g;

No. 4 Shengjiang (*Rhizoma Zingiberis Recens*) 15 g;

No. 5 Suye (*Folium Perillae*) 6 g.

Administration：Decoct the above ingredients in water for oral application.

Actions：Promoting the flow of qi to remove stagnation, descending the adverse flow of qi to eliminate phlegm.

Clinical Applicantion：This recipe is indicated for globus hystericus, marked by a subjective sensation as if something stuffed in the throat, which can neither be thrown up nor swallowed down, chest distress, cough or vomiting, greasy whitish fur, taut and smooth pulse. It is

【方解】　本方证由情志不遂，肝失疏泄，气郁不畅所致，治宜疏肝解郁，行气止痛之法。方中柴胡长于疏肝解郁，为君药。香附理气疏肝，川芎行气活血，共助柴胡以解郁止痛，为臣药。枳壳、橘皮理气行滞，芍药、甘草养血柔肝，缓急止痛，均为佐药。甘草并可调和药性，兼作使药。

半夏厚朴汤

【方源】　《金匮要略》。

【组成】　半夏12 g，厚朴9 g，茯苓12 g，生姜15 g，紫苏叶6 g。

【用法】　水煎服。

【功用】　行气散结，降逆化痰。

【临床应用】　适用于梅核气。症见咽中如有物阻，咯吐不出，吞咽不下，胸膈满闷，或咳或呕，舌苔白腻，脉弦滑。瘿病、胃神经官能症、慢性咽

applicable to hysteria, gastric neurosis, chronic pharyngitis, chronic bronchitis, and esophagismus, which pertain
to qi stagnation and phlegm accumulation with chief manifestations as sensation of something stuffed in the throat,
which can neither be spat out nor swallowed down, greasy
whitish fur, taut and smooth pulse. In case of excessive
stagnation of qi, add Xiangfu (*Rhizoma Cyperi*) and Yujin
(*Radix Curcumae*) to promote the effect of regulating flow
of qi. In case of hypochondriac pain, add Chuanlianzi (*Fructus Meliae Toosendan*) and Yanhusuo (*Rhizoma Corydalis*)
to disperse the stagnated liver-qi. In case of sore throat,
add Xuanshen (*Radix Scrophulariae*) and Jiegeng (*Radix Platycodi*) to eliminate toxin and promote the dispersive function of the lung for relieving sore throat.

Elucidation: The syndrome is caused by combined
stagnancy of phlegm and qi in the throat and disorder of
dispersing and descending functions of the lung and stomach. It should be treated by promoting the circulation of
qi, sending down the adversely rising qi and eliminating
phlegm. The first ingredient is capable of eliminating
phlegm, descending the adversely rising qi and regulating
the stomach. Ingredient No. 2 bears the effect of promoting the flow of qi and relieving fullness. Both act as monarch drugs, with one removing stagnation of qi and the
other eliminating phlegm. No. 3 has the function of invigorating the spleen and promoting diuresis, and helps No. 1
remove phlegm. Aromatic in nature and with diaphoretic
action, No. 5 can promote the effect of No. 2 in regulating
the flow of qi. Both function as minister drugs. No. 4 is
used as adjuvant drug, which regulates the stomach to relieve vomiting, and helps No. 1 send down the adversely
rising qi.

Cautions: Warm and dry in nature, this recipe
should not be used in case of fire transformation or lack of

炎、慢性支气管炎、食管痉挛
等以咽如物阻,吞吐不得,苔
白腻,脉弦滑为主症,属气滞
痰凝者,可用本方治疗。若气
郁较甚者,可加香附、郁金以
助行气解郁;若胁肋疼痛者,
可加川楝子、延胡索以疏肝理
气止痛;若咽痛者,可加玄参、
桔梗以解毒散结,宣肺利咽。

【方解】 本方证由痰气
互结咽喉,肺胃宣降失常所
致,治宜行气散结,降逆化痰
之法。方中半夏化痰散结,降
逆和胃;厚朴行气开郁,下气
除满,两药合用,一行气滞,一
化痰结,共为君药。茯苓健脾
渗湿,助半夏化痰;紫苏叶芳
香疏散,助厚朴理气,同为臣
药。生姜和胃止呕,助半夏和
中降逆,为佐药。

【注意事项】 本方药性
温燥,梅核气有化火之象,或

body fluid due to yin impairment.

由阴伤津少而致者,不宜使用。

Gualou Xiebai Baijiu Tang
(*Decoction of Trichosanthes and Macrostem with Liquor*)

瓜蒌薤白白酒汤

Source：*Jingui Yaolue*（*Synopsis of Prescriptions of the Golden Cabinet*）.

【方源】《金匮要略》。

Ingredients：

No. 1 Quangualou（*Fructus Trichosanthis*）12 g;

No. 2 Xiebai（*Bulbus Allii Macrostemi*）9 g;

No. 3 Liquor 30 - 60 ml.

【组成】　全瓜蒌12 g,薤白9 g,白酒30~60 ml。

Administration：Put in proper amount of water to decoct the above drugs for oral use.

【用法】　加水适量煎服。

Actions：Activating yang to remove stagnation, promoting the circulation of qi to eliminate phlegm.

【功用】　通阳散结,行气祛痰。

Clinical Applicantion：This recipe is indicated for chest bi-syndrome（obstruction of qi in the chest）, marked by vague pain over the chest, chest pain radiating to the back if severe, dyspnea, cough with sputum, shortness of breath, greasy whitish fur, deep and taut or tense pulse. It is applicable to angina pectoris of coronary heart disease, non-suppurative costochondritis, intercostal neuralgia, and other diseases, which pertain to obstruction of the chest-yang by phlegm and are chiefly manifested as chest pain, shortness of breath, whitish fur and taut pulse. In case of excessive phlegm with chest fullness and thick greasy fur, add Banxia（*Rhizoma Pinelliae*）to dispel phlegm, forming another recipe entitled Gualou Xiebai Banxia Tang. In case of excessive stagnation of qi with subjective sensation of qi rising upward, add Houpo（*Cortex Magnoliae Officinalis*）, Zhishi（*Fructus Aurantii Immaturus*）and Guizhi（*Ramulus Cinnamomi*）to regulate the flow of qi and check the adversely rising qi, which is known as Zhishi Xiebai Guizhi Tang. In case of

【临床应用】　适用于胸痹。症见胸部隐痛,甚至胸痛彻背,喘息咳唾,短气,舌苔白腻,脉沉弦或紧。冠心病心绞痛、非特异性肋软骨炎、肋间神经痛等以胸痛、短气、苔白、脉弦为主症,属痰气痹阻、胸阳不振者,可用本方治疗。或痰浊较甚,胸闷苔厚腻者,可加半夏以助祛痰散结之力,即瓜蒌薤白半夏汤;若气滞较甚,自觉气逆上冲者,可加厚朴、枳实、桂枝以行气降逆平冲,即枳实薤白桂枝汤;若寒邪较甚,胸背彻痛,脉沉迟者,可加干姜、桂枝、附子以通阳散寒。

dominant cold with manifestations as chest pain radiating to the back and deep slow pulse, add Ganjiang (*Rhizoma Zingiberis*), Guizhi (*Ramulus Cinnnamomi*) and Fuzi (*Radix Aconiti Praeparatae*) to activate yang and dispel cold.

Elucidation: The syndrome is caused by deficiency of chest-yang, leading to accumulation of phlegm in the interior and disorder of qi activity. It should be treated by activating yang, removing obstruction, promoting flow of qi and eliminating phlegm. The first ingredient is the monarch drug, which resolves phlegm, promotes the circulation of qi, and relieves stuffiness of the chest. No. 2 acts as minister drug, which activates yang and relieves stagnation, promotes the flow of qi and relieves pain. These two ingredients supplement each other and are used as primary drugs for treating obstruction of qi in the chest, with one removing stagnation of phlegm, and the other activating yang. Pungent and warm in nature, the last ingredient is capable of regulating qi and blood, performing its efficacy to strengthen the effect of activating the chest yang, and serves as adjuvant drug.

Cautions: If liquor is intolerable for the patient, it may either be applied with reduced amount or disused.

【方解】 本方证由胸阳不振,痰浊内阻,气机不畅所致,治宜通阳散结,行气祛痰之法。方中全瓜蒌化痰利气,宽胸散结,为君药。薤白通阳散结,行气止痛,为臣药。两药相配,一祛痰结,一通阳气,相辅相成,为治胸痹之要药。白酒辛温,和气血,行药势,以加强宣通胸阳之力,为佐使药。

【注意事项】 若病人不能饮酒,方中白酒可酌情减量或不用。

Zhishi Xiaopi Wan
(*Pill of Immature Bitter Orange for Relieving Stuffiness*)

Source: *Lanshi Micang (Secret Record of Orchids Cabinet)*.

Ingredients:

No. 1 Ganjiang (*Rhizoma Zingiberis*) 3 g;

No. 2 Zhigancao (*Radix Glycyrrhiae Praeparatae*) 6 g;

No. 3 Maiya (*Fructus Hordei Germinatus*) 6 g;

No. 4 Fuling (*Poria*) 6 g;

No. 5 Baizhu (*Rhizoma Atractylodis Macrocephalae*) 6 g;

枳实消痞丸

【方源】 《兰室秘藏》。

【组成】 干姜3g,炙甘草、麦芽、茯苓、白术各6g,半夏、人参各9g,厚朴12g,枳实、黄连各15g。

No. 6 Banxia (*Rhizoma Pinelliae*) 9 g;

No. 7 Renshen (*Radix Ginseng*) 9 g;

No. 8 Houpo (*Cortex Magnoliae Officinalis*) 12 g;

No. 9 Zhishi (*Fructus Aurantii Immaturus*) 15 g;

No. 10 Huanglian (*Rhizoma Coptidis*) 15 g.

Administration: Grind the above drugs into fine powder and make it into pills, take 6 - 9 g each time and twice or three times daily with warm boiled water. Or prepare the above drugs into decoction with dosages in proportion to the original recipe.

Actions: Promoting the circulation of qi to relieve fullness, and strengthening the spleen and harmonizing the stomach.

Clinical Applicantion: This recipe is indicated for syndromes of combination of cold and heat and qi stagnation due to deficiency of the spleen, marked by epigastric and abdominal fullness, no appetite, lassitude and weakness, loose stool, greasy yellowish fur, and thready pulse. It is applicable to chronic gastritis, chronic bronchitis, gastric neurosis and others, which are chiefly manifested as epigastric fullness, poor appetite, lassitude, and greasy yellowish fur, and are ascribed as simultaneous occurrence of cold and heat with excess and heat syndrome being dominant. In case of marked interior cold with preference for warmth and aversion to cold, reduce the dosage of the last ingredient and increase that of No. 1 instead or add Gaoliangjiang (*Rhizoma Alpiniae Officinarum*) and Rougui (*Cortex Cinnamomi*) to warm the middle-energizer and dispel cold.

Elucidation: The syndrome results from combination of cold and heat, and deficiency and excess. This is the result of deficiency of the spleen-yang and disorder of qi activity concomitant with damp heat. It should be treated by promoting the flow of qi to relieve fullness, and

【用法】　共研细末, 为丸。每次6~9 g, 温开水送下, 每日 2~3 次。亦可作汤剂, 用量按原方比例酌定。

【功用】　行气消痞, 健脾和胃。

【临床应用】　适用于脾虚气滞, 寒热错杂证。症见脘腹痞满, 不欲饮食, 倦怠乏力, 大便不调, 苔腻微黄, 脉细。慢性胃炎、慢性支气管炎、胃肠神经官能症等以心下痞满, 食少倦怠, 苔腻微黄为主症, 属脾虚气滞, 寒热错杂, 且实多虚少, 热重寒轻者, 可用本方治疗。若里寒较著, 喜温畏寒者, 可减黄连用量, 重用干姜, 或再加高良姜、肉桂以温中散寒。

【方解】　本方所治乃脾阳不足, 气机失畅, 兼挟湿热而成寒热互结、虚实错杂之证, 治宜行气消痞, 健脾和胃之法。方中枳实行气消痞, 为

strengthening the spleen and stomach. Ingredient No. 9 acts as monarch drug to promote the flow of qi and relieve fullness. No. 8 functions as minister drug with the effect of descending qi and relieve fullness. The combination of both is meant to double the effect of relieving fullness by regulating the circulation of qi. No. 10 is capable of clearing away heat and dampness, No. 6 regulating the stomach, and No. 1 warming the middle-energizer and dispelling cold, the combination of which achieves the result of adjusting cold and heat with pungent and bitter drugs. No. 3 possesses the action of promoting digestion and regulating the stomach, while No. 7, No. 5, No. 4 and No. 2 bear the effect of reinforcing the spleen, eliminating dampness and regulating the middle-energizer, the five drugs serving as adjuvant drugs. No. 2 also plays the role of guiding drug to mediate drug properties. The compatibility of all ingredients achieves the result of both reducing and reinforcement, both warming and clearing, with emphasis laid on reducing and clearing effects.

Cautions: This should not be used for qi stagnation of the spleen and stomach without manifestation as deficiency symptom of the middle-energizer.

Houpo Wenzhong Tang
(*Magnolia Decoction for Warming the Middle-energizer*)

Source: *Neiwaishang Bianhuo Lun* (*Differentiation on Endogenous and Exogenous Diseases*).

Ingredients:

No. 1 Houpo (*Cortex Magnoliae Officinalis*) 30 g;

No. 2 Jupi (*Pericarpium Citri Reticulatae*) 30 g;

No. 3 Zhigancao (*Radix Glycyrrhizae Praeparatae*) 15 g;

No. 4 Fuling (*Poria*) 15 g;

No. 5 Caodoukou (*Semen Alpiniae*) 15 g;

君药。厚朴下气除满,为臣药。两药合用以增强行气消痞除满之功。黄连清热燥湿,半夏和胃开结,干姜温中祛寒,三药相伍,辛开苦降,调其寒热;麦芽消食和胃,人参、白术、茯苓、炙甘草补中健脾,祛湿和中,俱为佐药。炙甘草调和药性,兼作使药。诸药配伍,消补兼施,温清并用,且消重于补,清大于温。

【注意事项】 脾胃气滞而无中虚之象者,不宜使用本方。

厚朴温中汤

【方源】 《内外伤辨惑论》。

【组成】 厚朴、橘皮各30 g,炙甘草、茯苓、草豆蔻、木香各15 g,干姜2 g。

No. 6 Muxiang (*Radix Aucklandiae*) 15 g;

No. 7 Ganjiang (*Rhizoma Zingiberis*) 2 g.

Administration：Grind the above drugs into fine powder, decoct 9 g each time in water for oral application with 3 slices of fresh ginger added.

Actions：Promoting flow of qi and warming the middle-energizer, drying dampness and relieving fullness.

Clinical Applicantion：This recipe is indicated for syndrome of qi stagnation due to accumulation of dampness, marked by epigastric and abdominal distension and fullness or pain, no appetite, greasy whitish fur, deep and taut pulse. It is applicable to chronic gastritis, chronic enteritis, gastric ulcer, leukorrhagia and others, which pertain to accumulation of dampness in the middle-energizer and qi stagnation of the spleen and stomach. If concomitant with heaviness of the body and limb edema, add Dafu-pi (*Pericarpium Arecae*) to descend qi and induce diuresis. In case of sharp pain with cold sensation in the abdomen, add Rougui (*Cortex Cinnamomi*) and Gaoliangjiang (*Rhizoma Alpiniae Officinarum*) to warm the middle-energizer and dispel cold so as to relieve pain.

Elucidation：The syndrome is caused by accumulation of cold and dampness in the middle-energizer and qi stagnation of the spleen and stomach. It should be treated by promoting flow of qi, warming the middle-energizer, drying dampness and relieving fullness. The first ingredient is capable of promoting circulation of qi and drying dampness, and used as monarch drug. No. 5 functions as minister drug, which warms the middle-energizer and dispels cold, drys dampness and activates the spleen. No. 2 and No. 6 help No. 1 relieve fullness, while No. 7 and fresh ginger assist No. 5 in warming the stomach and spleen to dispel cold and relieve pain. No. 4 has the function of reinforcing the spleen and promoting diuresis.

【用法】　共研粗末,每次9 g,加生姜3片,水煎服。

【功用】　行气温中,燥湿除满。

【临床应用】　适用于湿阻气滞证。症见脘腹胀满或疼痛,不思饮食,舌苔白腻,脉沉弦。慢性胃炎、慢性肠炎、胃溃疡、妇女带下量多等属湿阻中焦,脾胃气滞者,可用本方治疗。若兼身重肢体浮肿者,可加大腹皮以下气利水;若腹中冷痛较甚者,可加肉桂、高良姜以温中散寒止痛。

【方解】　本方证由寒湿中阻,脾胃气滞所致,治宜行气温中,燥湿除满之法。方中厚朴行气燥湿,为君药。草豆蔻温中散寒,燥湿运脾,为臣药。陈皮、木香助厚朴行气宽中以消胀除满;干姜、生姜助草豆蔻温胃暖脾以散寒止痛;茯苓健脾助运,渗利湿邪,俱为佐药。甘草调和药性,为使药。

These five ingredients together play the part of adjuvant drugs. No. 3 is used as guiding the to mediate the properties of other drugs.

Tiantai Wuyao San
(*Tiantai Powder of Linderae*)

Source: *Yixue Faming* (*Medical Inventions*).

Ingredients:

No. 1 Wuyao (*Radix Linderae*) 15 g;

No. 2 Muxiang (*Radix Aucklandiae*) 15 g;

No. 3 Xiaohuixiang (*Fructus Foeniculi*) 15 g;

No. 4 Qingpi (*Pericarpium Citri Reticulatae Viride*) 15 g;

No. 5 Gaoliangjiang (*Rhizoma Alpiniae Officinarum*) 15 g;

No. 6 Binglang (*Semen Arecae*) 9 g;

No. 7 Chuanlianzi (*Fructus Meliae Toosendan*) 12 g;

No. 8 Badou (*Fructus Crotonis*) 12 g.

Administration: Smash No. 8 slightly, then mix it with No. 7; roast the mixture with wheat bran till it turns black; after No. 8 and bran are removed from the mixture, the left is then mixed with other ingredients and ground into fine powder; take orally 3 g each time with warm wine. Or decoct the above drugs in water for oral application with dosages in proportion to the original recipe.

Actions: Dispersing stagnated liver-qi, dispelling cold to relieve pain.

Clinical Applicantion: This recipe is indicated for hernia of small intestines, marked by lower abdominal pain radiating to the testicle, swelling and falling to one side of the testicle, pale tongue with whitish fur, deep slow or taut pulse. It is applicable to orchitis, epididymitis, gastroduodenal ulcer, chronic gastritis and others, which are ascribed to accumulation of cold and stagnation of qi. In case of severe swelling and falling to one side,

天台乌药散

【方源】《医学发明》。

【组成】 乌药、木香、小茴香、青皮、高良姜各15 g,槟榔9 g,川楝子12 g,巴豆12 g。

【用法】 先将巴豆微打破,同川楝子用麸皮炒黑,去巴豆及麸皮不用,合余药共研细末,每次3 g,温酒调下。亦可作汤剂,用量按原方比例酌定。

【功用】 行气疏肝,散寒止痛。

【临床应用】 适用于小肠疝气。症见少腹痛引睾丸,偏坠肿胀,舌淡苔白,脉沉迟或弦。睾丸炎、附睾炎、胃及十二指肠溃疡、慢性胃炎等属寒凝气滞者,可用本方治疗。若偏坠肿胀较甚者,可加荔枝核、橘核以增强行气止痛之

add Lizhihe (*Semen Litchi*) and Juhe (*Semen Citri Reticulatae*) to enhance the effect of promoting the flow of qi and relieving pain. In case of severe local pain with cold sensation, add Rougui (*Cortex Cinnamomi*) and Wuzhuyu (*Fructus Evodiae*) to strengthen the effect of dispelling cold to relieve pain.

Elucidation：The syndrome is caused by cold accumulation in the liver meridian, leading to disorder of qi function. It should be treated by regulating the flow of qi and dispelling cold to relieve pain. The first ingredient has the function of promoting the flow of qi, dispelling cold and relieving pain and is used as monarch drug. Pungent, warm and aromatic in nature, No. 4 is capable of dispersing stagnated liver-qi, No. 2 promoting the flow of qi to relieve pain, No. 3 warming the liver to dispel cold, and No. 5 dispelling cold and relieving pain. They all function as minister drugs, and together enhance the effect of No. 1 in promoting the flow of liver-qi. Used as adjuvant drugs, No. 6 possesses the action of descending qi and remove stagnation, while No. 7 and No. 8 have their cold nature reduced and their action of promoting the flow of qi and removing stagnation strengthened after roasted together.

Cautions：This recipe bears a warm and dry nature, therefore, should not be used in case of pain from hernia due to downward flow of damp heat.

功；若局部冷痛较甚者，可加肉桂、吴茱萸以加强散寒止痛之力。

【方解】　本方证由寒凝肝脉，气机阻滞所致，治宜行气疏肝，散寒止痛之法。方中乌药行气疏肝，散寒止痛，为君药。青皮疏肝理气，木香行气止痛，小茴香暖肝散寒，高良姜散寒止痛，四药皆辛温芳香之品，合用以加强乌药的行气疏肝作用，同为臣药。槟榔下气导滞，川楝子与巴豆同炒后其寒性减而行气散结力增，均为佐药。

【注意事项】　本方药性温燥，若疝气疼痛属湿热下注者，不宜使用。

2.10.2　Prescriptions for Suppressing upward Adverse Flow of Qi

Suzi Jiangqi Tang
(*Decoction of Perilla Seed for Descending Qi*)

Source：*Taiping Huimin Hejiju Fang* (*Benevolent Prescriptions from Taiping Pharmaceutical Bureau*).

第二节　降气剂

苏子降气汤

【方源】　《太平惠民和剂局方》。

Ingredients:

No. 1 Suzi (*Fructus Perillae*) 75 g;

No. 2 Banxia (*Rhizoma Pinelliae*) 75 g;

No. 3 Danggui (*Radix Angelicae Sinensis*) 15 g;

No. 4 Zhigancao (*Radix Glycyrrhizae Praeparatae*) 60 g;

No. 5 Qianhu (*Radix Peucedani*) 30 g;

No. 6 Houpo (*Cortex Magnoliae Officinalis*) 30 g;

No. 7 Rougui (*Cortex Cinnamomi*) 30 g.

Administration: Grind the above drugs into fine powder, decoct 9 g each time in water with 2 slices of Shengjiang (*Rhizoma Zingiberis Recens*), 1 piece of Dazao (*Fructus Ziziphi Jujubae*) and small amount of suye (*Folium Perillae*) added to it. Or decoct all ingredients for oral application with dosages in proportion to the original recipe.

Actions: Descending the abnormally ascending qi to relieve dyspnea, eliminating phlegm to relieve cough.

Clinical Applicantion: This recipe is indicated for syndromes of cough and asthma with excess syndrome in the upper and deficiency syndrome in the lower, marked by cough, asthma, white sputum in large amount, fullness and choking sensation in the chest and hypochondrium, or lumbago and weakness of feet, or edema of limbs, white slippery or greasy fur, taut and smooth pulse. It is applicable to symptoms of chest distress, profuse white sputum, white slippery or greasy fur, as seen in chronic bronchitis, pulmonary emphysema and bronchial asthma. In case of difficulty in lying horizontally due to cough and asthma, add Chenxiang (*Lignum Aquilariae Resinatum*) to promote the effect of descending abnormally rising qi to relieve asthma. If concomitant with exterior syndrome as aversion to cold and fever, add Mahuang (*Herba Ephedrae*) and Xingren (*Semen Armeniacae Amarum*)

【组成】 苏子、半夏各75 g,当归15 g,炙甘草60 g,前胡、厚朴各30 g,肉桂30 g。

【用法】 共研粗末,每次9 g,加生姜2片,大枣1枚,苏叶适量,水煎服。亦可作汤剂,用量按原方比例酌定。

【功用】 降气平喘,祛痰止咳。

【临床应用】 适用于上实下虚之咳喘证。症见咳嗽气喘,痰多色白,胸膈满闷,或腰疼脚软,或肢体浮肿,舌苔白滑或白腻,脉弦滑。慢性支气管炎、肺气肿、支气管哮喘等见有胸闷痰多色白,苔白滑或白腻者,可用本方治疗。若咳喘难以平卧者,可加沉香以增强降气平喘之力;若兼有表证,恶寒发热者,可加麻黄、杏仁以宣肺平喘,疏散外邪;若兼气虚,倦息乏力者,可加人参、五味子以补益肺气;若无下虚之象者,可减去肉桂、当归,以专于祛邪治标。

to disperse the lung-qi for relieving asthma and eliminate exogenous pathogenic factors. If concomitant with qi deficiency, lassitude and weakness, add Renshen (*Radix Ginseng*) and Wuweizi (*Fructus Schisandrae*) to supplement the lung-qi. In the absence of deficiency syndrome in the lower, subtract No. 7 and No. 3 so as to focus on eliminating pathogenic factors and treating the secondary.

Elucidation: The syndrome results from excessive accumulation of phlegm and saliva, dysfunction of dispersing and descending of the lung and deficiency of kidney-yang, leading to failure of the kidney in receiving qi. That is why it is called "excess in the upper and deficiency in the lower". According to the principle of "treating the superficial symptoms at the onset of a disease", treatment of this syndrome should focus on descending the abnormally rising qi and eliminating phlegm to relieve asthma and cough. Ingredient No. 1 functions as monarch drug to send down qi and eliminate phlegm for relieving cough and asthma. Used as minister drugs, No. 2 is capable of drying dampness, eliminating phlegm and descending qi, No. 6 sending down qi, eliminating phlegm and relieving asthma, and No. 5 dispersing the lung-qi and eliminating phlegm to relieve cough. The monarch and minister drugs are aimed at dealing with excess syndrome in the upper. No. 7 can invigorate the kidney-yang to benefit the reception of qi and relieve asthma. No. 3 has the action of enriching blood, moistening dryness and relieving cough, and help No. 7 deal with deficiency syndrome in the lower. These two drugs play the part of adjuvant drug. No. 4 can mediate the properties of other drugs and is used as guiding drug. Shengjiang (*Rhizoma Zingeberis Recens*), Dazao (*Fructus Ziziphi Jujubae*) and Suye (*Folium Perillae*) added to the recipe are meant to regulate the

【方解】 本方证由痰涎壅肺,肺失宣降,兼肾阳不足,不能纳气化饮所致,故称之"上实下虚",根据"发时治标"的原则,以降气平喘,祛痰止咳为主。方中苏子降气化痰,止咳平喘,为君药。半夏燥湿化痰降逆,厚朴降气化痰平喘,前胡宣肺化痰止咳,三药合用,助苏子降气祛痰平喘,同为臣药。君臣相伍,以治上实。肉桂温补下元,纳肾气而平喘;当归养血润燥,助肉桂以治下虚,并能止咳,均为佐药。炙甘草调和药性,为使药。用时少加生姜、大枣、紫苏叶以和中祛痰,宣肺散寒。诸药配伍,标本兼顾,上下同治,而以治上治标为主。

stomach and eliminate phlegm, disperse the lung-qi and dispel cold. All together, they are to deal with both the superficial symptoms and root cause of the disease, both the upper and lower syndromes, with emphasis put on the upper and superficial.

Cautions: Most ingredients in this recipe are warm and dry in nature, so it is contraindicated for cough and asthma due to yin deficiency of the lung and kidney or asthma due to phlegm and lung heat.

【注意事项】 本方药物性多温燥,肺肾阴虚的咳喘,或肺热痰喘者禁用。

Dingchuan Tang
(*Asthma-relieving Decoction*)

Source: *Shesheng Zhongmiaofang* (*Effective Prescriptions for Health Conservation*).

Ingredients:

No.1 Baiguo (*Semen Ginkgo*) 9 g;

No.2 Mahuang (*Herba Ephedrae*) 9 g;

No.3 Suzi (*Fructus Perillae*) 6 g;

No.4 Gancao (*Radix Glycyrrhizae*) 3 g;

No.5 Kuandonghua (*Flos Farfarae*) 9 g;

No.6 Xingren (*Semen Armeniacae Amarum*) 9 g;

No.7 Sangbaipi (*Cortex Mori Radicis*) 9 g;

No.8 Huangqin (*Radix Scutellariae*) 6 g;

No.9 Banxia (*Rhizoma Pinelliae*) 9 g.

Administration: Decoct the above drugs in water for oral application.

Actions: Dispersing lung-qi and clearing away heat to resolve phlegm.

Clinical Applicantion: This recipe is indicated for asthma, marked by cough, dyspnea, chest distress and hypochondriac fullness, slight aversion to wind-cold, greasy yellowish fur, smooth and rapid pulse. It is applicable to bronchial asthma, chronic bronchitis and others, which chiefly manifest yellow sputum in large amount, greasy yellowish fur and smooth rapid pulse. In the ab-

定喘汤

【方源】 《摄生众妙方》。

【组成】 白果9 g,麻黄9 g,苏子6 g,甘草3 g,款冬花9 g,杏仁9 g,桑白皮9 g,黄芩6 g,半夏9 g。

【用法】 水煎服。

【功用】 宣降肺气,清热化痰。

【临床应用】 适用于哮喘。症见咳喘气急,痰多质稠色黄,胸膈胀闷,微恶风寒,舌苔黄腻,脉滑数。支气管哮喘、慢性支气管炎等以痰多色黄,苔黄腻,脉滑数为主症者,可用本方治疗。若无表证者,

sence of exterior syndrome, reduce the dosage of No. 2 to get the effect of dispersing the lung-qi and relieving asthma. In case of difficulty in expectoration, add Gualou (*Fructus Trichosanthis*) and Danxing (*Arisaema cum Bile*) to enhance the effect of clearing away heat and eliminating phlegm. In case of excessive heat in the lung, add Shigao (*Gypsum Fibrosum*) and Yuxingcao (*Herba Houttuyniae*) to purge away heat from the lung. In case of severe chest distress, add Zhike (*Fructus Aurantii*) and Houpo (*Cortex Magnoliae*) to regulate the flow of qi and relieve distress.

Elucidation: This syndrome results from dysfunction of the lung due to usual excess of phlegm-heat in the interior and attack by exogenous wind-cold. It should be treated by dispersing the lung-qi and clearing away heat to eliminate phlegm, and dispelling wind-cold as well. Ingredient No. 2 is capable of dispersing the lung-qi, relieving asthma and dispelling wind-cold, and No. 1 relieving asthma and eliminating phlegm with its astringent effect to the lung. Both are used as monarch drugs, one with dispersing effect and the other astringent effect, and can not only strengthen the effect of relieving asthma, but also prevent No. 2 from impairing the lung-qi because it is pungent and dispersing in nature. No. 6, No. 3, No. 5 and No. 9 can descend qi to remove asthma and eliminate phlegm to relieve cough, and are used as minister drugs to help monarch drugs resolve phlegm and relieve asthma. No. 7 and No. 8 act as adjuvant drugs, which purge away heat from the lung and eliminate phlegm to relieve asthma. No. 4 serves as guiding drug, mediating the properties of other drugs and stopping coughing.

Both this recipe and Suzi Jiangqi Tang possess the action of descending qi, revolving phlegm and relieving asthma, and are common prescriptions for cough and asthma.

麻黄可减量应用,取其宣肺定喘之功;若痰稠难出者,可加瓜蒌、胆星以增强清热化痰之力;若肺热重者,可加石膏、鱼腥草以清泄肺热;若胸闷较甚者,可加枳壳、厚朴以理气宽胸。

【方解】 本方证由素体痰热内蕴,又复外感风寒,肺失宣降所致,治宜宣降肺气,清热化痰为主,兼以疏风散寒。方中麻黄宣肺平喘而散风寒,白果敛肺定喘而化痰涎,两药相配,一散一收,既能增强平喘之功,又可防麻黄辛散太过耗伤肺气,共为君药。杏仁、苏子、款冬花、半夏降气平喘,化痰止咳,助君药祛痰平喘,同为臣药。桑白皮、黄芩清泄肺热,化痰平喘,均为佐药。甘草调和药性,且能止咳,为使药。

本方与苏子降气汤均有降气化痰平喘作用,皆为治疗咳喘证候的常用方剂。但苏

But the latter includes a compatibility of Suzi (*Fructus Perillae*) and Banxia (*Rhizoma Pinelliae*) with Rougui (*Cortex Cinnamomi*) and Danggui (*Radix Angelicae Sinensis*), which has the function of warming the kidney for the reception of qi and is fit for cough and asthma as the result of excessive cold-phlegm in the lung and deficiency in the lower, characterized by thin whitish sputum in large amount. However, this recipe has a compatibility of Mahuang (*Herba Ephedrae*) and Baiguo (*Semen Ginkgo*) with Sangbaipi (*Cortex Mori Radicis*) and Huangqin (*Radix Scutellariae*) which has the function of clearing away heat and relieving exterior syndrome. It is fit for asthma as the result of exterior cold and interior heat, which manifests chiefly the syndrome of interior accumulation of phlegm-heat and is characterized by cough, dyspnea, and thick yellowish sputum.

This recipe and Xiao Qinglong Tang are both capable of relieving exteriror syndrome and dispelling cold, dispersing the lung and resolving phlegm, and arresting cough and asthma and used in dealing with cough and asthma caused by retaining of wind-cold in the exterior and accumulation of phlegm in the lung. But the latter, with a compatibility of Mahuang (*Herba Ephedrae*) and Guizhi (*Ramulus Cinnamomi*) with Ganjiang (*Rhizoma Zingiberis*) and Xixin (*Herba Asari*), focuses on relieving exterior syndrome and dispelling cold, warming and resolving cold-phlegm and is fit for cough and asthma due to cold accumulation in the lung and excessive cold in the exterior, manifesting much clear thin and whitish sputum, and severe aversion to cold. The former, however, with a chief compatibility of Mahuang (*Herba Ephedrae*) and Baiguo (*Semen Ginkgo*) with Sangbaipi (*Cortex Mori Radicis*) and Huangqin (*Radix Scutellariae*), mainly functions to disperse the lung to expel cold, clear away

子降气汤以苏子、半夏与肉桂、当归相配,功兼温肾纳气,适用于寒痰壅肺,上实下虚而以痰涎壅肺为主的咳喘,以咳喘痰多,色白清稀为特点;本方则以麻黄、白果与桑白皮、黄芩为伍,功兼清热解表,适用于外寒内热以痰热内蕴为主的哮喘,以咳喘气急,痰黄质稠为特点。

本方与小青龙汤均有解表散寒,宣肺化痰,止咳平喘之功,皆可治疗风寒在表,痰浊壅肺之咳喘。但小青龙汤以麻黄、桂枝配伍干姜、细辛为主,功在解表散寒,温化寒饮,适宜于寒饮伏肺,表寒较重之咳喘,以痰多色白清稀,恶寒较甚为特点;而本方以麻黄、白果配伍黄芩、桑白皮为主,功在宣肺散寒,清肺化痰,适宜于痰热蕴肺,表寒较轻之哮喘,以痰多色黄粘稠,微恶风寒为特点。

heat from the lung to reduce phlegm and is fit for asthma
due to phlegm-heat in the lung and mild exterior cold,
which is characterized by much thick yellowish sputum and
slight aversion to wind-cold.

Cautions: This recipe is contraindicated for patients
with protracted asthma or yin deficiency of the lung and
kidney.

Xuanfu Daizhe Tang
(*Decoction of Inula and Hematitum*)

Source: *Shanghan Lun* (*Treatise on Exogenous
Febrile Diseases*).

Ingredients:

No. 1 Xuanfuhua (*Flos Inulae*) 9 g (wrapped with a
        piece of cloth while decocted);

No. 2 Daizheshi (*Ochra Haematitum*) 3 g;

No. 3 Renshen (*Radix Ginseng*) 6 g;

No. 4 Shengjiang (*Rhizoma Zingiberis Recens*) 15 g;

No. 5 Zhigancao (*Radix Glycyrrhizae Praeparatae*) 9 g;

No. 6 Banxia (*Rhizoma Pinelliae*) 9 g;

No. 7 Dazao (*Fructus Ziziphi Jujubae*) 4 pcs.

Administration: Decoct the above drugs in water
for oral application.

Actions: Descending the adverse flow of qi and resolving phlegm, invigorating qi and regulating the stomach.

Clinical Applicantion: This recipe is indicated for
syndromes with phlegm retention and reversed flow of qi
due to deficiency of the stomach, marked by frequent
belching, regurgitation, vomiting, epigastric fullness and
rigidity, pale tongue with whitish slippery fur, taut and
feeble pulse. It is applicable to such chief symptoms as
belching or hiccup ascribed to deficiency of the stomach
and phlegm retention as seen in gastric neurosis, chronic
gastritis, gastric dilatation, gastroduodenal ulcer, incomplete pylorochesis and neurotic hiccup. In absence of

【注意事项】 哮喘日久，肺肾阴虚者，禁用本方。

旋复代赭汤

【方源】《伤寒论》。

【组成】 旋复花9g(包煎)、代赭石3g，人参6g，生姜15g，炙甘草9g，半夏9g，大枣4枚。

【用法】 水煎服。

【功用】 降逆化痰，益气和胃。

【临床应用】 适用于胃虚痰阻气逆证。症见嗳气频作，反胃呕吐，心下痞硬，舌淡苔白滑，脉弦而虚。胃神经官能症、慢性胃炎、胃扩张、胃及十二指肠溃疡、幽门不全梗阻、神经性呃逆等以嗳气或呃逆为主要临床表现，证属胃虚痰阻者，可用本方治疗。若胃气不虚者，可去人参、大枣，且

deficient stomach-qi, subtract No. 3 and No. 7 and increase the dosage of No. 2 to enhance the effect of sending down the adversely rising qi. In case of vomiting with sputum and saliva, greasy and whitish fur, add Fuling (*Poria*) and Chenpi (*Pericarpium Citri Reticulatae*) to reduce phlegm and regulate the stomach. In case of cold syndrome of the stomach with preference for warmth, replace No. 4 with Ganjiang (*Rhizoma Zingiberis*) and add Dingxiang (*Flos Caryophylli*) and Shidi (*Calyx Kaki*) to warm the stomach and descend the adversely rising qi.

Elucidation: The syndrome results from the adversely rising stomach-qi due to deficiency of stomach qi and interior accumulation of phlegm. It should be treated by descending the reverse qi and reducing phlegm, supplementing qi and regulating the stomach. Ingredient No. 1 is capable of descending qi, reducing phlegm and arresting belching, and No. 2 descending adversely rising qi and relieving vomiting, both acting as monarch drugs. No. 6 possesses the action of drying dampness, reducing phlegm and descending reverse qi, and No. 4 warming the stomach, reducing phlegm and relieving vomiting. Both promote the function of the monarch drugs and play the part of minister drugs. No. 3, No. 7 and No. 5 can not only supplement qi, nourish and regulate the stomach, but also prevent No. 2 from impairing the stomach, all serving as adjuvant drugs. No. 5 also functions as guiding drug to mediate the properties of other drugs.

Jupi Zhuru Tang
(*Decoction of Tangerine Peel and Bamboo Shavings*)

Source: *Jingui Yaolue* (*Synopsis of Prescriptions of the Golden Cabinet*).

Ingredients:

No. 1 Jupi (*Pericarpium Citri Reticulatae*) 12 g;

加重代赭石用量,以增强重镇降逆之功;若呕吐痰涎,舌苔白腻者,可加茯苓、陈皮以助化痰和胃之力;若胃寒喜暖者,可将生姜易为干姜,并酌加丁香、柿蒂以温胃降逆。

【方解】 本方证由胃气虚弱,痰浊内阻,胃气上逆所致,治宜降逆化痰,益气和胃之法。方中旋复花降逆化痰止噫,代赭石重镇降逆止呕,共为君药。半夏燥湿化痰降逆,生姜温胃化痰止呕,助君药降逆气、化痰涎,同为臣药。人参、大枣、炙甘草益气补虚,养胃和中,又可防金石之品损伤胃气,为佐药。甘草调和药性,兼作使药。

橘皮竹茹汤

【方源】 《金匮要略》。

【组成】 橘皮12 g,竹茹12 g,生姜9 g,甘草6 g,人参

No. 2 Zhuru (*Caulis Bambusae in Taeniam*) 12 g;

No. 3 Shengjiang (*Rhizoma Zingiberis Recens*) 9 g;

No. 4 Gancao (*Radix Glycyrrhizae*) 6 g;

No. 5 Renshen (*Radix Ginseng*) 3 g;

No. 6 Dazao (*Fructus Ziziphi Jujubae*) 5 pcs.

Administration：Decoct the above drugs in water for oral application.

Actions：Dscending adversely rising qi and relieving hiccup, supplementing qi and clearing away heat.

Clinical Applicantion：This recipe is indicated for hiccup due to deficiency of the stomach with heat, marked by hiccup or retching, light red tongue, feeble and rapid pulse. It is applicable to vomitus gravidarum, incomplete pylorochesis, incessant hiccup after abdominal operation, and others, which pertain to deficiency of the stomach with heat. If concomitant with deficiency of stomach-yin, dry mouth and bright red tongue, add Maimendong (*Radix Ophiopogonis*) and Shihu (*Herba Dendrobii*) to nourish the stomach-yin. In the absence of deficient stomach-qi, subtract No. 5, No. 4 and No. 6 and add Shidi (*Calyx Kaki*) instead to strengthen the effect of descending the reverse qi and relieving hiccup.

Elucidation：The syndrome is caused by deficiency of the stomach with heat and reversely ascending stomach-qi. It should be treated by descending adverse flow of qi to relieve hiccup and supplementing qi and clearing away heat. Ingredient No. 1 is capable of promoting flow of qi and regulating the stomach to relieve hiccup and No. 2 clearing away heat from the stomach to relieve vomiting. Both act as monarch drugs and their combination can achieve the result of clearing away heat from the stomach and descending reverse qi. No. 5 has the function of invigorating the stomach and qi, and No. 3 regulating the stomach and relieving vomiting, both serving as minister

3 g,大枣 5 枚。

【用法】 水煎服。

【功用】 降逆止呃,益气清热。

【临床应用】 适用于胃虚有热之呃逆证。症见呃逆或干呕,舌嫩红,脉虚数。妊娠呕吐、幽门不全梗阻,以及腹部手术后呕逆不止等属胃虚有热者,可用本方治疗。若兼胃阴不足,口干舌光红者,可加麦门冬、石斛以滋养胃阴;若胃气不虚者,可去人参、甘草、大枣,加柿蒂以加强降逆止呃之效。

【方解】 本方证由胃虚有热,胃气上逆所致,治宜降逆止呃,益气清热之法。方中橘皮行气和胃以止呃,竹茹清热和胃以止呕,两药同用,清热和胃,降逆下气,共为君药。人参益胃补气,合橘皮行中有补;生姜和胃止呕,协竹茹清中有温,同为臣药。甘草、大枣益气和胃,助人参补益脾胃,又能调和药性,为佐使药。诸药配伍,清而不寒,补而不

drugs. No. 4 and No. 6 supplement qi and regulate the stomach, and help No. 5 reinforce the spleen and stomach. They can also mediate the properties of other drugs, functioning as adjuvant drugs. All the above drugs together bring about the effects of clearing away heat without causing cold, reinforcing qi without causing stagnation.

Cautions: This recipe is contraindicated for hiccup and vomiting accompanied by cold sensation and pain over the epigastrium, preference for warmth and aversion to cold.

滞,共成清补降逆之剂。

【**注意事项**】 若呃逆呕吐而胃脘冷痛,喜温畏寒者,禁用本方。

2.11 Prescriptions for Regulating Blood Circulation

第十一章
理血剂

Prescriptions for regulating blood circulation are chiefly composed of drugs that activate blood circulation. They bear the function of promoting blood circulation or arresting bleeding and are indicated for syndromes of blood stasis and hemorrhage.

Blood circulates incessantly in the vessels, but once the flow of blood is impeded, stagnation will be turned into stasis, blood will overflow from the vessels (namely bleeding syndrome). Therefore, this group of prescriptions is accordingly subdivided into prescriptions for activating blood flow to remove blood stasis and those for arresting bleeding.

The former mainly consists of drugs to activate blood flow and remove blood stasis and is indicated for blood accumulation and blood stasis syndrome due to stagnant blood in viscera or meridiens and collateralls. The latter, however, is chiefly composed of drugs with styptic action and fit for hemorrhage at various locations of diseases as the result of extravasation of blood.

The former mostly possesses drastic and purgative effect and is apt to consume blood and impair healthy qi and liable to cause blood and fetus disorder. Therefore drugs for removing blood stasis should not be used with an overdose, or it is advisable to use simultaneously drugs for building up body resistance to remove stagnant blood without impairing healthy qi. Besides, it should be used with

凡以理血药为主组成，具有活血或止血作用，用于治疗瘀血或出血病证的方剂，统称理血剂。

血液周流不息地循行于脉管之中，一旦血行不畅则凝滞成瘀，溢出脉外即为出血，因而理血剂相应地分为活血祛瘀剂与止血剂两类。

活血祛瘀剂由活血药为主组成，具有活血祛瘀作用，适用于瘀血阻于脏腑或经络而致的各种瘀血病证。止血剂由止血药为主组成，具有止血作用，适用于血液离经妄行而致的不同部位的出血病证。

活血祛瘀剂性多破泄，易于耗血伤正，并有动血、动胎之虞，使用时应当注意逐瘀不可过猛，或适当配伍扶正药物以使逐瘀而不伤正，月经过多及孕妇则应慎用。止血剂性多收涩，易于滞血留瘀，使用

great caution in women with profuse menstruation or at pregnancy. The latter usually has an astringent action and is liable to cause blood stagnation, so they should be combined with some drugs that activate blood flow and remove blood stasis to prevent stagnation of blood. In addition, whichever syndrome it is, it is certainly caused by cold and heat syndromes as well as excess and deficiency syndromes. Thus clinically, it is necessary to differentiate syndromes for etiology, distinguish between the primary and secondary aspects of the disease and determine severity of the disease. On this basis, therapeutic principle should be determined whether to treat the secondary or primary aspect, or deal with both simultaneously.

时宜适当配伍活血化瘀药物以防止血留瘀。此外,无论瘀血证或出血证,其成因均有寒热之分,虚实之异,治疗时宜审证求因,分清标本缓急,或治其标,或治其本,或标本兼顾。

2.11.1 Prescriptions for Promoting Blood Flow to Remove Stasis

Taohe Chengqi Tang
(Decoction of Peach Nucleus for Activating Qi)

Source: Shanghan Lun (Treatise on Exogenous Febrile Diseases).

Ingredients:

No. 1 Taoren (Semen Perisicae) 12 g;

No. 2 Dahuang (Radix et Rhizoma Rhei) 12 g;

No. 3 Guizhi (Ramulus Cinnamomi) 6 g;

No. 4 Zhigancao (Radix Glycyrrhizae Praeparatae) 6 g;

No. 5 Mangxiao (Natrii Sulfas) 6 g.

Administration: Decoct the first four ingredients in water; dissolve the last in this decoction after the residue is removed.

Actions: Purging away heat and removing blood stasis.

Clinical Application: This recipe is indicated for accumulation of heat in the lower-energizer, marked by

第一节　活血
祛瘀剂

桃核承气汤

【方源】《伤寒论》。

【组成】 桃仁12 g,大黄12 g,桂枝6 g,炙甘草6 g,芒消6 g。

【用法】 前四药水煎,汤成去滓,溶入芒消。

【功用】 泻热逐瘀。

【临床应用】 适用于瘀热结于下焦证。症见少腹疼

lower abdominal pain, normal urination, fever at night, or delirium, polydipsia, even dysphoria, or dysmenorrhea, amenia and postpartum lochiostasis, deep replete and uneven pulse. It is applicable to acute pelvic inflammation, retention of placenta, annexitis and others, which are ascribed to heat accumulation in the lower energizer. If concomitant with functional disorder of qi with severe flatulence and pain, add Xiangfu (*Rhizoma Cyperi*) and Wuyao (*Radix Linderae*) to promote the flow of qi and relieve pain. If the excessive heat invades upward manifesting headache and fullness of head, conjunctival congestion and flushed face, add Shengdihuang (*Radix Rehmanniae*) and Mudanpi (*Cortex Moutan Radicis*) to clear away heat from blood.

Elucidation：The syndrome is caused by heat accumulation in the lower energizer and its upward invasion to the mind. It should be treated by purging away heat stagnation. The first ingredient can remove blood stasis because of its potent properties, and No. 2 can remove stasis and purge away heat. Both are used as monarch drugs to deal with both stasis and heat and to lead heat downward. No. 3 is capable of promoting smooth flow of blood in the vessels and helps No. 1 remove blood stasis. While No. 5 bears the function of purging away heat stagnation and helping No. 2 remove blood stasis. No. 3 and No. 5 together play the part of minister drugs. No. 4 functions as adjuvant drug, which has the effect of supplementing qi and regulating the middle-energizer, and mediating the properties of other ingredients. It can also reduce the potent efficacy of other drugs and prevent them from impairing healthy qi.

Cautions：This recipe is drastic in effect and used to remove blood stasis. Therefore it should be applied carefully to patients with usual deficiency of the spleen and

痛,小便自利,至夜发热,或谵语烦渴,甚则狂躁不安,或妇女痛经、闭经、产后恶露不下,脉沉实而涩。急性盆腔炎、胎盘滞留、附件炎、肠梗阻等属瘀热内结下焦者,可用本方治疗。若兼气滞不畅,腹胀痛较甚者,可加香附、乌药以行气止痛;若兼瘀热上攻,头痛头胀,目赤面红者,可加生地黄、牡丹皮以清热凉血。

【方解】　本方证由瘀热结于下焦,上扰心神所致,治宜泻热逐瘀之法。方中桃仁破血祛瘀,大黄逐瘀泻热,两药合用,瘀热并治,导邪下行,共为君药。桂枝通行血脉,助桃仁活血化瘀;芒消泻热软坚,助大黄下瘀逐邪,同为臣药。炙甘草益气和中,缓诸药峻烈之性,以防逐瘀伤正,又能调和药性,为佐使药。

【注意事项】　本方为破血下瘀之剂,药性较为峻猛,素体脾虚便溏者慎用。

loose stool.

Xuefu Zhuyu Tang
(Decoction for Removing Blood Stasis in the Chest)

血府逐瘀汤

Source：*Yilin Gaicuo* (*Corrections on Medical Works*).

【方源】《医林改错》。

Ingredients：

No. 1 Taoren (*Semen Persicae*) 12 g;

No. 2 Honghua (*Flos Carthami*) 9 g;

No. 3 Danggui (*Radix Angelicae Sinensis*) 9 g;

No. 4 Shengdihuang (*Radix Rehmanniae*) 9 g;

No. 5 Chuanxiong (*Rhizoma Ligustici Chuanxiong*) 5 g;

No. 6 Chishaoyao (*Radix Paeoniae Rubra*) 6 g;

No. 7 Niuxi (*Radix Achyranthis Bidentatae*) 9 g;

No. 8 Jiegeng (*Radix Platycodi*) 5 g;

No. 9 Chaihu (*Radix Bupleuri*) 3 g;

No. 10 Zhike (*Fructus Aurantii*) 6 g;

No. 11 Gancao (*Radix Glycyrrhizae*) 3 g.

【组成】 桃仁12 g,红花、当归、生地黄各9 g,川芎5 g,赤芍药6 g,牛膝9 g,桔梗5 g,柴胡3 g,枳壳6 g,甘草3 g。

Administration：Decoct the above drugs in water for oral application.

【用法】 水煎服。

Actions：Promoting blood circulation to remove blood stasis, and promoting flow of qi to relieve pain.

【功用】 活血祛瘀,行气止痛。

Clinical Application：This recipe is indicated for blood stasis in the chest, marked by protracted chest pain and headache at fixed location as if pricked with needles, or protracted hiccup, or dysphoria due to interior heat, or palpitation, insomnia, irritability, hectic fever at dusk, dark-purple lips or blackish eyelids, deep-red tongue with ecchymoses, uneven or taut and tense pulse. It is applicable to chest pain as seen in angina pectoris of coronary heart disease, rheumatic heart disease, chest contusion and costal chondritis. It may also be used in headache, vertigo and mental depression as the result of sequelae of commotio cerebri, which are ascribed to blood stasis and

【临床应用】 适用于胸中血瘀证。症见胸痛、头痛日久,痛如针刺而有定处,或呃逆日久不止,或内热烦闷,或心悸失眠,急躁易怒,入暮潮热,唇暗或两目暗黑,舌黯红或有瘀斑,脉涩或弦紧。冠心病心绞痛、风湿性心脏病、胸部挫伤与肋软骨炎之胸痛,以及脑震荡后遗症之头痛、头晕、精神抑郁等属血瘀气滞,病位偏上者,可用本方治疗。

qi stagnation and affect the upper body. In case of abdominal mass, add Yujin (*Radix Curcumae*) and Danshen
(*Radix Saliviae Miltiorrhizae*) to promote blood flow
and remove stasis and mass.

Elucidation：This syndrome is the result of blood
stasis in the chest and disorder of qi activity. It should be
treated by promoting the circulation of blood and qi to remove stasis and relieve pain. The first two ingredients are
essential drugs for promoting blood circulation and removing blood stasis, which act as monarch drugs with doubled effect. Used as minister drugs, No. 6 has the action of
promoting blood flow and removing blood stasis, No. 5
promoting the flow of qi and blood, and No. 7 promoting
smooth flow of blood in vessels and causing blood stasis to
descend, which all help bring about the effect of monarch
drugs. No. 10 and No. 8 can regulate flow of qi and No. 9
disperse the stagnated liver-qi, whose combination constitutes the effects of regulating qi function of the liver and
gallbladder to promote blood circulation and remove blood
stasis. No. 4 and No. 3 nourish blood and yin and clear
away the latent heat in blood. The above five ingredients
play the part of adjuvant drugs. No. 11 serves as guiding
drug to mediate properties of other drugs. The compatibility of this recipe is meant to promote the circulation of
blood and nourish blood, to promote the flow of qi and
clear away heat simultaneously so as to prevent impairment of blood and accumulation of heat.

Fuyuan Huoxue Tang
(*Decoction for Recovery and*
Activating Blood Circulation)

Source：*Yixue Faming* (*Medical Inventions*).

Ingredients：

No. 1 Chaihu (*Radix Bupleuri*) 15 g;

No. 2 Tianhuafen (*Radix Trichosanthis*) 9 g;

若胁下有癥积者,可加郁金、
丹参以活血祛瘀,消癥化积。

【方解】 本方证由瘀血
阻于胸中,气机郁滞所致,治
宜活血祛瘀,行气止痛之法。
方中桃仁、红花均为活血祛瘀
要药,两药配伍,活血化瘀之
功相得益彰,共为君药。赤芍
药活血祛瘀,川芎行气活血;
牛膝通行血脉,导瘀血下行,
助君药以加强活血祛瘀之力,
同为臣药。枳壳、桔梗宽胸利
气,柴胡疏肝解郁,三药升降
并用,调畅胸中肝胆气机,使
气机畅行而利于行血消瘀;生
地黄、当归养血益阴,清血中
伏热,俱为佐药。甘草调和药
性,为使药。诸药配伍,活血
与养血并用,行气与清润并
施,则活血而不破血,行气而
不助热。

复元活血汤

【方源】 《医学发明》。

【组成】 柴胡15 g,天花
粉、当归各9 g,红花、甘草、穿
山甲(炮)各6 g,大黄(酒制)

No. 3 Danggui (*Radix Angelicae Sinensis*) 9 g;

No. 4 Honghua (*Flos Carthami*) 6 g;

No. 5 Gancao (*Radix Glycyrrhizae*) 6 g;

No. 6 Chuanshanjia (*Squama Manitis*) (roasted) 6 g;

No. 7 Dahuang (*Radix et Rhizoma Rhei*) (prepared with wine) 30 g;

No. 8 Taoren (*Semen Persicae*) (soaked in wine) 9 g.

Administration: Grind the above drugs into coarse powder; decoct 30 g of it with 30ml millet wine in water for oral application.

Actions: Promoting blood circulation to remove blood stasis, dispersing stagnated liver-qi to remove obstruction in the meridians.

Clinical Application: This recipe is indicated for blood stasis in hypochondriac region with unbearable pain due to injuries from falls, fractures, contusions and strains. It is applicable to chest and hypochondriac pain as seen in intercostal neuralgia and costal chondritis, which pertain to blood stasis and qi stagnation. In case of severe distension and pain due to qi stagnation, add Xiangfu (*Rhizoma Gyperi*) and Qingpi (*Pericarpium Citri Reticulatae Viride*) to promote flow of qi and relieve pain. In case of severe swelling and pain due to blood stasis, take orally the powder of Shensanqi (*Radix Notoginseng*), or add Ruxiang (*Olibanum*) and Moyao (*Myrrha*) to enhance the effect of removing blood stasis and relieving pain.

Elucidation: This syndrome is caused by trauma, which impairs the vessels and leads blood to flow outside the vessels and to retain in the chest and hypochondriac region. It should be treated by promoting blood circulation and dispersing the stagnated liver-qi to remove blood stasis and obstruction in the meridians. Ingredient No. 7 can remove blood stasis and lead pathogenic factors downward, and No. 1 regulate the flow of qi and guide other

30 g,桃仁(酒浸)9 g。

【用法】 共研粗末,每次30 g,加黄酒30 ml,水煎服。

【功用】 活血祛瘀,疏肝通络。

【临床应用】 适用于跌打损伤,瘀血留于胁下,痛不可忍。对于肋间神经痛、肋软骨炎等表现为胸胁疼痛,痛不可忍,属血瘀气滞者,亦可用本方治疗。若气滞胀痛较甚者,酌加香附、青皮以助行气止痛;若血瘀肿痛较甚者,可配合参三七末另吞,或酌加乳香、没药以增强化瘀止痛之效。

【方解】 本方证系外伤损络,血离经脉成瘀,停滞于胁肋而成,治宜活血祛瘀,疏肝通络之法。方中重用酒制大黄攻逐瘀血,导邪下行;柴胡疏肝理气,使气行血畅,并引诸药入肝经,两药配伍可攻逐胁下瘀血,共为君药。当

drugs to the liver meridian, both acting as monarch drugs. No. 3, No. 4 and No. 8 are used as minister drugs, which promote the circulation of blood to remove blood stasis and relieve swelling and pain. No. 6 has the function of removing blood stasis and obstruction in the collaterals, while No. 2 possesses the effect of clearing away heat from xuefen, removing heat accumulation and relieving swelling, both functioning as adjuvant drugs. No. 5 serves as guiding drug to mediate properties of other drugs. The wine added while drugs are decocted can strengthen the effect of promoting blood circulation and removing obstruction from collaterals.

Both this recipe and Xuefu Zhuyu Tang are used to treat swelling and pain of the chest and hypochondriac region. The former, with Dahuang (*Radix et Rhizoma Rhei*) and Chaihu (*Radix Bupleuri*) acting as monarch drugs, focuses on removing blood stasis in the hypochondriac region and includes such drugs capable of promoting blood flow and dealing with trauma as Chuanshanjia (*Squama Manitis*) and Tianhuafen (*Radix Trichosanthis*). Thus, it is mainly applied in chest and hypochondriac pain as the result of falls, fractures, contusions and strains. The latter, however, has a mild efficacy in removing blood stasis because it is composed of drugs capable of removing blood stasis, such as Taoren (*Semen Persicae*) and Honghua (*Flos Carthami*), and those of promoting the flow of qi. Thus it is widely used in syndrome of blood stasis and qi stagnation occurring in the chest and hypochondriac region as well as other locations of diseases.

Buyang Huanwu Tang
(*Decoction for Invigorating Yang and Recuperation*)

Source：*Yilin Gaicuo (Corrections on Medical Works*).

归、桃仁、红花活血祛瘀,消肿止痛,同为臣药。穿山甲破瘀通络;天花粉既能入血分凉血而续绝伤,又能清热散结以消肿,均为佐药。甘草调和药性,为使药。加酒煎药,可增强活血通络之力。

本方与血府逐瘀汤均可治疗胸胁瘀肿疼痛之证,但本方以大黄、柴胡共为君药,重在攻逐胁下瘀血,且方中配伍了穿山甲、天花粉等活血疗伤之品,因而主要用于跌打损伤所致的胸胁疼痛;血府逐瘀汤则以桃仁、红花等活血化瘀药配伍行气药为主,祛瘀之力较为和缓,广泛用于胸胁部位以及其他病变部位偏上的血瘀气滞证候。

补阳还五汤

【方源】《医林改错》。

Ingredients:

No. 1 Shenghuangqi (*Radix Astragali seu Hedysari*) 120 g;

No. 2 Dangguiwei (*tail of Radix Angelicae Sinensis*) 6 g;

No. 3 Chishaoyao (*Radix Paeoniae Rubra*) 6 g;

No. 4 Dilong (*Lumbricus*) 3 g;

No. 5 Chuanxiong (*Rhizoma Ligustici Chuanxiong*) 3 g;

No. 6 Honghua (*Flos Carthami*) 3 g;

No. 7 Taoren (*Semen Persicae*) 3 g.

Administration: Decoct the above drugs in water for oral application.

Actions: Invigorating qi, promoting blood circulation and removing blood stasis from the meridians.

Clinical Application: This recipe is indicated for sequelae of apoplexy, marked by hemiplegia, deviation of the eyes and mouth, involuntary drooling, frequent micturation or enuresis, deep-red tongue with thin whitish fur, and slow pulse. It is applicable to hemiplegia, paraplegia, and atrophy of the upper or lower limbs from sequelae of cerebrovascular accident or other reasons, which pertain to blood stasis due to qi deficiency. In case of excessive phlegm, add Zhibanxia (*Rhizoma Pinelliae Praeparatae*) and Tianzhuhuang (*Concretio Silicea Bambusae*) to dissolve phlegm. If concomitant with intricate and obscure speech, add Shichangpu (*Rhizoma Acori Graminei*), Yuanzhi (*Radix Polygalae*) and Fanyujin (*Radix Curcumae*) to restore consciousness and remove obstruction from collaterals. In case of deficient yang with aversion to cold and cold extremities, add Shufuzi (*Radix Aconiti Praeparatae*) to warm yang and dispel cold. In case of paralysis of the lower extremities, add Duzhong (*Cortex Eucommiae*) and Niuxi (*Radix Achyranthis Bidentatae*) to reinforce the liver and kidney and

【组成】 生黄芪120 g,当归尾6 g,赤芍药6 g,地龙3 g,川芎3 g,红花3 g,桃仁3 g。

【用法】 水煎服。

【功用】 补气活血通络。

【临床应用】 适用于中风后遗症。症见半身不遂,口眼歪斜,口角流涎,小便频数或遗尿不禁,舌黯淡,苔薄白,脉缓。脑血管意外后遗症及其他原因引起的偏瘫、截瘫,上肢或下肢痿软属气虚血瘀者,可用本方治疗。若痰多者,可加制半夏、天竺黄以化痰;若兼语言不利者,可加石菖蒲、远志、矾郁金以开窍通络;若阳气不足,畏寒肢冷者,可加熟附子以温阳散寒;若下肢瘫重者,可加杜仲、牛膝以补肝肾,强筋骨。

strengthen tendons and bones.

Elucidation：The syndrome arises when qi fails, due to deficiency, to promote the circulation of blood so that blood stasis occurs and tendons and muscles are in a state of malnutrition. This should be treated by supplementing qi, promoting blood flow and removing blood stasis from collaterals. Ingredient No. 1 in large dosage is used as monarch drug, which can replenish healthy qi so as to promote blood flow. No. 2 acts as minister drug, which can promote blood circulation and remove stasis from collaterals. No. 3, No. 5, No. 7 and No. 6 promote the effect of the minister drug, and No. 4 has the function of removing blood stasis from collaterals, all functioning as adjuvant drugs.

Cautions：The usual dosage for No. 1 is 30 - 60 g, which should be increased gradually if there is no marked effect. It should be taken continuously for a certain period of time after recovery so as to consolidate the therapeutic effect and prevent recurrence.

Wenjing Tang
(*Decoction for Warming Meridians*)

Source：*Jingui Yaolue* (*Synopsis of Prescriptions of the Golden Cabinet*).

Ingredients：

No. 1 Wuzhuyu (*Fructus Evodiae*) 9 g;

No. 2 Danggui (*Radix Angelicae Sinensis*) 6 g;

No. 3 Shaoyao (*Radix Paeoniae*) 6 g;

No. 4 Chuanxiong (*Rhizoma Ligustici Chuanxiong*) 6 g;

No. 5 Renshen (*Radix Ginseng*) 6 g;

No. 6 Guizhi (*Ramulus Cinnamomi*) 6 g;

No. 7 Ejiao (*Colla Corii Asini*) (melted) 6 g;

No. 8 Mudanpi (*Cortex Moutan Radicis*) 6 g;

No. 9 Shengjiang (*Rhizoma Zingiberis Recens*) 6 g;

No. 10 Gancao (*Radix Glycyrrhizae*) 6 g;

【方解】　本方证由气虚无力行血，以致脉络瘀阻，筋脉、肌肉失养而成，治宜补气活血通络之法。方中重用黄芪大补元气，令气旺以促血行，为君药。当归尾活血化瘀，使瘀去络通，为臣药。赤芍药、川芎、桃仁、红花助当归尾活血祛瘀，地龙通经活络以消脉络瘀滞，均为佐药。

【注意事项】　方中黄芪用量一般从 30～60 g开始，效果不显再逐渐增量。愈后还应继续服用一段时间，以巩固疗效，防止复发。

温经汤

【方源】　《金匮要略》。

【组成】　吴茱萸9 g,当归6 g,芍药6 g,川芎6 g,人参6 g,桂枝6 g,阿胶(烊冲)6 g,牡丹皮6 g,生姜6 g,甘草6 g,半夏6 g,麦门冬9 g。

No. 11 Banxia (*Rhizoma Pinelliae*) 6 g;

No. 12 Maimendong (*Radix Ophiopogonis*) 9 g.

Administration: Decoct the above drugs in water for oral application.

Actions: Warming the meridians and dispelling cold, removing blood stasis and nourishing blood.

Clinical Application: This recipe is indicated for deficiency-cold in the thoroughfare vessel and conception vessel and accumulation of blood stasis, marked by irregular menstruation, preceded or delayed menstrual cycle, or overdue or persistent menstrual duration, or repeated occurrence of menstruation within one month, or incessant metrostaxis, or dysmenorrhea, or amenorrhea, or failure to conceive due to cold in the uterine, and concomitant with fever at dusk, feverish sensation in palms, dry mouth and lips. It is applicable to dysfunctional uterine bleeding, chronic pelvic inflammation, infertility and others that have chief manifestations as irregular menstruation, lower abdominal pain with cold sensation and constant dysphoria. Baishaoyao (*Radix Paeoniae Alba*) could be used for the purpose of nourishing yin and blood and Chishaoyao (*Radix Paeoniae Rubra*) for clearing away heat and promoting blood circulation. In case of sharp pain of the lower abdomen with cold sensation, subtract No. 8 and No. 12 and add Aiye (*Folium Artemisiae Argyi*), or replace No. 6 with Rougui (*Cortex Cinnamomi*) to strengthen the effect of dispelling cold and relieving pain. If concomitant with qi stagnation, add Xiangfu (*Rhizoma Cyperi*) and Wuyao (*Radix Linderae*) to regulate the flow of qi and relieve pain. In case of persistent metrostaxis in light color, subtract No. 8 and add Aiye (*Folium Artemisiae Argyi*) and Shudihuang (*Radix Rehmanniae Praeparatae*) to warm meridians, nourish blood and arrest bleeding.

【用法】 水煎服。

【功用】 温经散寒，祛瘀养血。

【临床应用】 适用于冲任虚寒，瘀血阻滞证。症见妇女月经不调，或前或后，或逾期不止，或一月再行，或漏下不止，或痛经，或闭经，或宫冷不孕等，伴入暮发热，手心烦热，唇口干燥。功能性子宫出血、慢性盆腔炎、不孕症等以月经不调、小腹冷痛、时发烦热为主症者，可用本方治疗。方中芍药，如欲滋阴养血可用白芍药，欲清热活血可用赤芍药。若小腹冷痛较甚者，可去牡丹皮、麦门冬，加艾叶，或以肉桂易桂枝，以增强散寒止痛作用；若兼气滞者，可加香附、乌药以理气止痛；若漏下色淡不止者，可去牡丹皮，加艾叶、熟地黄以温经养血止血。

Elucidation：This syndrome is caused by deficiency-cold in the thoroughfare vessel and conception vessel and blood stasis，which further affects blood generation and leads to heat. It should be treated by means of warming meridians to dispel cold，removing stasis and nourishing blood and with supplementary method of nourishing yin and clearing away heat. Ingredient No. 1 and No. 6 act as monarch drugs，which can warm meridians，dispel cold，and promote blood circulation. No. 2，No. 4 and No. 3 are used as minister drugs to promote blood flow，remove blood stasis，nourish blood and regulate menstruation. No. 8 bears the action of promoting blood flow and removing blood stasis，and clearing away heat from blood，while No. 7 and No. 12 possess the function of nourishing blood and yin，moistening dryness and arresting bleeding. No. 5，No. 10，No. 11 and No. 9 can supplement qi and invigorate the spleen，warm the middle-energizer and regulate the stomach so as to promote transformation and digestion. The above seven ingredients play the part of adjuvant drugs. No. 10 also serves as guiding drug to mediate properties of other drugs. All ingredients together imply moistening action in warming action as well as tonic action in purgative action. Thus，this recipe is warm but not dry，and purgative but not drastic in nature.

Cautions：This syndrome belongs to simultaneous occurrence of cold and heat，deficiency and excess syndromes，manifesting chiefly cold accumulation and blood stasis. Thus this recipe is contraindicated for cases with excess heat marked by feverish sensation in palms，sores and chest，reddened tongue and rapid pulse.

Shenghua Tang
(*Decoction for Postpartum Troubles*)

Source：*Fu Qingzhu Nüke* (*Fu Qingzhu's Obstetrics and Gynecology*).

【方解】 本方证由冲任虚寒，瘀血阻滞，日久新血不生，阴虚生热所致，治宜温经散寒，祛瘀养血为主，兼以滋阴清热。方中吴茱萸、桂枝温经散寒，通行血脉，共为君药。当归、川芎、芍药活血祛瘀，养血调经，同为臣药。牡丹皮活血祛瘀，凉血退热；阿胶、麦门冬养血滋阴，润燥止血；人参、甘草、半夏、生姜益气补脾，温中和胃，以助生化，俱为佐药。甘草调和药性，兼作使药。诸药配伍，温中有润，通中寓补，故温而不燥，通而不峻。

【注意事项】 本方所治虽属寒热虚实错杂之证，但以寒凝血瘀为主，若瘀热较甚，五心烦热，舌红脉数者禁用。

生化汤

【方源】《傅青主女科》。

Ingredients：

No. 1 Quandanggui (*Radix Angelicae Sinensis*) 24 g;

No. 2 Chuanxiong (*Rhizoma Ligustici Chuanxiong*) 9 g;

No. 3 Taoren (*Semen Persicae*) 6 g;

No. 4 Paojiang (*Rhizoma Zingiberis Praeparatae*) 2 g;

No. 5 Zhigancao (*Radix Glycyrrhizae Praeparatae*) 2 g.

Administration：Decoct the above drugs in water or decoct them with millet wine for oral application.

Actions：Promoting blood circulation to remove blood stasis, warming the meridians to relieve pain.

Clinical Application：This recipe is indicated for abdominal pain due to postpartum blood stasis, marked by retention of lochia after delivery, lower abdominal pain with cold sensation. In case of mild abdominal pain, subtract No. 3. In case of sharp pain due to retention of blood mass, add Puhuang (*Pollen Typhae*), Wulingzhi (*Faeces Trogopterorum*) and Yanhusuo (*Rhizoma Corydalis*) to remove blood stasis and relieve pain. In case of sharp lower abdominal pain with cold sensation, add Rougui (*Cortex Cinnamomi*) and Xiaohuixiang (*Fructus Foeniculi*) to warm the meridians, dispel cold and relieve pain.

Elucidation：The syndrome is caused by deficient blood after delivery, cold accumulation and blood mass in the uterine. It should be treated by promoting blood flow, removing blood stasis, warming the meridians and relieving pain. Used in large dosage as monarch drug, No. 1 possesses the function of promoting blood circulation and removing blood stasis to promote blood regeneration. No. 2 and No. 3 respectively have the effect of promoting the circulation of blood and qi, and promoting blood flow to remove blood stasis, acting together as minister drugs. No. 4 is the adjuvant drug in the recipe, which can warm the meridains, dispel cold and relieve pain. No. 5 serves as guiding drug, capable of regulating the middle-energi-

【组成】 全当归24 g,川芎 9 g, 桃仁 6 g, 炮姜 2 g,炙甘草2 g。

【用法】 水煎或酌加黄酒同煎服。

【功用】 活血祛瘀,温经止痛。

【临床应用】 适用于产后瘀血腹痛证。症见恶露不行,小腹冷痛。若腹痛不甚者,可减去桃仁;若瘀块留滞,腹痛甚者,可加蒲黄、五灵脂、延胡索以祛瘀止痛;若小腹冷痛甚者,可加肉桂、小茴香以温经散寒止痛。

【方解】 本方证由产后血虚,寒凝血瘀,留阻胞宫所致,治宜活血祛瘀,温经止痛之法。方中重用当归补血活血,化瘀生新,为君药。川芎活血行气,桃仁活血祛瘀,同为臣药。炮姜温经散寒止痛,为佐药。炙甘草和中缓急,调和药性,为使药。加用黄酒同煎,意在取其温通血脉以助药力。

zer and relieving spasm as well as mediating the properties of other drugs. The millet wine used when decocting drugs, is meant to improve the properties of other drugs because it can warm the meridians and promote easy flow of blood.

Cautions: This recipe is contraindicated for retention of lochia after delivery, which is concomitant with fever, thirst, reddened tongue and ascribed to blood stasis due to blood heat.

Guizhi Fuling Wan
(*Pill of Cinnamon Twig and Poria*)

Source: *Jingui Yaolue* (*Synopsis of Prescriptions of the Golden Cabinet*).

Ingredients:

No. 1 Guizhi (*Ramulus Cinnamomi*);

No. 2 Fuling (*Poria*);

No. 3 Mudanpi (*Cortex Moutan Radicis*);

No. 4 Taoren (*Semen Persicae*);

No. 5 Shaoyao (*Radix Paeoniae*);

All in equal dosage.

Administration: Grind the above drugs into fine powder and make it into pills with honey; take 3 - 5 g each time and twice daily. Or decoct the above drugs with dosages in proportion to the original recipe.

Actions: Promoting blood circulation, removing blood stasis, and subduing abdominal mass.

Clinical Application: This recipe is indicated for stagnant blood in the uterine, marked by abdominal pain with tenderness, or incessant metrostaxis in dark purple color, or threatened abortion, dark-purple tongue and uneven pulse. It is applicable to endometrial inflammation, annexitis, hysteromyoma, oophoritic cyst and postpartum lochiostasis, which pertain to blood stasis in the uterine. Baishaoyao (*Radix Paeoniae Alba*) may be used for the

【注意事项】 产后恶露不行,伴发热、口渴、舌红等症,属血热而有瘀滞者,禁用本方。

桂枝茯苓丸

【方源】 《金匮要略》。

【组成】 桂枝、茯苓、牡丹皮、桃仁、芍药各等分。

【用法】 共研细末,炼蜜为丸,每次 3～5 g,每日 2 次。亦可作汤剂,用量按原方比例酌定。

【功用】 活血化瘀,缓消癥块。

【临床应用】 适用于瘀阻胞宫证。症见腹痛拒按,或漏下不止,血色紫黑晦暗,或妊娠胎动不安,舌质紫暗,脉涩。子宫内膜炎、附件炎、子宫肌瘤、卵巢囊肿,以及产后恶露不行等属瘀阻胞宫者,可用本方治疗。方中芍药,若欲

purpose of relieving spasm or pain and Chishaoyao (*Radix Paeoniae Rubra*) for clearing and purging away stagnant heat.

Elucidation: The syndrome is caused by stagnant blood retaining in the uterine, which may lead to metro-staxis due to failure of blood to circulate in the vessels, or threatened abortion due to lack of nutrients. Therefore therapeutic method for this syndrome is to promote blood flow and remove blood stasis so as to deal with the root cause of the syndrome. The first two ingredients are monarch drugs in the recipe, one for promoting blood cir-culation by warming and removing stasis from the vessels and the other promoting diuresis and eliminating mass. No. 4 is capable of eliminating blood stasis and abdominal mass, while No. 3 and No. 5 removing stasis and clearing away heat, which together strengthen the effect of mon-arch drugs as minister drugs. Honey is sweet, mild and moist in nature, and can reduce the drastic potency of other ingredients so that blood stasis is removed without impairing body resistance. The oral dosage is small so as to ensure an even milder efficacy in removing blood stasis.

2.11.2   Prescriptions for Arresting Bleeding

Shihui San
(*Powder Made of Ashes of Ten Drugs*)

Source: *Shiyao Shenshu* (*Miraculous Book on A-shes of Ten Prescriptions*).

Ingredients:

No. 1 Daji (*Herba seu Radix Cirsii Japonici*);

No. 2 Xiaoji (*Herba Cephalanoploris*);

No. 3 Heye (*Folium Nelumbinis*);

No. 4 Cebaiye (*Cacumen Biotae*);

缓急止痛,可用白芍药;若欲清泄瘀热,则用赤芍药。

【方解】 本方所治诸证均由瘀血阻于胞宫而成,或因血不归经而漏下不止,或因胎失所养而胎动不安,治宜活血化瘀以除病本。方中桂枝温通血脉以行瘀滞,茯苓利水渗湿以助消癥,共为君药。桃仁破瘀血,消癥积;牡丹皮、芍药破瘀血,清瘀热,均可助君药以加强活血消癥之力,为臣佐药。白蜜甘缓而润,以之为丸可缓和诸药破泄之力,使祛瘀而不伤正,加之服药剂量极轻,使本方祛瘀之力更为和缓。

第二节　止血剂

十灰散

【方源】 《十药神书》。

【组成】 大蓟、小蓟、荷叶、侧柏叶、白茅根、茜草根、栀子、大黄、丹皮、棕榈皮各等分。

No. 5 Baimaogen (*Rhizoma Imperatae*);

No. 6 Qiancaogen (*Radix Rubiae*);

No. 7 Zhizi (*Fructus Gardeniae*);

No. 8 Dahuang (*Radix et Rhizoma Rhei*);

No. 9 Mudanpi (*Cortex Moutan Radicis*);

No. 10 Zonglupi (*Petiolus Trachycarpi*);

All in equal dosage.

Administration: Each ingredient is burned with its nature maintained and then ground into powder. A Chinese ink stick is properly ground in an adequate amount of juice of lotus root or carrot. 9 - 15 g of the powder is taken with the juice containing Chinese ink each time. If the above drugs is made into pills, it is named "Shihui Wan". And in this case, take 9 g each time orally and twice or 3 times daily with warm boiled water.

Actions: Removing heat from blood to arrest bleeding.

Clinical Application: This recipe is indicated for bleeding syndrome due to blood heat, marked by hematemesis, hemoptysis, and epistaxis with bright red, reddened tongue with yellowish fur, rapid pulse. It is applicable to such diseases with the above symptoms as hemorrhage of digestive tract, bronchiectasis and hemoptysis from tuberculosis. In case of excessive heat in the blood, make the above drugs into decoction instead of powder and increase the dosage of No. 8 and No. 7, and add Niuxi (*Radix Achyranthis Bidentatae*) and Daizheshi (*Ochra Haematitum*) as well to make heat descend.

Elucidation: The syndrome arises when the flare up of fire and qi scorches blood vessels and forces blood to go astray. It should be treated by removing heat from blood to arrest bleeding. This recipe is chiefly composed of such drugs with the action of cooling blood and stopping bleeding as No. 1, No. 2, No. 3, No. 4, No. 5 and No. 6. Ingredient No. 10 has both astringent and styptic actions. No. 7

【用法】　各药炒炭存性，共研细末，藕汁或萝卜汁磨京墨适量，调服 9～15 g。如制成丸剂，名十灰丸，每次9 g，温开水送下，每日 2～3 次。

【功用】　凉血止血。

【临床应用】　适用于血热妄行证。症见吐血、咯血、嗽血、衄血，血色鲜红，舌红苔黄，脉数。消化道出血、支气管扩张以及肺结核咯血等见有上述特征者，可用本方治疗。若血热较盛者，可将本方改作汤剂使用，并重用大黄、栀子，酌加牛膝、代赭石等镇降之品，以引血热下行。

【方解】　本方证由气火上炎，灼伤血络，迫血妄行所致，治宜凉血止血之法。方中以大蓟、小蓟、荷叶、茜草、侧柏叶、白茅根等凉血止血药为主，配以棕榈皮收涩止血，再配伍栀子清热泻火，大黄导热

is capable of purging away fire, and No. 8 descending heat so as to restore normal circulation of blood. No. 9 possesses the function of clearing away heat and cooling blood and can arrest bleeding and remove blood stasis when combined with No. 8. All ingredients are charred so as to enhance the astringent and styptic action. The lotus root or carrot juice and Chinese ink are meant to strengthen the effect of clearing away heat from blood and arresting bleeding. This is commonly used in rescue work for stopping bleeding, which involves both removing heat from blood and purging away heat, both astringent effect and removing blood stasis.

Cautions: This recipe can only be used to treat the superficial symptoms of bleeding. Therefore after bleeding is arrested, the root cause of the syndrome should be dealt with. Besides, this recipe is contraindicated for bleeding with deficiency cold syndrome.

Kexue Fang
(*Prescription for Treating Hemoptysis*)

Source: *Danxi Xinfa* (*Danxi's Experiential Therapy*).

Ingredients:

No. 1 Qingdai (*Indigo Naturalis*) (ground in water) 6 g;

No. 2 Gualouren (*Semen Trichosanthis*) 9 g;

No. 3 Hezi (*Fructus Chebulae*) 6 g;

No. 4 Haifushi (*Pumex*) 9 g;

No. 5 Zhizi (*Fructus Gardeniae*) (parched black) 9 g.

Administration: Grind the above drugs into fine powder and make it into pills with honey and ginger juice; dissolve in the mouth 9 g each time and twice daily. Or decoct the above drugs with proper dosages in proportion to the original recipe.

Actions: Expelling fire from the liver and lung, eliminating heat from blood and arresting bleeding.

下行,使气火下降而血不妄行;并用牡丹皮清热凉血,配大黄活血祛瘀,可使血止而不留瘀。方中诸药皆炒炭使用,以加强收涩止血作用。以藕汁或萝卜汁磨京墨调服,意在增强清热凉血止血之功。全方凉血与清降并用,收涩与化瘀兼施,为急救止血的常用方剂。

【注意事项】 本方为止血治标之剂,血止后当治其病本。虚寒性出血禁用本方。

咳血方

【方源】《丹溪心法》。

【组成】 青黛(水飞)6 g,瓜蒌仁9 g,诃子6 g,海浮石9 g,栀子(炒黑)9 g。

【用法】 共研细末,以蜜同姜汁为丸。每次9 g,嚼化,每日2次。亦可作汤剂,用量按原方比例酌定。

【功用】 清肝宁肺,凉血止血。

Clinical Application：This recipe is indicated for hemoptysis due to invasion of the lung by liver-fire, marked by cough, thick sputum with blood streaks, difficult expectoration, vexation and irritability, chest and hypochondriac pain, dry throat and bitter mouth, flushed face, constipation, reddened tongue with yellow fur, taut and rapid pulse. It is applicable to hemoptysis as seen in bronchiectasis and tuberculosis, which pertains to liver-fire invading the lung. In case of yin impairment by fire, add Shashen (*Radix Adenophorae Strictae*) and Maimendong (*Radix Ophiopogonis*) to moisten the lung and nourish yin. In case of severe cough with much sputum, add Zhebeimu (*Bulbus Fritillariae Thunbergii*), Tianzhuhuang (*Concretio Silicea Bambusae*) and Pipaye (*Folium Eriobotryae*) to remove heat from the lung so as to resolve phlegm and relieve cough. In case of bleeding in large amount, add Xianhecao (*Herba Agrimoniae*) and Baimaogen (*Rhizoma Imperatae*) or use this recipe together with Shihui San.

Elucidation：The syndrome results from liver-fire scorching the lung, which leads to impairment of the lung collaterals, and is known as "Wood-fire impairs metal". It should be treated by clearing away heat from the liver and lung and eliminating heat from blood to arrest bleeding. Ingredient No. 1 can eliminate heat from the liver and blood and No. 5 purge away fire to relieve vexation, both used as monarch drugs to purge away the liver-fire. No. 2 can clear away heat and dissolve phlegm, moisten the lung and relieve cough, while No. 4 clears away heat from the lung and eliminates phlegm, both functioning as minister drugs. No. 3 has an astringent effect on the lung and acts as adjuvant drug. Although this recipe is named "recipe for treating hemoptysis" in Chinese, it comprises none styptic drug. Thus it shows that this recipe is formulated

【临床应用】 适用于肝火犯肺之咳血证。症见咳嗽痰稠带血，咯吐不爽，心烦易怒，胸胁作痛，咽干口苦，颊赤便秘，舌红苔黄，脉弦数。支气管扩张、肺结核等病的咳血，属肝火犯肺而致者，可用本方治疗。若火热伤阴者，可加沙参、麦门冬以润肺养阴；若咳甚痰多者，可加浙贝母、天竺黄、枇杷叶以清肺化痰止咳；若出血量多者，可加仙鹤草、白茅根或合十灰散同用。

【方解】 本方证由肝火灼肺，肺络受损所致，又称"木火刑金"，治宜清肝宁肺，凉血止血之法。方中青黛清肝凉血，栀子泻火除烦，合用以泻肝火之本，共为君药。瓜蒌仁清热化痰，润肺止咳；海浮石清肺泻热，软坚化痰，同为臣药。诃子敛肺止咳，为佐药。本方名为"咳血方"，却未用一味止血药物，可见其立方之意在于通过清肝泻火，清肺止咳治本而达止血之目的。

in light of the principle of purging away liver-fire and removing heat from the lung to relieve cough so that bleeding will be arrested.

Cautions: This recipe is contraindicated for hemoptysis due to yin deficiency of the lung and kidney or that concomitant with loose stool due to spleen deficiency.

Xiaoji Yinzi
(*Small Thistle Decoction*)

Source: *Jisheng Fang* (*Prescriptions for Saving Lives*).

Ingredients:

No. 1 Shengdihuang (*Radix Rehmanniae*) 120 g;

No. 2 Xiaoji (*Herba Cephalanoploris*) 15 g;

No. 3 Huashi (*Talcum Pulveratum*) 15 g;

No. 4 Mutong (*Caulis Akebiae*) 6 g;

No. 5 Puhuang (*Pollen Typhae*) (parched) 9 g;

No. 6 Danzhuye (*Herba Lophatheri*) 9 g;

No. 7 Oujie (*Nodus Nelumbinis Rhizomatis*) 9 g;

No. 8 Danggui (*Radix Angelicae Sinensis*) 6 g;

No. 9 Zhizi (*Fructus Gardeniae*) (parched) 9 g;

No. 10 Zhigancao (*Radix Glycyrrhizae Praeparata*) 6 g.

Administration: Grind the above drugs into coarse powder and decoct 12 g each time in water for oral application.

Actions: Removing heat from blood to arrest bleeding, inducing diuresis to treat stranguria.

Clinical Application: This recipe is indicated for blood-stranguria, marked by haematuria, frequent, dribbling and painful urination, reddened tongue and rapid pulse. It is applicable to urinary infection and calculi in urinary system with the above manifestations, which pertain to heat syndrome of the urinary bladder. It is advisable to replace No. 10 with Shenggancao (*Radix Glycyrrhizae*), aiming to clearing and purging away heat. In case of excessive

【注意事项】 咳血由肺肾阴虚而致者,或兼脾虚便溏者,禁用本方。

小蓟饮子

【方源】 《济生方》。

【组成】 生地黄120 g,小蓟15 g,滑石15 g,木通6 g,炒蒲黄9 g,淡竹叶9 g,藕节9 g,当归6 g,炒栀子9 g,炙甘草6 g。

【用法】 共研粗末,每次12 g,水煎服。

【功用】 凉血止血,利尿通淋。

【临床应用】 适用于血淋证。症见尿中带血,小便频数,赤涩热痛,舌红,脉数。急性泌尿系感染以及泌尿系结石等见有上述表现,属下焦膀胱有热者,可用本方治疗。方中炙甘草宜改为生甘草,取其有清热泻火作用。若下焦邪

heat in the lower energizer, add Huangbai (*Cortex Phello-dendri*), Pugongying (*Herba Taraxaci*) and Shiwei (*Folium Pyrrosiae*) to clear away heat and induce diuresis. In case of pain of the penis as if stabbed, add Hupo (*Succinum*) and Haijinsha (*Spora Lygodii*) to treat stranguria and relieve pain. In case of impairment of both qi and yin due to long course of illness, subtract No. 3 and No. 4 and add Dangshen (*Radix Codonopsis Pilosulae*), Huangqi (*Radix Astragali seu Hedysari*) and Ejiao (*Colla Corii Asini*) to supplement qi and nourish yin.

Elucidation：The syndrome results from heat accumulation in the urinary bladder, causing impairment of the blood vessels and disturbance of qi transformation of the urinary bladder. It should be treated by removing heat from blood to arrest bleeding and inducing diuresis to treat stranguria. The first two ingredients clear away heat from blood and arrest bleeding and function as monarch drugs. No. 5 and No. 7 can not only clear away heat from blood, but also remove blood stasis, acting as minister drugs. No. 3, No. 4 and No. 6 possess the function of clearing and purging away heat and inducing diuresis, while No. 9 has the effect of purging away fire from the triple energizer and descending heat. No. 8 can nourish yin and blood in combination with No. 1 so as to induce diuresis without impairing yin, and can prevent ingredients of cold or cool nature from causing blood stasis because it has a warm nature. These five ingredients together play the part of adjuvant drugs. No. 10 is used as guiding drug to regulate the middle-energizer and mediate drug properties.

Cautions：This recipe is contraindicated for hematuria without manifestations due to pathogenic heat.

Huangtu Tang
(*Decoction of Baked Yellow Earth*)
Source：*Jingui Yaolue* (*Synopsis of Prescrip-*

【方解】　本方证由热聚膀胱，损伤血络，膀胱气化失司所致，治宜凉血止血，利尿通淋之法。方中小蓟、生地黄清热凉血止血，共为君药。藕节、蒲黄凉血止血，并能化瘀，可使血止而不留瘀，同为臣药。滑石、木通、淡竹叶清热泻火，利尿通淋；栀子清泄三焦之火，导热下行；当归与生地黄相伍滋阴养血，以使利水而不伤阴，且当归性温又可防寒凉滞血，均为佐药。甘草和中调药，为使药。

【注意事项】　尿中带血而无热象者，禁用本方。

黄土汤

【方源】《金匮要略》。

tions of the Golden Cabinet).

Ingredients：

No. 1 Gancao (*Radix Glycyrrhizae*) 9 g;

No. 2 Gandihuang (*Radix Rehmanniae*) 9 g;

No. 3 Baizhu (*Rhizoma Atractylodis Macrocephalae*) 9 g;

No. 4 Paofuzi (*Radix Aconiti Lateralis Praeparata*) 9 g;

No. 5 Ejiao (*Colla Corii Asini*) 9 g;

No. 6 Huangqin (*Radix Scutellariae*) 9 g;

No. 7 Zaoxintu (*Terra Flava Vsta*) 30 g.

Administration：Decoct No. 7 first in water to get its decoction, in which other ingredients are decocted for oral application.

Actions：Warming yang and invigorating the spleen, nourishing blood and arresting bleeding.

Clinical Application：This recipe is indicated for bleeding syndrome due to yang deficiency, marked by hematochezia, or hematemesis, epistaxis, or metrorrhagia with dark-red blood, cold limbs, sallow complexion, pale tongue with whitish fur, deep thready and feeble pulse. It is applicable to chronic hemorrhage of gastrointestinal tract, dysfunctional uterine bleeding, and others attributable to deficiency of spleen-yang. In case of poor appetite, replace No. 5 with Ejiaozhu (*Colla Corii Asini*) (Pearled and parched ass-hide gelatin with talc powder) to reduce its greasy nature. In case of excessive deficiency of qi with lassitude and weakness, add Renshen (*Radix Ginseng*) to supplement qi so as to control blood. In case of excessive hemorrhage, add Shensanqi (*Radix Notoginseng*) and Baiji (*Rhizoma Bletillae*) to strengthen the styptic action.

Elucidation：The syndrome is caused by deficiency of the spleen-yang, deficiency-cold of the middle-energizer

【组成】 甘草、干地黄、白术、炮附子、阿胶、黄芩各9 g,灶心黄土(包煎)30 g。

【用法】 以灶心黄土先煎取汁,再入余药煎服。

【功用】 温阳健脾,养血止血。

【临床应用】 适用于阳虚出血证。症见大便下血,或吐血、衄血,或妇人崩漏,血色暗淡,四肢不温,面色萎黄,舌淡苔白,脉沉细无力。慢性胃肠道出血以及功能性子宫出血属脾阳不足者,可用本方治疗。若胃纳差者,阿胶可改为阿胶珠,以减其滋腻之性;若气虚较甚,倦怠乏力者,可加人参以益气摄血;若出血量多者,可加参三七、白及等止血药以加强止血作用。

【方解】 本方证由脾阳不足,中焦虚寒,统摄无力所

and dysfunction of the spleen in controlling blood. It should be treated by warming the spleen-yang and nourishing blood to stop bleeding. No. 7 (also called Fulonggan) functions as monarch drug to warm and nourish the middle-energizer and arrest bleeding. No. 3 and No. 4 can warm the spleen-yang so as to restore its function of controlling blood and are used as minister drugs. Both monarch and minister drugs bring about the result of treating both the superficial symptoms as well the root cause of the syndrome. No. 2 and No. 5 act as adjuvant drugs, which can, on the one hand, nourish yin and blood so as to make up the deficiency of both yin and blood as the result of bleeding and on the other, function together with No. 6 to restrict the excessive warm and dry nature of No. 3 and No. 4 so as to prevent disturbance or impairment of blood. Meanwhile, No. 3 and No. 4 can restrict the greasy nature of No. 2 and No. 5. Thus it can be seen they are both opposite and supplementary to each other. No. 1 is used as guiding drug to supplement qi, invigorate the spleen and mediate the properties of the other drug as well. These ingredients together form a recipe with both cold and warm natures, treating both the primary and the secondary by coordinating potent and mild drugs. So it is warm but not dry and tonic but not greasy.

Cautions: This recipe is contraindicated for hemorrhage with bright red, dry mouth and reddened tongue.

致,治宜温阳健脾,养血止血之法。方中灶心黄土(即伏龙肝)温养中焦,收涩止血,为君药。白术、附子温阳健脾,以恢复脾之阳气统摄血液作用,与君药相伍,标本兼治,为臣药。干地黄、阿胶滋阴养血止血,以补益由于出血而致阴血之不足,并与寒凉之黄芩共同制约白术、附子过于温燥之性,以防动血伤血,均为佐药。与此同时,白术、附子又可制约地黄、阿胶滋腻碍胃之性,两者相反相成。甘草益气补脾,调和药性,为使药。诸药配伍,寒热并用,标本兼顾,刚柔相济,故温而不燥,补而不腻。

【注意事项】 出血而色鲜红,口干舌红者,禁用本方。

2.12 Prescriptions for Treating Wind Syndrome

第十二章

治风剂

Prescriptions that are mainly composed of drugs pungent in flavor and disperse in nature for dispelling exogenous wind or subduing endogenous wind to relieve convulsion and used for syndromes due to wind are known as prescriptions for treating wind syndrome.

Wind syndrome refers to those caused by pathogenic wind. Since pathogenic wind includes exogenous wind and endogenous wind, this group of prescriptions is subdivided correspondingly into prescriptions for dispelling exogenous wind and those for subduing endogenous wind.

The former is mainly made up of pungent and disperse drugs with the effect of dispelling pathogenic wind and used for treating diseases as the result of attack of muscles, meridians and collaterals, tendons and joints by exogenous wind. The latter, however, consists chiefly of drugs with the action of checking liver-yang to stop endogenous wind and is applied to diseases caused by liver-wind stirring inside the body.

In the application of this group of prescriptions, first of all, it is essential to differentiate between exogenous and endogenous wind, between cold and heat syndrome as well as between deficiency and excess syndrome. Exogenous wind should be dispelled and endogenous wind subdued. If wind is complicated with pathogenic cold, heat, dampness or phlegm, it is necessary to adopt the method of expelling cold, clearing away heat, inducing diuresis or eliminating phlegm simultaneously. In addition, in case of

凡以辛散祛风或熄风止痉药为主组成,具有疏散外风或平熄内风作用,用于治疗风病的方剂,统称治风剂。

风病是指由风邪而致的一类疾病。由于风邪有从外感者,亦有从内生者,因而治风剂相应地分为疏散外风剂与平熄内风剂两类。

疏散外风剂由辛散祛风药为主组成,具有疏风散邪作用,适用于风邪外袭,侵入肌肉、经络、筋骨、关节等处所致诸病。平熄内风剂由平肝熄风药为主组成,具有平肝熄风作用,适用于肝风内动所致诸病。

使用治风剂时,首先必须辨别风病的属内、属外,分别其寒、热、虚、实。若属外风,则宜疏散;属于内风,则宜平熄。如风邪挟寒、挟热、挟湿、挟痰者,应与祛寒、清热、化湿、化痰等法结合运用。此外,对于外风与内风兼挟为患者,应当加以兼顾,但须分清

exogenous wind concomitant with endogenous wind, it is necessary to differentiate the primary from the secondary syndrome. In doing so, prescriptions are formed rationally.

主次,合理组方。

2.12.1 Prescriptions for Dispelling Exogenous Wind

Chuanxiong Chatiao San (*Powder of Ligusticum*)

Source: *Taiping Huimin Hejiju Fang* (*Benevolent Prescriptions from Taiping Pharmaceutical Bureau*).

Ingredients:

No.1 Chuangxiong (*Rhizoma Ligustici Chuanxiong*) 120 g;

No.2 Jingjie (*Herba Schizonepetae*) 120 g;

No.3 Baizhi (*Radix Angelicae Dahuricae*) 60 g;

No.4 Qianghuo (*Rhizoma seu Radix Notopterygii*) 60 g;

No.5 Zhigancao (*Radix Glycyrrhizae Praeparatae*) 60 g;

No.6 Xixin (*Herba Asari*) 30 g;

No.7 Fangfeng (*Radix Ledebouriellae*) 45 g;

No.8 Bohe (*Herba Menthae*) 240 g.

Administration: Grind the above drugs into fine powder, take 6 g each time and twice daily with tea. Or decoct the above drugs in water with dosages in proportion to the original recipe.

Actions: Dispelling wind to relieve pain.

Clinical Application: This recipe is indicated for headache due to attack of exogenous wind, marked by headache, hemicrania, or pain on top of the head, aversion to cold with fever, dizziness, nasal obstruction, thin whitish fur, and superficial pulse. It is applicable to headache generated from migraine, angioneurotic headache or chronic rhinitis that is accompanied by nasal obstruction and superficial pulse and ascribed to attack by exogenous

第一节 疏散外风剂

川芎茶调散

【方源】《太平惠民和剂局方》。

【组成】 川芎、荆芥各120 g,白芷、羌活、炙甘草各60 g,细辛30 g,防风45 g,薄荷240 g。

【用法】 共研细末,每次6 g,清茶调下,每日 2 次。亦可作汤剂,用量按原方比例酌定。

【功用】 疏风止痛。

【临床应用】 适用于外感风邪头痛证。症见偏正头痛或巅顶作痛,恶寒发热,目眩鼻塞,舌苔薄白,脉浮。偏头痛、血管神经性头痛、慢性鼻炎所引起的头痛,伴有鼻塞、脉浮属外感风邪而致者,可用本方治疗。若因外感风

wind. In case of attack by wind-cold with aversion to cold, increase the dosage of No. 1 and add Suye (*Folium Perillae*) and Shengjiang (*Rhizoma Zingiberis Recens*) to enhance the effect of dispelling wind and cold. In case of attack by wind-heat with fever or dry mouth and reddened tongue, subtract No. 4 and No. 6 and add Manjingzi (*Fructus Viticis*) and Juhua (*Flos Chrysanthemi*) to expel wind-heat. In case of protracted headache, add Quanxie (*Scorpio*), Jiangcan (*Bombyx Batryticatus*) and Taoren (*Semen Perisicae*) to expel wind and promote blood circulation for alleviating pain.

Elucidation: The syndrome arises when exogenous wind invades head and obstructs the lucid yang-qi. It should be treated by dispelling wind and alleviating pain. No. 1, No. 3 and No. 4 have the effect of expelling wind and alleviating pain, among which No. 1 is good at relieving pain and treating headache of shaoyang meridian or jueyin meridian (i. e. pain on top of the head or in the temples), No. 4 is effective for headache of taiyang meridian (pain on the rear of the head radiating to the neck) and No. 3 is specially good for headache of yangming meridian (pain over the forehead). These three drugs supplement one another in effect and function as monarch drugs. No. 6 is capable of dispelling cold and alleviating pain and No. 8 expelling wind and refreshing mind, acting as minister drugs. No. 2 and No. 7 strengthen the effect of both monarch and minister drugs in dispelling wind and are used as adjuvant drugs. No. 5 is the guiding drug, which mediates the properties of othe drugs. Since most ingredients are warm or dry with expelling effect, tea is used to prevent impairment of body fluid and consumption of qi because tea is cold and bitter in nature with descending effect. This makes the recipe warm but not dry, has ascending and descending effects, and expels pathogenic

寒而起，恶寒明显者，可重用川芎，酌加苏叶、生姜以加强祛风散寒之效；若由外感风热而致，发热明显或口干舌红者，可去羌活、细辛，加蔓荆子、菊花以疏散风热；若头痛久而不愈者，可配全蝎、僵蚕、桃仁以搜风活血止痛。

【方解】 本方证由外感风邪，循经上犯头部，阻遏清阳之气所致，治宜疏风止痛之法。方中川芎、白芷、羌活疏风止痛，其中川芎长于止痛，尤善治少阳、厥阴经头痛（头顶痛或两侧头痛），羌活善治太阳经头痛（后头痛牵连项部），白芷善治阳明经头痛（前额部），三药相辅相成，共为君药。细辛散寒而长于止痛，薄荷疏风并清利头目，助君药疏风散邪，同为臣药。荆芥、防风疏散风邪，协君、臣则更增疏散风邪之力，为佐药。炙甘草调和药性，为使药。由于方中药物大多升散温燥，故以清茶调服，取其寒凉苦降以防温燥伤津、升散耗气之弊，从而使本方温而不燥，升中有降，祛邪而不伤正气。

factors without impairing healthy qi.

Cautions：This recipe is contraindicated for headache due to deficiency of qi and blood, or due to wind generated from hyperactive yang.

Xiaofeng San
(*Powder for Dispersing Pathogenic Wind*)

Source：*Waike Zhengzong* (*Orthodox Manual of
External Diseases*).

Ingredients：

No. 1 Jingjie (*Herba Schizonepetae*) 9 g;

No. 2 Fangfeng (*Radix Ledebouriellae*) 9 g;

No. 3 Niubangzi (*Fructus Arctii*) 9 g;

No. 4 Chantui (*Periostracum Cicadae*) 3 g;

No. 5 Cangzhu (*Rhizoma Atractylodis*) 6 g;

No. 6 Kushen (*Radix Sophorae Flavescentis*) 6 g;

No. 7 Shigao (*Gypsum Fibrosum*) 15 g;

No. 8 Zhimu (*Rhizoma Anemarrhenae*) 9 g;

No. 9 Danggui (*Radix Angelicae Sinensis*) 9 g;

No. 10 Humaren (*Semen Sesami*) 9 g;

No. 11 Shengdihuang (*Radix Rehmanniae*) 12 g;

No. 12 Mutong (*Caulis Akebiae*) 1.5 g;

No. 13 Gancao (*Radix Glycyrrhizae*) 1.5 g.

Administration：Decoct the above drugs in water
for oral application.

Actions：Dispelling wind and nourishing blood,
clearing away heat and removing dampness.

Clinical Application：This recipe is indicated for
rubella and eczema, marked by red skin rash or dots and
spots over the whole body with pruritus, exudation of
body fluid after scratching, whitish or yellowish fur, superficial and rapid pulse. It is applicable to urticaria, allergic dermatitis, paddy field dermatitis, dermatitis medi-
camentosa, neurodermatitis, and others, which are characterized by red skin rashes with pruritus and caused by

【注意事项】　头痛因气
血不足或阳亢风动而致者,禁
用本方。

消风散

【方源】《外科正宗》。

【组成】　荆芥、防风、牛
蒡子各9 g,蝉蜕3 g,苍术、苦
参各6 g,石膏15 g,知母、当
归、胡麻仁各9 g,生地黄12 g,
木通、甘草各1.5 g。

【用法】　水煎服。

【功用】　疏风养血,清热
除湿。

【临床应用】　适用于风
疹、湿疹。症见皮肤疹出色
红,或遍身云片斑点,瘙痒,抓
破后渗出津水,苔白或黄,脉
浮数。荨麻疹、过敏性皮炎、
稻田性皮炎、药物性皮炎、神
经性皮炎等以疹出色红而痒
为特点,属风湿热邪为患者。

pathogenic wind, dampness or heat. In case of feverish body and thirst due to dominant wind-heat, add Jinyinhua (*Flos Lonicerae*) and Lianqiao (*Fructus Forsythiae*) to dispel wind and clear away heat. In case of dominant damp heat with fullness or stuffiness in chest or epigastrium, heaviness and weakness of the body, thick and greasy yellowish fur, add Difuzi (*Fructus Kochiae*), Cheqianzi (*Semen Plantaginis*) and Zhizi (*Fructus Gardeniae*) to clear away heat and induce diuresis. In case of excessive heat in xuefen with feverish sensation in palms and sores, reddened or deep-red tongue, add Chishaoyao (*Radix Paeoniae Rubra*), Mudanpi (*Cortex Moutan Radicis*) and Zicao (*Radix Arnebiae seu Lithospermi*) to clear away heat from blood and cool the blood.

Elucidation: The syndrome is caused by wind-heat or wind-dampness retaining in the skin and interstitial space. It should be treated by dispelling wind and nourishing blood as well as clearing away heat and inducing diuresis. The first four ingredients are the monarch drugs in the recipe, which can dispel wind from the superficies and relieve itching. No. 5 has the function of expelling wind and dampness, No. 6 clearing away heat and dampness, No. 12 clearing away damp heat by promoting diuresis, and No. 8 and No. 7 clearing away heat and purging away fire, which altogether eliminate damp heat retaining in the superficies and function as minister drugs. No. 9, No. 11 and No. 10 serve as adjuvant drugs, capable of nourishing blood and promoting circulation of blood. They can not only prevent wind from impairing blood but also prevent drugs of bitter and dry nature from impairing yin and consuming blood. The last ingredient possesses the effect of purging away fire and mediating drug properties and plays the role of guiding drug.

Cautions: During the application of this recipe,

可用本方治疗。若风热偏盛而身热、口渴者,可加金银花、连翘以疏风清热解毒;若湿热偏盛,胸脘痞满,身重乏力,舌苔黄厚而腻者,可加地肤子、车前子、栀子以清热利湿;若血分热甚,五心烦热,舌红或绛者,可加赤芍药、牡丹皮、紫草以清热凉血。

【方解】 本方证由风热或风湿之邪侵袭人体,浸淫血脉,郁于肌肤腠理之间所致,治宜疏风养血,清热除湿之法。方中荆芥、防风、牛蒡子、蝉蜕疏风止痒,以祛除在表之风邪,为君药。苍术祛风燥湿,苦参清热燥湿,木通清利湿热,知母、石膏清热泻火,共同祛除在表之湿热,同为臣药。当归、生地黄、胡麻仁养血活血,一则防风邪浸淫血脉,损伤阴血,二则可防诸苦燥渗利之品伤阴耗血之弊,均为佐药。生甘草清热泻火,调和药性,为使药。

【注意事项】 服用本方

patients should refrain from pungent flavor, meat, strong tea, cigarettes and liquor. Otherwise, the therapeutic effect may be weakened.

Xiao Huoluo Dan
(*Bolus for Activating Meridians*)

Source: *Taiping Huimin Hejiju Fang* (*Benevolent Prescriptions from Taiping Pharmaceutical Bureau*).

Ingredients:

No. 1 Zhichuanwu (*Radix Aconiti Praeparatae*) 180 g;

No. 2 Zhicaowu (*Radix Aconiti Kusnezoffii Praeparatae*) 180 g;

No. 3 Paotiannanxing (*Rhizoma Arisaematis*) (prepared) 180 g;

No. 4 Dilong (*Lumbricus*) 180 g;

No. 5 Ruxiang (*Olibanum*)(ground) 66 g;

No. 6 Moyao (*Myrrha*)(ground) 66 g.

Administration: Grind the above drugs into fine powder and make it into boluses with honey, weighing 3 g each; take one bolus at one time and twice daily with mellow wine or warm boiled water or schizonepeta tea.

Actions: Dispelling wind-dampness, removing phlegm and activating the collaterals, promoting blood circulation and relieving pain.

Clinical Application: This recipe is indicated for arthralgia due to wind, cold and dampness, marked by contracture or pain of limbs, muscles and tendons, difficult movement of joints, migratory pain, aversion to cold and preference for warmth, pale tongue or purplish tongue, whitish fur, deep and thready pulse. It is applicable to rheumatic arthritis, rheumatoid arthritis, hyperosteogeny, and others that are characterized by contracture and pain of limbs, preference for warmth and aversion to cold, pale tongue with whitish fur. In case of long-term illness concomitant with the deficiency of qi and blood as

期间,忌食辛辣、鱼腥、烟酒、浓茶等,以免影响疗效。

小活络丹

【方源】 《太平惠民和剂局方》。

【组成】 制川乌、制草乌、炮天南星、地龙各180 g,乳香(研)、没药(研)各66 g。

【用法】 上研细末,炼蜜为丸,每丸重3 g,每次 1 丸,以陈酒或温开水或荆芥茶送下,每日 2 次。

【功用】 祛风除湿,化痰通络,活血止痛。

【临床应用】 适用于风寒湿痹。症见肢体筋脉挛痛,关节屈伸不利,疼痛游走不定,恶寒喜暖,舌淡或有紫气,舌苔白,脉沉细。风湿性关节炎、类风湿关节炎、骨质增生症等以肢体挛痛,喜温畏寒,舌淡苔白为特点者,可用本方治疗。若病久而兼肝肾气血不足者,可配合独活寄生丸同服。

well as the liver and kidney, use Duhuo Jisheng Wan simultaneously.

Elucidation: The syndrome arises when wind, cold and dampness retain in the meridians and collaterals for so long that qi and blood fail to circulate normally, and phlegm and blood stasis are generated. It should be treated by eliminating wind, cold and dampness to remove phlegm and blood stasis and activating the collaterals. The first two ingredients act as monarch drugs to dispel wind, cold and dampness, warm meridians and relieve pain. No. 3 can dry dampness, resolve phlegm, expel wind and activate the meridians and collaterals, acting as minister drug. No. 5 and No. 6 are used as adjuvant drugs to promote the circulation of qi and blood and alleviate pain. No. 4 has the function of activating the meridians and collaterals and leading other drugs to the collaterals so as to eliminate pathogenic factors, and plays the part of guiding drug. Mellow wine can enhance the efficacy of drugs, promote the flow of qi and blood, and activate the meridians and collaterals. Schizonepeta tea can strengthen the effect of dispelling wind and cold. Therefore clinically they should be applied properly according to the actual condition.

Cautions: This recipe is warm and dry in nature and drastic in potency, thus fit for patients with strong constitution and excess syndrome. It should be used with caution for those with heat syndrome due to yin deficiency or for pregnant women.

2.12.2 Prescriptions for Calming Endogenous Wind

Lingjiao Gouteng Tang
(**Decoction of Antelop's Horn and Uncaria Stem**)

Source: *Chongding Tongsu Shanghan Lun* (*Re*

【方解】 本方证由风寒湿邪滞留经络,日久气血失于流畅,津液凝聚为痰,血行痹阻为瘀,以致风寒湿与痰瘀痹阻经络,治宜祛风散寒,除湿化痰,活血通络之法。方中制川乌、制草乌祛风散寒,除湿通络,温经止痛,为君药。天南星燥湿化痰,祛风通络,为臣药。乳香、没药行气活血,通络止痛,为佐药。地龙通经活络,并引诸药入络祛邪,为佐使药。以陈酒服药,可助药势,行气血,通经络;若以荆芥泡茶服药,则可助发散风寒之效,临证可视病证酌情选用。

【注意事项】 本方药性温燥,药力峻烈,适宜于体壮气实邪甚者,若阴虚有热或孕妇慎用。

第二节 平熄
内风剂

羚角钩藤汤

【方源】《重订通俗伤寒

vised Edition of Popular Treatise on Exogenous Febrile Diseases).

Ingredients：

No. 1 Lingyangjiaopian (*Cornu Saigae Tataricae*) [presently replaced by Shanyangjiao (*horn of goat*)]4.5 g;

No. 2 Gouteng (*Ramulus Uncariae cum Uncis*)(to be decocted later) 9 g;

No. 3 Juhua (*Flos Chrysanthemi*) 9 g;

No. 4 Sangye (*Folium Mori*) 6 g;

No. 5 Xianshengdihuang (*Radix Rehmanniae*) 15 g;

No. 6 Baishaoyao (*Radix Paeoniae Alba*) 9 g;

No. 7 Chuanbeimu (*Bulbus Fritillariae Cirrhosae*) 12 g;

No. 8 Xianzhuru (*Caulis Bambusae in Taenis*)(fresh) 15 g;

No. 9 Fushenmu (*Radix Pini Sclerotium Poriae*) 9 g;

No. 10 Shenggancao (*Radix Glycyrrhizae Recens*) 2.4 g.

Administrations：Decoct No. 1 and No. 8 first, then decoct the rest in their decoction for oral application.

Actions：Removing heat from the liver and subduing endogenous wind, increasing body fluid and activating muscles and tendons.

Clinical Application：This recipe is indicated for wind due to excessive heat, marked by unrelieved high fever, irritability, tic of hands and feet, deep-red and dry tongue, or parched and prickled tongue, taut and rapid pulse. It is applicable to headache, vertigo and convulsion caused by eclampsia gravidarum, epidemic encephalitis B and hypertension, and others, which are concomitant with high fever, taut and rapid pulse and ascribed to excessive heat in the liver meridian. In case of excessive heat with coma, use Zixue (*Powder*) and Angong Niuhuang Wan simultaneously to induce resuscitation. In case of severe convulsion, add Quanxie (*Scorpio*), Chantui (*Periostra-*

论》。

【组成】 羚羊角片（现用山羊角替代）4.5 g，钩藤（后下）、菊花各9 g，桑叶6 g，鲜生地黄15 g，白芍药9 g，川贝母12 g，鲜竹茹15 g，茯神木9 g，生甘草2.4 g。

【用法】 竹茹与羚羊角先煎代水，再入余药煎服。

【功用】 凉肝熄风，增液舒筋。

【临床应用】 适用于热盛动风证。症见高热不退，烦闷躁扰，手足抽搐，舌绛而干，或舌焦起刺，脉弦而数。妊娠子痫、流行性乙型脑炎以及高血压病引起的头痛、眩晕、抽搐等伴有高热，脉弦数，属肝经热盛者，可用本方治疗。若热邪内闭，神志昏迷者，可配合紫雪、安宫牛黄丸等清热开窍药同用；若抽搐甚者，可加全蝎、蝉蜕、蜈蚣等以加强熄

cum Cicadae) and Wugong (*Scolopendra*) to enhance the effect of subduing endogenous wind and relieving convulsion.

Elucidation：The syndrome arises when heat invades jueyin and causes excessive heat in the liver meridian and extreme heat producing wind. Simultaneously pathogenic heat scorches body fluid, resulting in producing phlegm and disturbing the mind. These should be treated by eliminating heat from the liver meridian and subduing endogenous wind, increasing body fluid and activating muscles and tendons. The first two ingredients function as monarch drugs with the effect of removing heat from the liver and subduing endogenous wind, clearing away heat and relieving convulsion. No. 3 and No. 4 are pungent and cool in nature and used as minister drugs to promote the effect of the monarch drugs. No. 5, No. 6 and No. 10, sour and sweet in nature, bear the function of nourishing yin and increasing body fluid, nourishing the liver and activating tendons. No. 7 and No. 8 are capable of clearing away heat and eliminating phlegm, while No. 9 checking hyperfunction of the liver and tranquilizing mind. These six ingredients play the part of adjuvant drugs. No. 10 also serves as guiding drug, which mediates the properties of other drugs.

Cautions：This recipe is contraindicated for hyperactivity of endogenous wind due to yin deficiency at the late stage of febrile diseases.

Zhengan Xifeng Tang
(*Decoction for Tranquilizing Liver-wind*)

Source：*Yixue Zhongzhong Canxi Lu* (*Discourse on Integrated Traditional Chinese and Western Medicine*).

Ingredients：

No. 1 Huainiuxi (*Radix Achyranthis Bidentatae*) 30 g；

风止痉之功。

【方解】 本方证由邪热传入厥阴,肝经热盛,热极动风,同时热邪灼津炼液成痰,扰及心神所致,治宜凉肝熄风,增液舒筋之法。方中羚羊角、钩藤凉肝熄风,清热解痉,共为君药。桑叶、菊花辛凉疏泄,助君药清热熄风,为臣药。鲜生地黄、白芍药、生甘草酸甘化阴,滋阴增液,柔肝舒筋,川贝母、鲜竹茹清热化痰,茯神木平肝宁心安神,俱为佐药。甘草调和药性,兼作使药。

【注意事项】 热病后期阴虚风动者,禁用本方。

镇肝熄风汤

【方源】《医学衷中参西录》。

【组成】 怀牛膝、代赭石各30 g,龙骨、牡蛎、龟版、白芍

No. 2 Daizheshi (*Ochra Haematitum*) 30 g;

No. 3 Longgu (*Os Draconis*) 15 g;

No. 4 Muli (*Concha Ostreae*) 15 g;

No. 5 Guiban (*Plastrum Testudinis*) 15 g;

No. 6 Baishaoyao (*Radix Paeoniae Alba*) 15 g;

No. 7 Xuanshen (*Radix Scrophulariae*) 15 g;

No. 8 Tianmendong (*Radix Asparagi*) 15 g;

No. 9 Chuanlianzi (*Fructus Meliae Toosendan*) 6 g;

No. 10 Shengmaiya (*Fructus Hordei Germinatus*) 6 g;

No. 11 Yinchen (*Herba Artemisiae Capillaris*) 6 g;

No. 12 Gancao (*Radix Glycyrrhizae*) 4.5 g.

Administration：Decoct the above drugs in water for oral application.

Actions：Tranquilizing the liver, calming endogenous wind, nourishing yin and suppressing hyperactive yang.

Clinical Application：This recipe is indicated for apoplectic stroke (apoplexy due to endogenous wind) marked by vertigo, ocular distension, tinnitus, pain and feverish sensation in the head, restlessness, flushed face, or frequent belching, or gradually-limited movement of limbs, wry mouth; or falling down from faint in serious cases, loss of consciousness, coming around when moved; or failing to recover after awake, taut and forceful pulse. It is applicable to hypertension and vascular headache, and others that pertain to yin deficiency of the liver and kidney and hyperactivity of the liver-yang. In case of extreme heat in the heart, add Shengshigao (*Gypsum Fibrosum*) to clear away heat. In case of excessive phlegm, add Danxing (*Arisaema cum Bile*) to clear away heat and eliminate phlegm. In case of feeble *chi* pulse when pressed, add Shudihuang (*Radix Rehmanniae Praeparatae*) and Shanzhuyu (*Fructus Corni*) to reinforce the liver and kidney.

药、玄参、天门冬各15 g，川楝子、生麦芽、茵陈各6 g，甘草4.5 g。

【用法】　水煎服。

【功用】　镇肝熄风，滋阴潜阳。

【临床应用】　适用于类中风。症见头目眩晕，目胀耳鸣，脑部热痛，心中烦热，面色如醉，或时常噫气，或肢体渐觉不利，口角渐形歪斜；甚或眩晕颠仆，昏不知人，移时始醒；或醒后不能复原，脉弦长有力。高血压病、血管性头痛等属肝肾阴亏，肝阳上亢者，可用本方治疗。若心中热甚者，可加生石膏以清热泻火；若痰多者，可加胆星以清热化痰；若尺脉重按虚者，可加熟地黄、山茱萸以补益肝肾。

Elucidation: The syndrome is caused by yin deficiency of the liver and kidney, hyperactivity of the liver-yang and disturbance of qi and blood circulation causing blood to flow upward. It should be treated by expelling endogenous wind from the liver, nourishing yin and suppressing hyperactive yang, and causing blood to flow downward. With a large dosage No. 1 functions as monarch drug to lead blood downward and nourish the liver and kidney. No. 2, No. 3 and No. 4 are capable of descending qi, suppressing hyperactive yang and expelling endogenous wind and used as minister drugs. No. 5, No. 6, No. 7 and No. 8 possess the effect of nourishing yin and clearing away heat so as to suppress the hyperactive yang, while No. 9, No. 10 and No. 11 bear the action of clearing away heat from the liver and regulating liver-qi, the seven drugs serving as adjuvant drugs. Used as guiding drug, No. 12 can mediate drug properties on the one hand, and regulate the stomach on the other when in compatibility with No. 10 so as to prevent mineral or stone drugs from impairing the stomach. This recipe aims primarily to cause blood to circulate downward and suppress the hyperactive yang, and simultaneously to reinforce the liver and kidney and disperse the stagnated liver-qi.

Cautions: This recipe is drastic in its effect of expelling endogenous wind and suppressing hyperactive yang, thus can only be applied to severe syndromes with hyperactive liver-yang and reversed flow of qi and blood.

Tianma Gouteng Yin
(*Decoction of Gastrodia and Uncaria*)

Source: *Zabing Zhengzhi Xinyi* (*New Concepts for Diagnosis and Treatment of Miscellaneous Diseases*).

Ingredients:

No. 1 Tianma (*Rhizoma Gastrodiae*) 9 g;

No. 2 Gouteng (*Ramulus Uncariae cum Uncis*)(to

【方解】 本方证由肝肾阴虚,肝阳上亢,气血逆乱,血气并走于上所致,治宜镇肝熄风,滋阴潜阳,引血下行之法。方中重用怀牛膝以引血下行,并可补益肝肾,为君药。代赭石、龙骨、牡蛎重镇降逆,潜阳熄风,为臣药。龟版、白芍药、玄参、天门冬滋阴清热以制亢阳,茵陈、川楝子、生麦芽清肝泄热,条达肝气,以利于肝阳的潜降,均为佐药。甘草调和药性,与生麦芽相配,还能和胃调中,防止金石药物损伤胃气,为佐使药。诸药配伍,以引血下行、重镇潜阳为主,兼以滋补肝肾、疏肝达郁。

【注意事项】 本方为镇肝潜阳重剂,非肝阳上亢,气血上逆之重证不宜使用。

天麻钩藤饮

【方源】 《杂病证治新义》。

【组成】 天麻9 g,钩藤(后下)12 g,石决明(先煎)18 g,栀子、黄芩各9 g,川牛膝

be decocted later) 12 g;

No. 3 Shijueming (*Concha Haliotidis*)(to be decocted first) 18 g;

No. 4 Zhizi (*Fructus Gardeniae*) 9 g;

No. 5 Huangqin (*Radix Scutellariae*) 9 g;

No. 6 Chuanniuxi (*Radix Achyranthis Bidentatae*) 12 g;

No. 7 Duzhong (*Cortex Eucommiae*) 9 g;

No. 8 Yimucao (*Herba Leonuri*) 9 g;

No. 9 Sangjisheng (*Ramulus Loranthi*) 9 g;

No. 10 Yejiaoteng (*Caulis Polygoni Multiflori*) 9 g;

No. 11 Fushen (*Sclerotium Poriae Circum Radicem Pini*) 9 g.

Administration: Decoct the above drugs in water for oral application.

Actions: Calming the liver to stop endogenous wind, clearing away heat and promoting blood circulation, nourishing the liver and kidney.

Clinical Application: This recipe is indicated for syndrome of hyperactive liver-yang and upward disturbance of liver-wind, marked by headache, vertigo, insomnia, reddened tongue with yellowish fur, taut pulse. It is applicable to hypertension with the above symptoms. In case of severe headache and vertigo, add Shanyangjiao (*horn of goat*) and Daizheshi (*Ochra Haematitum*) to strengthen the effect of suppressing the hyperactive yang and expelling endogenous wind.

Elucidation: The syndrome is caused by deficiency of the liver and kidney, hyperactive liver-yang and liver-wind stirring in the body, and disturbance of the mind. It should be treated by expelling liver-wind, clearing away heat, promoting blood flow, and reinforcing the liver and kidney. The first two ingredients are used as monarch drugs to expel the liver-wind. No. 3 and No. 6 act as min-

12 g,杜仲、益母草、桑寄生、夜交藤、茯神各9 g。

【用法】　水煎服。

【功用】　平肝熄风,清热活血,补益肝肾。

【临床应用】　适用于肝阳偏亢,肝风上扰证。症见头痛,眩晕,失眠,舌红苔黄,脉弦。高血压病患者出现上述症状者,可用本方治疗。如头痛眩晕较甚者,可加山羊角、代赭石以加强潜阳熄风之力。

【方解】　本方证由肝肾不足,肝阳偏亢,肝风内动,心神失宁所致,治宜平肝熄风,清热活血,补益肝肾之法。方中天麻、钩藤为平肝熄风要药,共为君药。石决明平肝潜阳,川牛膝引血下行,两药合

ister drugs, the former is capable of expelling endogenous wind and suppressing hyperactive yang and the latter leading blood downward. The two is used together to enhance the monarch drugs in suppressing hyperactive yang, sending down reversed flow of qi, and expelling endogenous wind. The rest serves as adjuvant drug, of which No. 4 and No. 5 clear away heat from the liver meridian, No. 8 promotes blood flow and induces diuresis so as to check the hyperactive and adverse ascent yang. No. 7 and No. 9 can reinforce the liver and kidney, which are the root cause of this syndrome, and No. 10 and No. 11 can tranquilize the mind.

Da Dingfeng Zhu
(*Bolus for Serious Endogenous Wind Syndrome*)

Source: *Wenbing Tiaobian* (*Treatise on Differentiation and Treatment of Seasonal Febrile Diseases*).

Ingredients:

No. 1 Baishaoyao (*Radix Paeoniae Alba*) 18 g;

No. 2 Gandihuang (*Radix Rehmanniae*) 18 g;

No. 3 Maimendong (*Radix Ophiopogonis*) 18 g;

No. 4 Guiban (*Plastrum Testudinis*) 12 g;

No. 5 Biejia (*Carapax Trionycis*) 12 g;

No. 6 Muli (*Concha Ostreae*) 12 g;

No. 7 Zhigancao (*Radix Glycyrrhizae Praeparatae*) 12 g;

No. 8 Ejiao (*Colla Corii Asini*) (melted) 9 g;

No. 9 Humaren (*Semen Lini*) 6 g;

No. 10 Wuweizi (*Fructus Schisandrae*) 6 g;

No. 11 Jizihuang (*fresh yolk*) 2.

Administration: Decoct the above drugs except No. 8 and No. 11 in water, then remove the residue from the decoction and dissolve No. 8 in it; put No. 11 into it and stir evenly before it is taken warm.

Actions: Nourishing yin and subduing wind.

用以加强君药潜阳降逆,平肝熄风之力,同为臣药。栀子、黄芩清热泻火以除肝经之热,益母草活血利水以降亢逆之阳,杜仲、桑寄生补益肝肾以治发病之本,夜交藤、朱茯神宁神定志以安心神之乱,均为佐药。

大定风珠

【方源】《温病条辨》。

【组成】 白芍药、干地黄、麦门冬各18 g,龟版、鳖甲、牡蛎、炙甘草各12 g,阿胶(烊冲)9 g,胡麻仁、五味子各6 g,鸡子黄2个。

【用法】 上药除阿胶、鸡子黄外,水煎去滓,入阿胶烊化,再入鸡子黄搅匀温服。

【功用】 滋阴熄风。

Clinical Application：This recipe is indicated for stirring endogenous wind due to yin deficiency, marked by lassitude and clonic convulsion at later stage of febrile diseases, feeble pulse, deep-red tongue with little fur, susceptibility to prostration. It is applicable to epidemic encephalitis B, epidemic cerebrospinal meningitis, and others that belong to severe inpairment of yin fluid and stirring-up of deficiency-wind during the recovery period of febrile diseases.

Elucidation：The syndrome is caused by impairment of genuine yin due to protracted febrile diseases, or extreme deficiency of genuine yin due to erroneous application of diaphoretic or purgative methods. These cause malnutrition of the liver-meridians and deficiency-wind to stir in the interior. It should be treated by nourishing yin and subduing wind. No.8 and No.11 function as monarch drugs to nourish yin and expel endogenous wind. No.1, No.2 and No.3 are capable of nourishing yin and the liver and No.4 and No.5 nourishing yin and suppressing yang, all playing the role of minister drugs. Both monarch and minister drugs, strong in flavor and greasy in nature, are used for nourishing yin, suppressing yang and dispelling wind. Acting as adjuvant drugs, No.9 has the function of nourishing yin and moistening dryness, No.6 subduing wind and suppressing yang, while No.10 in combination No.7, sour and sweet in nature, can increase yin fluid so as to strengthen the effect of nourishing yin and subduing wind. No.7 also serves as guiding drug to mediate the properties of other drugs.

Cautions：This recipe aims chiefly to replenish yin, thus it is contraindicated for yin deficiency with prevalence of excessive heat.

【临床应用】　适用于阴虚动风证。症见温病后期，神倦瘛疭，脉气虚弱，舌绛苔少，有时时欲脱之势。流行性乙型脑炎、流行性脑脊髓膜炎等热病恢复期阴液重伤，虚风内动者，可用本方治疗。

【方解】　本方证由温病迁延日久，邪热灼伤真阴，或因误汗、妄攻、重伤阴液以致真阴大亏，肝脉失养，虚风内动，治宜滋阴熄风之法。方中鸡子黄、阿胶滋养阴液以熄内风，共为君药。白芍药、干地黄、麦门冬滋阴柔肝，龟版、鳖甲滋阴潜阳，同为臣药。君臣相合，味厚滋腻，有填补真阴，潜阳熄风之功。胡麻仁养阴润燥，牡蛎平肝潜阳，五味子与炙甘草相配，酸甘化阴，以加强滋阴熄风之效，均为佐药。炙甘草调和药性，兼作使药。

【注意事项】　本方重在滋补真阴，若阴液虽亏而邪热犹盛者禁用。

2.13 Prescriptions for Eliminating Dampness

第十三章
祛湿剂

Prescriptions for eliminating dampness are mainly composed of diuretic drugs with effects of eliminating dampness, inducing diuresis, relieving stranguria and discharging turbidity, and are suitable for pathogenic dampness.

Dampness may be generated either exteriorly or interiorly, and located either in the superficies or the interior, either in the upper or in the lower. Dampness also differs in nature as cold or heat. Therefore, prescriptions for eliminating dampness are subdivided accordingly to prescriptions for drying dampness and regulating the stomach, those for clearing away heat and dampness, those for promoting diuresis and eliminating dampness, those for warming and eliminating water-dampness, and those for explelling wind and eliminating dampness.

Prescriptions for drying dampness and regulating the stomach chiefly consist of drugs with bitter and warm nature, which possess the effects of drying dampness, invigorating the spleen, promoting the flow of qi and regulating the stomach and are applied to syndrome of dampness retention in the middle-energizer. Prescriptions for clearing away heat and dampness are composed of drugs with the effects of clearing away heat and toxins and inducing diuresis and used for syndrome of damp heat accumulation in the interior. Prescriptions for promoting diuresis and eliminating dampness are made up of drugs with the effect of promoting diuresis and eliminating damphess, which

凡以祛湿药为主组成,具有化湿利水,通淋泄浊作用,用于治疗湿邪为病的方剂,统称祛湿剂。

湿邪之成有外感内生之分,病位有表里上下之别,性质有属寒属热之异。因而祛湿剂相应地分为燥湿和胃剂、清热祛湿剂、利水渗湿剂、温化水湿剂与祛风胜湿剂五类。

燥湿和胃剂由苦温燥湿药为主组成,具有燥湿健脾,行气和胃作用,适用于湿阻中焦之证。清热祛湿剂由清热祛湿药为主组成,具有清热解毒,利湿化浊作用,适用于湿热内蕴之证。利水渗湿剂由淡渗利湿药为主组成,具有通利小便,利水消肿作用,适用于水湿壅盛之证。温化水湿剂由温阳药配伍利湿药为主组成,具有温阳祛寒,利水渗

can promote urination and relieve swelling and are fit for excessive retention of water-dampness. Prescriptions for warming and eliminating water-dampness consist of drugs with the effect of warming yang and removing cold, inducing diuresis and eliminating dampness, which can warm yang and are suitable for syndrome of phlegm retention due to cold-dampness. Prescriptions for explelling wind and eliminating dampness possess the effects of dispelling wind and cold, eliminating dampness and relieving pain and are applied to obstruction of meridians and collaterals by dampness.

This group of prescriptions is apt to consume and impair body fluid because they are mostly composed of drugs that are aromatic, warm, dry, sweet and bland and can promote diuresis. For this reason, they should be cautiously used for patients with usual deficiency of yin and body fluid, or those with weak constitution after illness, or pregnant women.

2.13.1　Prescriptions for Eliminating Dampness and Regulating the Stomach

Pingwei San
(*Powder for Regulating Stomach Function*)

Source：*Taiping Huimin Hejiju Fang* (*Benevolent Prescriptions from Taiping Pharmaceutical Bureau*).

Ingredients：

No. 1 Cangzhu (*Rhizoma Atractylodis*) 2 500 g；

No. 2 Houpo (*Cortex Magnoliae Officinalis*) 1 560 g；

No. 3 Chenpi (*Pericarpium Citri Reticulatae*) 1 560 g；

No. 4 Zhigancao (*Radix Glycyrrhizae Praeparatae*) 900 g.

湿作用,适用于寒湿痰饮之证。祛风胜湿剂由祛风湿药为主组成,具有祛风散寒,胜湿止痛作用,适用于湿阻经络之证。

祛湿剂多由芳香温燥或甘淡渗利之药组成,易于耗伤阴津,故素体阴虚津亏,病后体弱以及孕妇等慎用。

第一节　燥湿和胃剂

平胃散

【方源】《太平惠民和剂局方》。

【组成】苍术2 500 g,厚朴、陈皮各1 560 g,炙甘草900 g。

Administration: Grind the above drugs into fine powder; then decoct 6 - 9 g at one time with 2 slices of fresh ginger and 2 pieces of Chinese dates in water for oral application.

Actions: Drying dampness and invigorating the spleen, promoting the flow of qi and regulating the stomach.

Clinical Application: This recipe is indicated for dampness retention in the spleen and stomach, marked by abdominal fullness, anorexia, tastelessness, nausea and vomiting, belching and regurgitation, heaviness of the body, lassitude and sleepiness, thick greasy whitish fur, slow pulse. It is applicable to chronic gastritis, dysfunction of digestive tract, gastroduodenal ulcer, and others that have chief manifestations as abdominal fullness and greasy whitish fur and are ascribed to dampness retention in the spleen and stomach. In case of heat transformed from dampness with bitter and dry mouth and greasy yellowish fur, add Huanglian (*Rhizoma Coptidis*) and Huangqin (*Radix Scutellariae*) to clear away heat-dampness. If concomitant with interior cold syndrome manifesting cold sensation in the abdomen, loose stool, and aversion to cold with preference for warmth, add Ganjiang (*Rhizoma Zingiberis*) and Caodoukou (*Semen Alpiniae Katsumadai*) to warm and dispel cold-dampness. If concomitant with disharmony between the spleen and stomach manifesting poor digestion, add Shenqu (*Massa Fermentata Medicinalis*), Shanzha (*Fructus Crataegi*) and Maiya (*Fructus Hordei Germinatus*) to promote digestion. In case of diarrhea due to excessive dampness, add Fuling (*Poria*) and Zexie (*Rhizoma Alismatis*) to promote diuresis and relieve diarrhea.

Elucidation: The syndrome is caused by dampness in the middle energizer, disorder of qi function, dysfunction of

【用法】　共研细末,每次 6～9 g,加生姜 2 片、大枣 2 枚,水煎服。

【功用】　燥湿健脾,行气和胃。

【临床应用】　适用于湿滞脾胃证。症见脘腹胀满,不思饮食,口淡无味,恶心呕吐,嗳气吞酸,肢体沉重,怠惰嗜卧,舌苔白腻而厚,脉缓。慢性胃炎、消化道功能紊乱、胃及十二指肠溃疡等以腹胀、苔白腻为主症,属湿滞脾胃者,可用本方治疗。若湿蕴化热,口苦而干,舌苔黄腻者,可加黄连、黄芩以清热燥湿;若兼里寒,腹冷便溏,畏寒喜温者,可加干姜、草豆蔻以温化寒湿;若兼脾胃不和,饮食难消者,可加神曲、山楂、麦芽以消食化滞;若湿盛泄泻者,可加茯苓、泽泻以利湿止泻。

【方解】　本方证由湿阻中焦,气机不畅,脾失健运,胃

the spleen and stomach. It should be treated by drying dampness and reinforcing the spleen, promoting flow of qi and regulating the stomach. With large dosage, No. 1 is used as monarch drug to eliminate dampness and activating the spleen. No. 2 has the function of eliminating dampness and promoting the circulation of qi and functions as minister drug, which can not only enhance the effect of the monarch drug but also relieve abdominal fullness. As adjuvant drug, No. 3 promotes the flow of qi and regulates the stomach. It assists No. 2 in promoting the flow of qi to relieve abdominal fullness and strengthens the effect of No. 1 in eliminating dampness and regulating the middle-energizer. No. 4 serves as guiding drug, mediating the properties of other drugs. Fresh ginger and Chinese dates are meant respectively to regulate the stomach and reinforce the spleen so that the effect of regulating the spleen and stomach is further enhanced.

Cautions: This recipe is contraindicated for those with deficiency of the spleen and stomach or usual deficiency of yin.

Huoxiang Zhengqi San
(Powder of Agastachis for Restoring Vital Qi)

Source: *Taiping Huimin Hejiju Fang* (*Benevolent Prescriptions from Taiping Pharmaceutical Bureau*).

Ingredients:

No. 1 Huoxiang (*Herba Agastachis*) 90 g;

No. 2 Suye (*Folium Perillae*) 30 g;

No. 3 Baizhi (*Radix Angelicae Dahuricae*) 30 g;

No. 4 Dafupi (*Pericarpium Arecae*) 30 g;

No. 5 Fuling (*Poria*) 30 g;

No. 6 Banxiaqu (*Rhizoma Pinelliae*) 60 g;

No. 7 Baizhu (*Rhizoma Atractylodis Macrocephalae*) 60 g;

No. 8 Chenpi (*Pericarpium Citri Reticulatae*) 60 g;

失和降所致,治宜燥湿健脾,行气和胃之法。方中重用苍术燥湿运脾,为君药。厚朴燥湿行气,既可协苍术加强燥湿作用,又能理气以除脘腹胀满,为臣药。陈皮行气和胃,合厚朴以助行气除满之力,合苍术更增燥湿和中之功,为佐药。炙甘草调和药性,为使药。用时少加生姜以和胃,加大枣以补脾,从而进一步加强了本方调和脾胃的作用。

【注意事项】　脾胃虚弱或素体阴虚者,慎用本方。

藿香正气散

【方源】　《太平惠民和剂局方》。

【组成】　藿香 90 g,苏叶、白芷、大腹皮、茯苓各30 g,半夏曲、白术、陈皮、厚朴、桔梗各 60 g,炙甘草 75 g。

No. 9 Houpo (*Cortex Magnoliae Officinalis*) 60 g;

No. 10 Jiegeng (*Radix Platycodi*) 60 g;

No. 11 Zhigancao (*Radix Glycyrrhizae Praeparatae*) 75 g.

Administration: Grind the above drugs into fine powder; decoct 6 - 9 g in water at one time with 3 slices of fresh ginger and 1 pieces of Chinese dates for oral application.

Actions: Relieving exterior syndrome, eliminating dampness and regulating qi and the middle-energizer.

Clinical Application: This recipe is indicated for exogenous wind-cold and interior impairment and dampness retention, marked by aversion to cold with fever, headache, abdominal pain, vomiting and diarrhea, greasy whitish fur, superficial or soft pulse. It is applicable to acute gastroenteritis and gastrointestinal type cold occurring in summer, which manifest chiefly vomiting and diarrhea due to pathogenic cold-heat as well as greasy whitish fur and pertain to exterior cold and interior dampness. In case of prevalence of exterior pathogenic factors manifesting aversion to cold without perspiration, add Xiangru (*Herba Elsholtziae seu Moslae*) to help relieve exterior syndrome. In case of sharp pain or fullness of the abdomen due to stagnated qi, add Muxiang (*Radix Aucklandiae*) and Yanhusuo (*Rhizoma Corydalis*) to promote the circulation of qi and relieve pain.

Elucidation: The syndrome is caused by exogenous wind and cold, stagnant wei-yang, and dampness in the middle-energizer. It should be treated by relieving exterior syndrome, eliminating dampness, and regulating qi and the middle-energizer. As monarch drug, No. 1 can dispel wind and cold, eliminate dampness, regulate the middle-energizer and stop vomiting. No. 2 and No. 3, pungent and aromatic in nature with dispersive action, can promote the action of the monarch drug in dispelling wind-

【用法】 共研细末,每次 6～9 g,加生姜 3 片、大枣 1 枚,水煎服。

【功用】 解表化湿,理气和中。

【临床应用】 适用于外感风寒,内伤湿滞证。症见恶寒发热,头痛,脘腹疼痛,呕吐泄泻,舌苔白腻,脉浮或濡。急性胃肠炎、夏季胃肠型感冒等以寒热吐泻,舌苔白腻为主症,属外寒内湿者,可用本方治疗。若表邪偏重,恶寒无汗者,可加香薷以助解表之功;若气滞脘腹胀痛较甚者,可加木香、延胡索以行气止痛。

【方解】 本方证由外感风寒,卫阳被郁,湿浊中阻,脾胃不和,升降失常所致,治宜解表化湿,理气和中之法。方中藿香散风寒,化湿浊,和中止呕,为君药。苏叶、白芷辛香发散,助藿香外解风寒,芳香化湿,同为臣药。茯苓、白术健脾运湿,和中止泻;半夏、

cold and eliminating dampness and act as minister drugs. No. 5 and No. 7 have the function of invigorating the spleen, regulating the middle-energizer and stopping vomiting, while No. 6 and No. 8 eliminating dampness, regulating the stomach, descending the adverse qi and relieving vomiting. No. 9 and No. 4 can promote the circulation of qi, eliminate dampness and relieve fullness, and No. 10 is effective in relieving exterior syndrome and inducing diuresis. These seven ingredients function as adjuvant drugs. No. 11 plays the role of guiding drug, mediating drug properties. All in combination makes it possible to dispel wind and cold in the exterior and eliminate dampness in the interior so that normal circulation of qi and function of the spleen and stomach are restored.

　　This recipe and Pingwei San both possess the function of drying dampness, promoting the flow of qi, and regulating the spleen and stomach. They are used for treating abdominal pain, vomiting and diarrhea due to dampness retention in the spleen and stomach. However, this recipe is fit for exogenous wind-cold and interior impairment and dampness retention because it is good at promoting the circulation of qi and inducing diuresis and can relieve exterior syndrome and regulate the middle-energizer. The latter has a better effect in drying dampness and activating the spleen and is indicated for disharmony between the spleen and stomach due to dampness retention in the middle-energizer. Therefore the chief factor in distinguishing the two is whether it possesses the functions of relieving exterior syndrome and dispersing cold, and whether dampness retention in the spleen and stomach is complicated with exterior syndrome.

　　Cautions：Ingredients in this recipe are mostly aromatic and pungent, so they should not be decocted for a long time.

陈皮燥湿和胃，降逆止呕；厚朴、大腹皮行气化湿，畅中除满；桔梗宣肺利膈，既利于解表，又利于化湿，俱为佐药。炙甘草调和药性，为使药。诸药配伍，使风寒外散，湿浊内化，则气机通畅，清升浊降，脾胃运纳复常。

　　本方与平胃散均有燥湿行气，健脾和胃之功，可用于治疗湿滞脾胃腹痛吐泻。然本方理气化湿力强，且能解表和中，适宜于外感风寒，内伤湿滞证；平胃散则专于燥湿运脾，而无解表之功，主治湿邪中阻，脾胃失和证。因此，有无解表散寒作用，主治湿滞脾胃是否兼有表证是两方的主要区别。

　　【注意事项】　本方药物大多芳香辛散，入汤剂不宜久煎。

2.13.2 Prescriptions for Clearing away Heat and Dampness

Yinchenhao Tang
(*Oriental Wormwood Decoction*)

茵陈蒿汤

Source：*Shanghan Lun* (*Treatise on Exogenous Febrile Diseases*).

【方源】　《伤寒论》。

Ingredients：

No. 1 Yinchenhao (*Herba Artemisiae Capillaris*) 18 g;

No. 2 Zhizi (*Fructus Gardeniae*) 9 g;

No. 3 Dahuang (*Radix et Rhizoma Rhei*) 6 g.

【组成】　茵陈蒿 18 g,栀子 9 g,大黄 6 g。

Administration：Decoct the above drugs in water for oral application.

【用法】　水煎服。

Actions：Clearing away heat, removing dampness, and relieving jaundice.

【功用】　清热利湿退黄。

Clinical Application：This recipe is indicated for jaundice due to damp heat, marked by bright yellowish skin and eyes, slight fullness in the abdomen, thirst, difficult urination, greasy and yellowish fur, deep and rapid pulse. It is applicable to jaundice as seen in acute icteric hepatitis, cholecystitis, cholelithiasis and leptospirosis, which pertains to accumulation of damp heat in the interior and is characterized by bright yellowish skin and greasy yellowish fur. In case of excessive dampness, add Fuling (*Poria*) and Zexie (*Rhizoma Alismatis*) to promote diuresis. In case of excessive heat, add Huangbai (*Cortex Phellodendri*) and Longdancao (*Radix Gentianae*) to clear away heat. In case of hypochondriac pain, add Chaihu (*Radix Bupleuri*) and Chuanlianzi (*Fructus Mediae Toosendan*) to disperse the stagnated liver-qi.

【临床应用】　适用于湿热黄疸。症见一身面目俱黄,黄色鲜明,腹微满,口渴,小便不利,舌苔黄腻,脉沉数。急性黄疸型肝炎、胆囊炎、胆石症、钩端螺旋体病等引起的黄疸,以黄色鲜明,舌苔黄腻为特点,属湿热内蕴者,可用本方治疗。若湿重者,可加茯苓、泽泻以利水渗湿;若热重者,可加黄柏、龙胆草以清热祛湿;若胁痛明显者,可加柴胡、川楝子以疏肝理气。

Elucidation：The syndrome is caused by accumulation of dampness and heat in the interior, causing heat to fail to disperse out and dampness fail to be excreted. It

【方解】　本方所治黄疸由湿热与瘀热蕴结于里,热不得外越,湿不得下泄,湿热交

should be treated by clearing away heat and removing dampness. No. 1 is monarch drug with the effect of clearing away heat and promoting diuresis. No. 2 can purge away intense heat and eliminate damp heat through urination, acting as minister drug. No. 3 is capable of removing heat accumulation through defication and used as adjuvant drug. The three together can eliminate dampness and heat separately through urination or defication so that jaundice will disappear.

Cautions：This recipe is contraindicated for patients with yin jaundice.

Sanren Tang
(*Decoction of Three Kinds of Kernels*)

Source：*Wenbing Tiaobian* (*Treatise on Differentiation and Treatment of Febrile Diseases*).

Ingredients：

No. 1 Xingren (*Semen Armeniacae Amarum*) 15 g;

No. 2 Huashi (*Talcum*) 18 g;

No. 3 Tongcao (*Tetrapanacis*) 6 g;

No. 4 Baidoukou (*Semen Amoni Cardamoni*) 6 g;

No. 5 Zhuye (*Herba Lophatheri*) 6 g;

No. 6 Houpo (*Cortex Magnoliae Officinalis*) 6 g;

No. 7 Yiyiren (*Semen Coicis*) 18 g;

No. 8 Banxia (*Rhizoma Pinelliae*) 15 g.

Administration：Decoct the above drugs in water for oral application.

Actions：Promoting qi function and eliminating dampness and heat.

Clinical Application：This recipe is indicated for the initial stage of damp-warm syndrome and summer-warm syndrome complicated with dampness, marked by headache, aversion to cold, heaviness and pain of the body, sallow complexion, chest distress, anorexia, afternoon fever, whitish fur, absence of thirst, taut thready

蒸而成,治宜清热利湿退黄之法。方中茵陈蒿清热利湿,为退黄疸之要药;栀子清热降火,通利三焦,引湿热自小便而出,为臣药。大黄泻热逐瘀,通利大便,导瘀热由大便而下,为佐药。三药合用,可使湿热之邪从二便分消,湿热得除,瘀热得下,则黄疸自退。

【注意事项】　黄疸属阴黄者,禁用本方。

三仁汤

【方源】《温病条辨》。

【组成】　杏仁 15 g,滑石 18 g,通草、白豆蔻、竹叶、厚朴各 6 g,薏苡仁 18 g,半夏 15 g。

【用法】　水煎服。

【功用】　宣畅气机,清利湿热。

【临床应用】　适用于湿温初起及暑温挟湿。症见头痛恶寒,身重疼痛,面色淡黄,胸闷不饥,午后身热,苔白不渴,脉弦细而濡。肠伤寒、肾盂肾炎、风湿性关节炎等属湿

and soft pulse. It is applicable to typhoid fever, pyelone-phritis, rheumatic arthritis, and others that pertain to accumulation of damp heat in the interior with dampness prevailing over heat. In case of marked exterior syndrome at the initial stage of damp heat syndrome, add Huoxiang (*Herba Agastachis*) and Xiangru (*Herba Elsholtziae seu Moslae*) to relieve exterior syndrome and eliminate dampness. In case of alternating chills and fever, add Qinghao (*Herba Artemisiae Chinghao*) and Caoguo (*Fructus Tsaoko*) to eliminate dampness.

Elucidation: The syndrome is caused by the initial stage of damp-warm syndrome with more dampness than heat, leading to retention of heat due to obstruction of dampness. It should be treated by promoting qi function and eliminating damp heat. No. 1 can help disperse lung-qi in the upper-energizer. The lung controls qi of the whole body, qi transformation leads to dampness transformation. No. 4 is aromatic and can eliminate dampness and promote the flow of qi of the spleen and stomach, while No. 7 is bland and can remove dampness through urination. The three eliminate damp heat separately from the three energizers, and serve together as monarch drugs. No. 8 and No. 6 possess the actions of promoting the circulation of qi and eliminating dampness, while No. 4 and the above two ingredients together regulate the stomach, the three being minister drugs. No. 5, No. 3 and No. 2 are capable of clearing away heat and eliminating dampness and help No. 7 eliminate damp heat, acting as adjuvant drugs.

Cautions: This recipe is not applicable for cases with bitter and dry mouth and greasy and yellowish fur.

Ganlu Xiaodu Dan
(*Sweet Dew for Detoxification*)

Source: *Wenre Jingwei* (*Compendium on Seasonal Febrile Diseases*).

热内蕴,湿重于热者,可用本方治疗。若湿温初起,卫分表证较为明显者,可加藿香、香薷以解表化湿;若寒热往来者,可加青蒿、草果以和解化湿。

【方解】 本方证由湿温初起,湿重热轻,湿遏热伏所致,治宜宣畅气机,清利湿热之法。方中杏仁宣利上焦肺气,盖肺主一身之气,气化则湿亦化;白豆蔻芳香化湿,行气宽中,畅中焦脾胃之气;薏苡仁淡渗利湿,使湿热从小便而去,三药合用,宣上畅中渗下,使湿热从三焦分消,共为君药。半夏、厚朴行气化湿,合白豆蔻畅中和胃,同为臣药。竹叶、通草、滑石清热利湿,助薏苡仁渗利湿热,均为佐药。

【注意事项】 口干而苦,舌苔黄腻者,禁用本方。

甘露消毒丹

【方源】 录自《温热经纬》。

Ingredients：

No. 1 Huashi（*Talcum*）450 g;

No. 2 Yinchenhao（*Herba Artemisiae Scopariae*） 330 g;

No. 3 Huangqin（*Radix Scutellariae*）300 g;

No. 4 Shichangpu（*Rhizoma Acori Graminei*）180 g;

No. 5 Chuanbeimu（*Bulbus Fritillariae*）150 g;

No. 6 Mutong（*Caulis Akebiae*）150 g;

No. 7 Huoxiang（*Herba Agastachis*）120 g;

No. 8 Shégan（*Rhizoma Belamcandae*）120 g;

No. 9 Lianqiao（*Fructus Forsythiae*）120 g;

No. 10 Bohe（*Herba Menthae*）120 g;

No. 11 Baidoukou（*Semen Amomi Cardamomi*）120 g.

Administration：Grind the above drugs into fine powder, take orally 9 g of the powder each time, and twice daily with warm boiled water. Or prepare it with Shenqu（*Massa Fermentata Medicinalis*）as pasted pills and take with boited water, or prepare the drugs directly into decoction with dosages in proportion to the original recipe.

Actions：Eliminating dampness and turbidity, and clearing away heat and toxins.

Indications：This recipe is indicated for seasonal damp heat diseases, marked by fever, lassitude, chest distress, abdominal fullness, thirst, sore throat, yellow skin and eyes, scanty dark urine, diarrhea and turbid urine, pale or thick greasy or dry yellowish fur. It is applicable to typhoid fever, infectious icterohepatitis, cholecystitis, leptospirosis, and others, which pertain to retention of both dampness and heat in the interior with equal predominance. It is especially used in summer. In case of evident jaundice, add Zhizi（*Fructus Gardeniae*）and Dahuang（*Radix et Rhizoma Rhei*）to eliminate damp heat. In case of severe swelling and pain of the throat,

【组成】　滑石 450 g,茵陈蒿 330 g,黄芩 300 g,石菖蒲 180 g,川贝母、木通各 150 g,藿香、射干、连翘、薄荷、白豆蔻各 120 g。

【用法】　共研细末,每次 9 g,温开水调服,每日 2 次。亦可以神曲糊丸,开水化服。若作汤剂,用量按原方比例酌定。

【功用】　利湿化浊,清热解毒。

【临床应用】　适用于湿温时疫。症见发热倦怠,胸闷腹胀,口渴咽痛,身目发黄,小便短赤,泄泻淋浊,舌苔淡白或厚腻或干黄。肠伤寒、黄疸型传染性肝火、胆囊炎、钩端螺旋体病等属湿热内蕴,湿热并重者,可用本方治疗,夏令暑热季节尤为常用。若黄疸明显者,可加栀子、大黄以清泄湿热;若咽喉肿痛较甚者,可加山豆根、板蓝根以解毒消

add Shandougen (*Radix Sophorae Subprostratae*) and Banlangen (*Radix Isatidis*) to eliminate toxin, relieve swelling and sore throat.

Elucidation: The syndrome is caused by exogenous dampness and heat retaining in qifen and interacting on each other. It should be eliminated by promoting diuresis and clearing away heat and toxins. No. 1 can clear away heat, induce diuresis and remove summer-heat, No. 2 can clear away heat, induce diuresis and relieve jaundice, and No. 3 can eliminate heat and dampness and purge away fire, the three being monarch drugs. No. 4 and No. 7 are aromatic with the effect of inducing diuresis, removing turbid substances and regulating the middle-energizer. No. 11 bears the function of promoting the flow of qi, inducing diuresis, regulating the stomach and stopping vomiting. No. 6 is capable of eliminating damp heat and leading it downward. These four drugs play the role of minister drugs. No. 9, No. 8, No. 5 and No. 10 possess the effect of removing toxin, relieving sore throat, removing mass and subduing swelling, serving as adjuvant drugs.

Lianpo Yin

(*Decoction of Coptis Rhizome and Bark of Officinalis Magnolia*)

Source: *Huoluan Lun* (*Treatise on Cholera Morbus*).

Ingredients:

No. 1 Houpo (*Cortex Magnoliae Officinalis*) 6 g;

No. 2 Huanglian (*Rhizoma Coptidis*) (baked with ginger juice) 3 g;

No. 3 Shichangpu (*Rhizoma Acori Tatarinowii*) 3 g;

No. 4 Banxia (*Rhizoma Pinelliae*) 3 g;

No. 5 Dandouchi (*Semen Sojae Praeparatum*) 9 g;

No. 6 Jiaozhizi (*Fructus Gardeniae*) (parched) 9 g;

No. 7 Lugen (*Rhizoma Phragmitis*) 60 g.

肿利咽。

【方解】 本方证由外感湿热,邪留气分,湿热交蒸所致,治宜利湿化浊,清热解毒之法。方中重用滑石清热利湿解暑,茵陈蒿清热利湿退黄,黄芩清热燥湿泻火,三药合用,清热除湿之功尤佳,共为君药。石菖蒲、藿香芳香化湿,辟秽和中;白豆蔻行气化湿,和胃止呕;木通清利湿热,导邪下行,同为臣药。连翘、射干、川贝母、薄荷解毒利咽,散结消肿,均为佐药。

连朴饮

【方源】 《霍乱论》。

【组成】 厚朴 6 g,黄连(姜汁炒)、石菖蒲、半夏各 3 g,淡豆豉、焦栀子各 9 g,芦根 60 g。

Administration：Decoct the above drugs in water for oral application.

Actions：Eliminating heat-dampness, regulating the flow of qi and activating the middle energizer.

Clinical Application：This recipe is indicated for vomiting and diarrhea due to damp heat, marked by vomiting and diarrhea, chest and epigastric fullness, vexation, scanty dark urine, greasy yellowish fur, smooth pulse. It is applicable to acute gastroenteritis, typhoid fever, paratyphoid and others, which are characterized by vomiting and diarrhea, chest and epigastric fullness, and greasy yellowish fur and ascribed to accumulation of damp heat in the middle-energizer with both heat and dampness equal predominance. This recipe is very effective in regulating the stomach and stopping vomiting. But in case of serious diarrhea it is necessary to add Biandou (*Semen Dolichoris*) and Yiyiren (*Semen Coicis*) so as to enhance the effect of inducing diuresis and relieving diarrhea.

Elucidation：The syndrome is caused by disturbance in ascending and descending function of the spleen and stomach qi due to accumulation of damp heat in the interior. It should be treated by clearing away heat, drying dampness and regulating the middle-energizer. Bitter and cold in nature, No. 2 can eliminate heat and dry dampness and regulate the stomach. No. 1, pungent and warm, can promote the flow of qi, eliminate dampness and send down the adverse flow of qi. As monarch drugs, both bring about the result of eliminating heat-dampness and regulating the middle energizer. No. 6 assists No. 2 to clear away heat, No. 3 helps No. 1 eliminate dampness, and No. 4 promotes the function of the monarch drugs to regulate the stomach and relieve vomiting, the three playing the role of minister drugs. No. 5, in combination with No. 6, can clear away heat from the chest and epigastrium so as

【用法】　水煎服。

【功用】　清热燥湿，理气和中。

【临床应用】　适用于湿热吐泻证。症见上吐下泻，胸脘痞闷，心烦躁扰，小便短赤，舌苔黄腻，脉滑。急性胃肠炎、肠伤寒、副伤寒等上吐下泻，以胸脘痞闷，舌苔黄腻为特点，属湿热中阻，湿热并重者，可用本方治疗。本方和胃止呕之功较著，若腹泻明显者，宜加扁豆、薏苡仁以加强利湿止泻作用。

【方解】　本方证由湿热内蕴，脾胃升降失常所致，治宜清热燥湿，理气和中之法。方中黄连苦寒清热燥湿和胃，厚朴辛温行气化湿降逆，两药并用，辛开苦降，清热燥湿，理气和中，共为君药。栀子助黄连以清热，石菖蒲助厚朴以化湿，半夏助君药以和胃止呕，共为臣药。淡豆豉配栀子可清宣胸脘郁热而除烦闷，芦根可清热止呕生津，以防吐泻太过伤津之虞，均为佐药。

to relieve restlessness with oppressive feeling. No. 7 is capable of clearing away heat, relieving vomiting and increasing body fluid so as to prevent the impairment of body fluid caused by excessive vomiting and diarrhea. No. 5 and No. 7 act as adjuvant drugs.

Bazheng San
(*Eight Health-restoring Powder*)

Source: *Taiping Huimin Hejiju Fang* (*Benevolent Prescriptions from Taiping Pharmaceutical Bureau*).

Ingredients:

No. 1 Cheqianzi (*Semen Plantaginis*) 500 g;

No. 2 Qumai (*Herba Dianthi*) 500 g;

No. 3 Bianxu (*Herba Polygoni Avicularis*) 500 g;

No. 4 Huashi (*Talcum*) 500 g;

No. 5 Zhiziren (*Semen Gardeniae*) 500 g;

No. 6 Zhigancao (*Radix Glycyrrhizae Praeparatae*) 500 g;

No. 7 Mutong (*Caulis Akebiae*) 500 g;

No. 8 Dahuang (*Radix et Rhizoma Rhei*) 500 g.

Administration: Grind the above drugs into fine powder; decoct 6 –9 g of the powder together with a little Dengxincao (*Medulla Junci*) in water for oral application.

Actions: Clearing away heat and purging fire, inducing diuresis and relieving stranguria.

Clinical Application: This recipe is indicated for stranguria due to dampness and heat, marked by frequency and urgency of urination with pain, urinary stuttering and bradyuria, turbid and dark urine, even uroschesis, stuffiness of the lower abdomen, dry mouth and throat, greasy yellowish fur, smooth and rapid pulse. It is applicable to cystitis, urethritis, acute prostatitis, calculi of the urinary system, pyelonephritis and others, which chiefly manifest frequency and urgency of urination with pain, reddened tongue with yellowish fur and pertain to

八正散

【方源】 《太平惠民和剂局方》。

【组成】 车前子、瞿麦、萹蓄、滑石、栀子仁、炙甘草、木通、大黄各500 g。

【用法】 共研粗末,每次6～9 g,加灯心草少许,水煎服。

【功用】 清热泻火,利水通淋。

【临床应用】 适用于湿热淋证。症见尿频尿急,溺时涩痛,淋沥不畅,尿色浑赤,甚则癃闭不通,小腹急满,口燥咽干,舌苔黄腻,脉滑数。膀胱炎、尿道炎、急性前列腺炎、泌尿系结石、肾盂肾炎等以尿频急涩痛,舌红苔黄为主症,属下焦湿热者,可用本方治疗。本方又是治疗湿热下注

accumulation of dampness and heat in the lower energizer. This recipe is commonly used for various types of stranguria due to downward flow of damp-heat. In case of stranguria with blood in urine, add Shengdihuang (*Radix Rehmanniae*), Xiaoji (*Herba Cephalanoploris*) and Baimaogen (*Rhizoma Imperatae*) to remove heat from blood and cool blood. In case of stranguria caused by urinary stone, add Jinqiancao (*Herba Lysimachiae*) and Haijinsha (*Spora Lygodii*) to remove stone and relieve stranguria. In case of stranguria marked by chyluria, add Bixie (*Rhizoma Dioscoreae*) and Shichangpu (*Rhizoma Acori Tatarinowii*) to separate the clear from the turbid.

Elucidation: The syndrome is caused by flow of dampness-heat down to the urinary bladder and obstructed urination. It should be treated by clearing away heat and purging fire, inducing diuresis and relieving stranguria. This recipe is very effective in eliminating dampness and heat because it comprises many diuretics as No. 7, No. 4, No. 1, No. 2 and No. 3. Ingredient No. 5 is capable of removing damp heat from the three energizers and No. 8 purging away heat and fire. No. 6 mediates the effects of other drugs and Dengxincao (*Medulla Junci*) leads heat downward.

Cautions: This recipe consists of diuretics with bitter and cold nature and is fit for syndrome with excess fire. Thus it should be used with great caution in those with weak constitution or pregnant women.

Liuyi San
(*Liuyi Powder*)

Source: *Shanghan Zhige* (*Formulas for Exogenous Febrile Diseases*).

Ingredients:

No. 1 Huashi (*Talcum*) 180 g;

No. 2 Shenggancao (*Radix Glycyrrhizae Recens*) 30 g.

而致各种淋证的通用方：若血淋尿血者,可加生地黄、小蓟、白茅根以凉血止血;若石淋涩痛者,可加金钱草、海金沙以化石通淋;若膏淋混浊者,可加草薢、石菖蒲以分清化浊。

【方解】 本方证由湿热下注膀胱,水道不利所致,治宜清热泻火,利水通淋之法。方中集木通、滑石、车前子、瞿麦、萹蓄诸利水通淋之品,清利湿热之功颇著。栀子清泄三焦湿热,大黄泄热降火,甘草调和药性,用时少加灯心草以导热下行。

【注意事项】 本方苦寒通利,适用于实火之证,若淋证日久,体质虚弱,以及孕妇等慎用。

六一散

【方源】 《伤寒直格》。

【组成】 滑石 180 g,生甘草 30 g。

Administration：Grind the above drugs into fine powder; decoct 9 g each time after wrapped with a piece of cloth or take orally with warm boiled water; three times daily.

Actions：Clearing away heat and eliminating dampness.

Clinical Application：This recipe is indicated for damp heat syndrome of the lower-energizer, marked by feverish body, polydipsia, bradyuria, or frequency and urgency of urination with pain, or diarrhea, reddened tongue with greasy yellowish fur, rapid pulse. It is applicable to cystitis, urethritis, acute enteritis and others, which pertain to damp heat syndrome. Since this recipe is mild in action, it is seldom used singly and often wrapped with a piece of cloth and decocted with some recipe with the function of clearing away heat and promoting diuresis.

Elucidation：The syndrome is caused by downward flow of damp heat to the urinary bladder, which either causes difficulty in urination, or retains in the intestines, and leads to dysfunction in transportaion. It should be treated by clearing away heat and eliminating dampness. Huashi (*Talcum*) in the recipe is sweet, bland and cold in nature — bland nature can eliminate dampness, cold nature clear away heat, and smoothness promoting defecation and urination. It is good at clearing away heat, relieving vexation, inducing diuresis and relieving stranguria and is used as monarch drug. No. 2 functions as adjuvant drug, which is capable of clearing away heat and purging fire, mediating drug properties and preventing No. 1 from impairing the middle-energizer. This recipe is a common one for clearing away heat and inducing diuresis, which is cold in nature but does not impair the middle-energizer, induces diuresis but without drastic potency.

Cautions：This recipe is contraindicated for patients

【用法】 共研细末,每次 9 g,包煎或温开水调下,每日 3 次。

【功用】 清热利湿。

【临床应用】 适用于下 焦湿热证。症见身热烦渴,小 便不利,或尿频急涩痛,或泄 泻,舌红苔黄腻,脉数。膀胱 炎、尿道炎、急性肠炎等属湿 热证者,可用本方治疗。本方 药少力薄,较少单独使用,多 以纱布包后加入清热利湿方 剂中煎服。

【方解】 本方证由湿热 下注所致,或注于膀胱,水道 不利,或渗于肠道,传导失司, 治宜清热利湿之法。方中滑 石甘淡而寒,淡能渗湿,寒能 清热,滑能利窍,功擅清热除 烦,利水通淋,为君药。生甘 草清热泻火,调和药性,并可 防滑石寒凉伤中,为佐使药。 两药配伍,寒凉而不伤中,利 水而不峻利,为清利湿热的常 用方剂。

【注意事项】 素体阴虚

with usual yin deficiency or without heat syndrome.

Ermiao San
(*Powder of Two Wonderful Drugs*)

Source：*Danxi Xinfa* (*Danxi's Experiential Therapy*).

Ingredients：

No.1 Huangbai (*Cortex Phellodendri*) (backed)；

No.2 Cangzhu (*Rhizoma Atractylodis*) (backed)；

In equal dosage.

Administration：Grind the above drugs into fine powder；take orally 6 g each time with 2 drops of ginger juice and warm boiled water. Or prepare it into pills entitled Ermiao Wan and take 6 g each time with warm boiled water.

Actions：Clearing away heat and drying dampness.

Clinical Application：This recipe is indicated for downward flow of dampness and heat, marked by painful tendons and bones, or flaccid feet, or swelling and painful feet and knees, or leukorrhagia, or eczema of genitals, scanty dark urine, greasy yellowish fur, soft and rapid pulse. It is applicable to arthritis, eczema of scrotum, vaginitis and other diseases that affect the lower body and pertain to damp heat syndrome. In case of numbness and flaccidity of feet and knees, Niuxi (*Radix Achyranthis Bidentatae*) may be added to reinforce the joints, waist and knees, and if made into pills, they are named Sanmiao Wan. If the above syndrome is concomitant with swelling and pain of feet and knees, difficulty in bending and stretching movement, Yiyiren (*Semen Coicis*) can also be added to induce diuresis and activate tendons, forming another recipe entitled Simiao Wan. In case of eczema of the genitals, add Chixiaodou (*Semen Phaseoli*) and Fuling (*Poria*) to clear away heat and dampness as well as relieve eczema.

或无热象者,禁用本方。

二妙散

【方源】《丹溪心法》。

【组成】 炒黄柏、炒苍术各等分。

【用法】 共研细末,每次6 g,加姜汁2滴,温开水调服。或制成丸剂,称二妙丸,每次6 g,温开水送下。

【功用】 清热燥湿。

【临床应用】 适用于湿热下注证。症见筋骨疼痛,或两足痿软,或足膝红肿疼痛,或湿热带下,或下部湿疮,小便短赤,舌苔黄腻,脉濡数。关节炎、阴囊湿疹、阴道炎等病位偏下,属湿热证者,可用本方治疗。若脚膝麻木,痿软无力者,可加牛膝以利关节,强腰膝,制成丸剂即三妙丸;若又兼足膝肿痛,屈伸不利者,可再加薏苡仁以利湿舒筋,制成丸剂即四妙丸;若下部湿疮,可加赤小豆、赤茯苓以清湿热,解疮毒。

Elucidation: All the syndromes are caused by damp-ness and heat, which either flows into tendons, or mus-cles, or genitals or muscular striae. It should be treated by clearing away heat and drying dampness. No.1, bitter and cold in nature, is used as monarch drug to remove dampness and heat from the lower energizer. No. 2 is warm and bitter in nature, so it can dry dampness and re-inforce the spleen to make dampness off without genera-ting again. Simple but effective, this recipe is commonly used for treating damp heat syndrome of the lower-energi-zer.

Cautions: This recipe has an equal efficacy both in clearing away heat and eliminating dampness, thus it is not suitable for syndrome with more dampness than heat.

2.13.3 Prescriptions for Promoting Diuresis and Eliminating Dampness

Wuling San
(*Powder of Five Drugs Containing Poria*)

Source: *Shanghan Lun* (*Treatise on Exogenous Febrile Diseases*).

Ingredients:

No.1 Zhuling (*Polyporus*) 9 g;

No.2 Zexie (*Rhizoma Alismatis*) 15 g;

No.3 Baizhu (*Rhizoma Atractylodis*) 9 g;

No.4 Fuling (*Poria*) 9 g;

No.5 Guizhi (*Ramulus Cinnamomi*) 6 g.

Administrations: Grind the above drugs into fine powder; take orally 6 g each time and 3 times daily with warm boiled water. Or prepare them into decoction, with dosages in proportion to the original recipe.

Actions: Inducing diuresis, eliminating dampness, warming yang and promoting qi function.

【方解】 本方所治诸证皆为湿热下注所致,或流注筋骨,或注于筋脉,或下注前阴,或蕴于肌腠,故治宜清热燥湿之法。方中黄柏苦寒,善祛下焦湿热,为君药。苍术苦温,燥湿健脾,使湿去而不再生。二药配伍,药简力专,为治疗下焦湿热诸证的常用方剂。

【注意事项】 本方清热祛湿之功并重,若湿重热轻者不宜使用。

第三节　利水
渗湿剂

五苓散

【方源】《伤寒论》。

【组成】 猪苓 9 g,泽泻15 g,白术 9 g,茯苓 9 g,桂枝6 g。

【用法】 共研细末,每次6 g,温开水调下,每日 3 次。亦可作汤剂,用量按原方比例酌定。

【功用】 利水渗湿,温阳化气。

Clinical Application：This recipe is indicated for syndrome of fluid retention in the interior, marked by edema, diarrhea, dysuria, pale tongue with glossy whitish fur, soft pulse. It is applicable to edema from nephritis and cirrhosis, acute enteritis, uroschesis, hydrocephalus and others, which pertain to fluid-retention and dampness in the interiror. In case of excessive retention of fluid, Wupi San〔Chenpi (*Pericarpium Citri Reticulatae*), Fulingpi (*Cortex Sclerotii Poriae*), Shengjiangpi (*Exocarpium Zingiberis Recentis*), Sangbaipi (*Cortex Mori Radicis*) and Dafupi (*Pericarpium Arecae*)〕may be used simultaneously to enhance the effect of inducing diuresis and relieving swelling.

Elucidation：The syndrome is caused by dysfunction of the spleen in transportation and transformation, leading to retention of fluid in the interiror and dysfunction of qi transformation of the bladder. It should be treated by inducing diuresis and warming yang to promote qi function. With a large dosage, No. 2 is effective in inducing diuresis and used as monarch drug. No. 4 and No. 1 are sweet and mild in nature and function as minister drugs, which can promote diuresis and enhance the effect of the monarch drug in relieving swelling. No. 3 in combination with No. 4 futher strengthens the function of reinforcing the spleen and inducing diuresis, while No. 5 promotes the function of the bladder in excretion of urine. No. 3 and No. 5 together play the role of adjuvant drugs. Originally this recipe was used for treating retention of fluid manifesting dysfunction of the bladder in excretion of urine and braduria, which are caused by the unrelieved exogenous pathogenic factors retaining in taiyang meridian. Thus it can be inferred that No. 5 also bears the effect of relieving exterior syndrome and eliminating pathogenic factors. This recipe is mainly to invigorate the spleen and induce diure-

【临床应用】　适用于水湿内停证。症见水肿，泄泻，小便不利，舌淡，苔白滑，脉濡。肾炎、肝硬化所引起的水肿，急性肠炎、尿潴留、脑积水等属水湿内停者，可用本方治疗。若水湿壅盛者，可与五皮散（陈皮、茯苓皮、生姜皮、桑白皮、大腹皮）合用以增强利水消肿之效。

【方解】　本方证由脾失健运，水湿内停，膀胱气化不利所致，治宜利水渗湿，温阳化气之法。方中重用泽泻利水渗湿，为君药。茯苓、猪苓甘淡利湿，茯苓又能健脾，两药协助君药加强利水消肿之功，同为臣药。白术合茯苓则健脾运湿之力更著，桂枝助膀胱之气化，均为佐药。原书以本方治疗太阳表邪未解，内传膀胱以致气化不行，小便不利的蓄水证，故用桂枝还有解表散邪之意。诸药配伍，重在健脾利水，故凡脾失健运，水湿内停之证皆可治之。

sis and, thus, fit for retention of fluid due to dysfunction of the spleen.

Cautions: Warm in nature as this recipe is, it should not be used for the case of heat transformed from water-dampness.

Zhuling Tang
(*Umbellate Pore Decoction*)

Source: *Shanghan Lun* (*Treatise on Exogenous Febrile Diseases*).

Ingredients:

No. 1 Zhuling (*Polyporus*) 9 g;

No. 2 Zexie (*Rhizoma Alismatis*) 9 g;

No. 3 Fuling (*Poria*) 9 g;

No. 4 Ejiao (*Colla Corri Asini*) (melted) 9 g;

No. 5 Huashi (*Talcum*) 9 g.

Administration: Decoct the above drugs in water for oral application.

Actions: Promoting diuresis, eliminating dampness, clearing away heat and nourishing yin.

Clinical Application: This recipe is indicated for yin impairment by retention of water and heat, marked by dysuria, fever, thirst with desire for drinking, or vexation, insomnia, or concomitant with vomiting and diarrhea, or stranguria with blood in urine, reddened tongue with whitish or yellowish fur, thready and rapid pulse. It is applicable to such cases associated with dysuria as infection of the urinary system, nephritis and others, which pertain to retention of water and heat concomitant with yin deficiency. If concomitant with frequency and urgency of urination with pain, add Zhizi (*Fructus Gardeniae*) and Cheqianzi (*Semen Plantaginis*) to clear away heat and induce diuresis for treating stranguria. In case of stranguria with blood in urine or hematuria, add Baimaogen (*Rhizoma Imperatae*) and Xiaoji (*Herba Cephalanoploris*)

猪苓汤

【方源】 《伤寒论》。

【组成】 猪苓、泽泻、茯苓、阿胶(烊化)、滑石各9 g。

【用法】 水煎服。

【功用】 利水渗湿,清热养阴。

【临床应用】 适用于水热互结伤阴证。症见小便不利,发热,口渴欲饮,或心烦不寐,或兼呕吐泄泻,或发为血淋,舌红苔白或微黄,脉细数。泌尿系感染、肾炎等小便不利,属水热互结又兼阴虚者,可用本方治疗。若兼尿频急涩痛者,可加栀子、车前子以清热利水通淋;若血淋或血尿者,可加白茅根、小蓟以凉血止血。

to remove heat from blood and stop bleeding.

Elucidation：This syndrome is caused by fluid-retention and heat retaining in the lower energizer，leading to yin impairment and dysfunction of qi transformation of the bladder. It should be treated by inducing diuresis，clearing away heat and nourishing yin. No. 1 and No. 3 function as monarch drugs，which can induce diuresis and invigorate the spleen. No. 2 is used as minister drug，which further enhances the effect of inducing diuresis in combination with the monarch drugs. No. 5 and No. 4 act as adjuvant drugs，the former capable of clearing away heat，promoting diuresis and treating stranguria and the latter nourishing yin and blood and arresting bleeding. All ingredients as a whole bring about the result of promoting diuresis without impairing yin and nourishing yin without retaining pathogenic factors so that dampness and heat are eliminated，yin fluid restored and all the symptoms relieved.

Both this recipe and Wuling San possess diuretic function and are used for the treatment of dysuria. The latter is specially fit for dysuria due to dysfunction of the spleen in transportation，retention of dampness and dysfunction of qi transformation of the bladder. That is why Zexie（*Rhizoma Alismatis*），Zhuling（*Polyporus*）and Fuling（*Poria*）are used in compatibility with Guizhi（*Ramulus Cinnamomi*）to activate yang and with Baizhu（*Rhizoma Atractylodis Macrocephalae*）to promote the spleen in transportation. It is formed with the effects of warming yang，promoting qi transformation and the excretion of urine. The former，however，is suitable for dysuria as the result of retention of fluid and heat concomitant with yin impairment and includes a compatibility of Zexie（*Rhizoma Alismatis*），Zhuling（*Polyporus*）and Fuling（*Poria*）with Huashi（*Talcum*）to clear away heat and treat stranguria and with Ejiao（*Colla Corri Asi-*

【方解】 本方证由水热结于下焦，日久耗伤阴液，膀胱气化不行所致，治宜利水渗湿，清热养阴之法。方中猪苓、茯苓利水渗湿，健脾助运，共为君药。泽泻淡渗利水，与二苓同用，则利水渗湿之功益著，为臣药。滑石清热利水通淋，阿胶滋阴养血止血，均为佐药。诸药配伍，利水渗湿与清热养阴并进，利水而不伤阴，滋阴而不敛邪，使水湿去，邪热清，阴津复，诸证自解。

本方与五苓散同为利水渗湿之剂，均可治疗水湿内停的小便不利。但五苓散证属脾失健运，水湿停蓄，膀胱气化不利之小便不利，故方用泽泻、猪苓、茯苓配桂枝以通阳化气，伍白术以健脾助运以制水，合成温阳化气利水之剂。猪苓汤证属水热互结兼有阴伤之小便不利，故以猪苓、茯苓、泽泻配滑石以清热通淋，配伍阿胶滋阴润燥，合成清热滋阴利水之剂。

ni) to nourish yin and moisten dryness, which bears the function of clearing away heat, nourishing yin and inducing diuresis.

Cautions: This recipe is mainly for inducing diuresis, consequently contraindicated for cases with excessive heat or serious impairment of yin fluid.

Fangji Huangqi Tang
(*Decoction of Tetrandra and Astragalus*)

Source: *Jingui Yaolue* (*Synopsis of Prescriptions of the Golden Cabinet*).

Ingredients:
No. 1 Fangji (*Radix Stephaniae Tetrandrae*) 12 g;
No. 2 Huangqi (*Radix Astragali seu Hedysari*) 15 g;
No. 3 Zhigancao (*Radix Glycyrrhizae Praeparatae*) 6 g;
No. 4 Baizhu (*Rhizoma Atractylodis Macrocephalae*) 9 g.

Administration: Add to the above drugs 4 slices of fresh ginger and 2 pieces of Dazao (*Fructus Ziziphi Jujubae*) and decoct them in water for oral application.

Actions: Invigorating qi and dispelling wind, reinforcing the spleen and inducing diuresis

Clinical Application: This recipe is indicated for wind-edema or wind-dampness syndrome (rheumatism), marked by perspiration with aversion to wind, heaviness of the body, edema of limbs, dysuria, pale tongue with whitish fur, superficial pulse. It is applicable to chronic glomerulonephritis, cardiac edema, rheumatic arthritis and others, which pertain to exterior-deficiency and excessive dampness. In case of severe edema, add Fuling (*Poria*) and Zexie (*Rhizoma Alismatis*) to strengthen the effect of inducing diuresis and relieving edema. In case of chest fullness and abdominal flatulence, add Chenpi (*Pericarpium Citri Reticulatae*) and Zhike (*Fructus Aurantii*) to promote the flow of qi and relieve fullness.

Elucidation: The syndrome results from attack by

【注意事项】 本方重在利水,若邪热较盛或阴津大亏者禁用。

防己黄芪汤

【方源】 《金匮要略》。

【组成】 防己 12 g,黄芪 15 g,炙甘草 6 g,白术 9 g。

【用法】 加生姜 4 片,大枣 2 枚,水煎服。

【功用】 益气祛风,健脾利水。

【临床应用】 适用于风水或风湿。症见汗出恶风,身重,肢体浮肿,小便不利,舌淡苔白,脉浮。慢性肾小球肾炎、心源性水肿、风湿性关节炎等属表虚湿盛者,可用本方治疗。若水肿较甚者,可加茯苓、泽泻以加强利水消肿之效;若胸腹胀满者,可加陈皮、枳壳以行气宽中。

【方解】 本方证由表虚

exogenous wind due to exterior-deficiency, retention of dampness in the muscular striae, meridians and collaterals. It should be treated by invigorating qi, dispelling wind, reinforcing the spleen and inducing diuresis. No. 1 has the function of dispelling wind and eliminating dampness, while No. 2 possesses the effect of invigorating qi to strengthen the superficial resistance and inducing diuresis to relieve edema. The two together can dispel wind and promote diuresis without imparing the superficial resistance as well as strengthen body resistance without retaining pathogenic wind, playing the part of monarch drugs. Used as minister drug, No. 4 is capable of invigorating qi, reinforcing the spleen and inducing diuresis and further enhances the effect of the monarch drugs. No. 3 has the function of invigorating qi and reinforcing the middle-energizer as well as mediating drug properties and functions as adjuvant drug. The fresh ginger and Chinese dates can not only regulate and nourish the spleen and stomach so as to build up body resistance, but also regulate *ying* and *wei* to promote the effect of relieving exterior syndrome and eliminating pathogenic wind.

Cautions: This recipe is contraindicated for excessive fluid retention and dampness without exterior-deficiency.

不固,外受风邪,水湿郁于肌表经络之间所致,治宜益气祛风,健脾利水之法。方中防己疏风散邪,祛湿利水;黄芪益气固表,行水消肿,两药配伍,祛风行水而不伤表,扶正固表而不留邪,共为君药。白术补气健脾祛湿,配黄芪可加强益气固表之力,伍防己可加强祛湿行水之功,为臣药。炙甘草益气补中,调和药性,为佐使药。煎加生姜、大枣既可调补脾胃以助补虚扶正,又能调和营卫以助解表散邪。

【注意事项】　水湿壅盛而无表虚之象者,禁用本方。

2.13.4　Prescriptions for Warming and Eliminating Water-dampness

第四节　温化水湿剂

Linggui Zhugan Tang
(*Decoction of Poria, Bighead Atractylodes, Cinnamom and Licorice*)

苓桂术甘汤

Source: *Jingui Yaolue* (*Synopsis of Prescriptions of the Golden Cabinet*).

【方源】　《金匮要略》。

Ingredients:

No. 1 Fuling (*Poria*) 12 g;

【组成】　茯苓 12 g,桂枝 9 g,白术 9 g,甘草 6 g。

No. 2 Guizhi (*Ramulus Cinnamoni*) 9 g;

No. 3 Baizhu (*Rhizoma Atractylodis Macrocephalae*) 9 g;

No. 4 Gancao (*Radix Glycyrrhizae*) 6 g.

Administration: Decoct the above drugs in water for oral application.

Actions: Warming yang and relieving phlegm retention, reinforcing the spleen and inducing diuresis.

Clinical Application: This recipe is indicated for syndrome of phlegm retention, marked by chest and hypochondriac fullness, vertigo, palpitation, short breath with cough, whitish glossy fur, taut and smooth pulse. It is applicable to such cases associated with edema as chronic bronchitis, bronchial asthma, cardiogenic glomerulonephritis or chronic glomerulonephritis, and others, which pertains to retention of water-dampness due to yang deficiency. In case of cough with much sputum, add Banxia (*Rhizoma Pinelliae*) and Chenpi (*Pericarpium Citri Reticulatae*) to eliminate dampness and phlegm. In case of flatulence or borborygmus, add Zhishi (*Furctus Aurantii Immaturus*) to promote the flow of qi and diuresis. In case of marked deficiency of the spleen with poor appetite and loose stool, add Dangshen (*Radix Codonopsis Pilosulae*) and Huangqi (*Radix Astragali seu Hedysari*) to invigorate qi and reinforce the spleen.

Elucidation: The syndrome is caused by yang deficiency of the middle-energizer, leading to dysfunction of the spleen, and failure of qi to dissolve fluid-retention retaining in the heart. It should be treated by warming yang and activating the spleen. No. 1 is the monarch drug with the function of reinforcing the spleen and inducing diuresis. Acting as minister drug, No. 2 is capable of warming yang and can remove phlegm when in combination with No. 1. Ingredient No. 3 functions as adjuvant drug, which can invigorate the spleen, eliminate dampness and prevent

【用法】 水煎服。

【功用】 温阳化饮,健脾渗湿。

【临床应用】 适用于痰饮病。症见胸胁胀满、眩晕心悸,短气而咳,舌苔白滑,脉弦滑。慢性支气管炎、支气管哮喘、心源性或慢性肾小球肾炎等见有水肿,属阳虚水湿不化者,可用本方治疗。若咳嗽痰多者,可加半夏、陈皮以燥湿化痰;若脘腹胀满或腹中有水声,可加枳实以行气利水;若脾虚明显,食少便溏者,可加党参、黄芪以益气补脾。

【方解】 本方证由中阳不足,脾失健运,气不化水,饮停心下而成,治宜温阳化饮,健脾渗湿之法。方中茯苓健脾渗湿利水,为君药。桂枝温阳化气,配茯苓可温化痰饮,为臣药。白术健脾燥湿助运,除生痰之源,为佐药。炙甘草健脾补中,调和药性,为使药。诸药配伍,温而不热,利而不

generation of phlegm. No. 4 plays the role of guiding drug with the effect of reinforcing the spleen and mediating drug properties. All ingredients together form a recipe to warm yang without generating heat and induce diuresis without causing drastic purgation. It is a mild recipe of warming yang and dissolving phlegm-fluid.

Zhenwu Tang
(Decoction for Strengthening Spleen-kidney-yang)

Source：*Shanghan Lun* (*Treatise on Exogenous Febrile Diseases*).

Ingredients：

No. 1 Fuling (*Poria*) 9 g；

No. 2 Shaoyao (*Radix Paeoniae*) 9 g；

No. 3 Baizhu (*Rhizoma Atractylodis Macrocephalae*) 6 g；

No. 4 Shengjiang (*Rhizoma Zingiberis Recens*) 9 g；

No. 5 Paofuzi (*Radix Aconiti Praeparatae*) 9 g.

Administration：Decoct the above drugs in water for oral application.

Actions：Warming yang and inducing diuresis.

Clinical Application：This recipe is indicated for retention of water-dampness in the interior due to yang deficiency of the spleen and kidney, marked by edema of limbs, dysuria, or abdominal pain and diarrhea, whitish and glossy fur, deep pulse; or excessive diaphoresis of taiyang diseases, unrelieved fever after perspiration, palpitation, vertigo, twitching of the body and restlessness. It is applicable to chronic glomerulonephritis, cardiac edema, hypothyroidism, chronic bronchitis, chronic enteritis, Meniere's syndrome and others, which chiefly manifest dysuria, heaviness or edema of the limbs, whitish fur and deep pulse and pertain to excessive water-dampness due to yang deficiency of the spleen and kidney. Clinically Baishaoyao (*Radix Paeoniae Alba*) is often used. If con-

峻，为温化痰饮的平和之剂。

真武汤

【方源】《伤寒论》。

【组成】　茯苓 9 g,芍药 9 g,白术 6 g,生姜 9 g,炮附子 9 g。

【用法】　水煎服。

【功用】　温阳利水。

【临床应用】　适用于脾肾阳虚,水湿内停证。症见肢体浮肿,小便不利,或腹痛泄泻,舌苔白滑,脉沉;或太阳病过汗,以致汗出不解,仍发热,心悸头眩,身𝑚动,振振欲擗地。慢性肾小球肾炎、心源性水肿、甲状腺功能低下、慢性支气管炎、慢性肠炎、梅尼埃综合征等以小便不利,肢体沉重或浮肿,苔白脉沉为主症,属脾肾阳虚,水湿内盛者,可用本方治疗。方中芍药,现临床多用白芍药。若兼咳嗽者,

comitant with cough, add Ganjiang (*Rhizoma Zingiberis*), Xixin (*Herba Asari*) and Wuweizi (*Fructus Schisandrae*) to warm the lung and remove phlegm. In case of severe diarrhea, subtract No. 2 and add, instead, Ganjiang (*Rhizoma Zingiberis*) and Yizhiren (*Fructus Alpiniae Oxyphyllae*) to warm the middle-energizer and relieve diarrhea. If concomitant with vomiting, add Wuzhuyu (*Fructus Evodiae*) and Banxia (*Rhizoma Pinelliae*) to warm the stomach and relieve vomiting.

Elucidation: The syndrome is caused by retention of water-dampness in the interior due to yang-deficiency of the spleen and kidney, which fail to promote flow of qi and induce diuresis. Or it may also result from yang impairment due to excessive diaphoresis, and fluid-retention due to yang deficiency. It should be treated by warming yang and inducing diuresis. No. 4 acts as monarch drug, which can warm the kidney-yang, promote the flow of qi and induce diuresis on the one hand, and warm the spleen-yang on the other so as to promote the transportation and transformation of water-dampness. No. 1 and No. 3 function as minister drugs with the action of reinforcing the spleen and inducing diuresis to subdue edema. Pungent and warm in nature and with dispersing action, No. 4 can promote the effect of No. 5 in warming yang and dispelling cold and assist No. 1 and No. 3 in eliminating water-dampness. No. 2 possesses the functions of promoting diuresis, nourishing the liver to relieve abdominal pain and preserving yin and relaxing the tendons so as to relieve muscular twitching and cramp. These two ingredients serve as adjuvant drugs.

Shipi San
(*Powder for Reinforcing the Spleen*)

Source: *Chongding Yanshi Jisheng Fang (Revised Edition of Yan's Prescriptions for Saving Lives)*.

加干姜、细辛、五味子以温肺化饮;若腹泻较重者,可去芍药之寒,加干姜、益智仁以温中止泻;若兼呕吐者,可加吴茱萸、半夏以温胃止呕。

【方解】 本方证由脾肾阳虚,不能化气行水,以致水湿内停,或过汗伤阳,阳虚水泛所致,治宜温阳利水之法。方中附子温肾助阳,化气行水,兼暖脾阳,以助运化水湿,为君药。茯苓、白术健脾运湿,利水消肿,同为臣药。生姜辛温而散,助附子温阳祛寒,协茯苓、白术温散水湿。芍药之功有三:一者利小便以行水气,二者柔肝以止腹痛,三者敛阴舒筋以止筋惕肉瞤,同为佐药。

实脾散

【方源】《重订严氏济生方》。

Ingredients:

No. 1 Houpo (*Cortex Magnoliae Officinalis*) 30 g;

No. 2 Baizhu (*Rhizoma Atractylodis Macrocephalae*) 30 g;

No. 3 Mugua (*Fructus Chaenomelis*) 30 g;

No. 4 Muxiang (*Radix Aucklandiae*) 30 g;

No. 5 Caoguo (*Fructus Tsaoko*) 30 g;

No. 6 Binglang (*Semen Arecae*) 30 g;

No. 7 Paofuzi (*Radix Aconiti Praeparatae*) 30 g;

No. 8 Baifuling (*Poria*) 30 g;

No. 9 Ganjiang (*Rhizoma Zingiberis*) 30 g;

No. 10 Gancao (*Radix Glycyrrhizae*) 15 g.

Administration: Grind the above drugs into fine powder; take 12 g each time and add to it 5 slices of fresh ginger and 1 piece of Chinese date before decocting in water for oral application.

Actions: Warming yang and reinforcing the spleen, promoting the flow of qi and inducing diuresis.

Clinical Application: This recipe is indicated for edema due to yang deficiency, marked by severe swelling of the lower body, cold extremities, non-thirstiness, chest and abdominal fullness, large and pale tongue with greasy whitish fur, deep and slow pulse. It is applicable to edema from chronic glomerulonephritis, cardiac edema, ascites due to cirrhosis and others, which pertain to fluid-retention due to yang deficiency. In case of severe edema with dysuria, add Zhuling (*Polyporus*) and Zexie (*Rhizoma Alismatis*) to enhance the effect of inducing diuresis and relieving edema. In case of loose stool, replace No. 6 with Dafupi (*Pericarpium Arecae*) so as to reduce the effect of descending qi. In case of constipation, add Qianniuzi (*Semen Pharbitidis*) to strengthen the purgative and diuretic action.

Elucidation: The syndrome is caused by yang-defi-

【组成】　厚朴、白术、木瓜、木香、草果、槟榔、炮附子、白茯苓、干姜各 30 g，甘草 15 g。

【用法】　共研粗末，每次 12 g，加生姜 5 片，大枣 1 枚，水煎服。

【功用】　温阳健脾，行气利水。

【临床应用】　适用于阳虚水肿。症见半身以下肿甚，手足不温，口中不渴，胸腹胀满，舌淡胖苔白腻，脉沉迟。慢性肾小球肾炎的水肿、心源性水肿、肝硬化腹水等属阳虚水泛者，可用本方治疗。若水肿较甚，小便不利者，可加猪苓、泽泻以增强利水消肿之效；若大便溏泄者，可去槟榔而改用大腹皮，以减其下气之力；若大便秘结者，可加牵牛子以增泻下逐水之功。

【方解】　本方证由脾肾

ciency of the spleen and kidney, which fail to transport and transform fluid and dampness, leading to fluid-dampness retaining in the muscles. It should be treated by warming yang and invigorating the spleen, promoting the flow of qi and inducing diuresis. No. 7 is effective in warming kidney-yang and No. 9 in warming the spleen-yang, both helpful in promoting the circulation of qi to induce diuresis and activating yang to inhibit yin and used as monarch drugs. No. 8 functions as minister drug to reinforce the spleen, induce diuresis and relieve edema. The combined application of the monarch and minister drugs can deal with both the superficial symptoms and the root cause of the syndrome, aimed at warming yang and promoting diuresis. No. 3 can eliminate water-dampness through urination in combination with No. 8. Ingredients No. 1, No. 4, No. 6 and No. 5 have the function of descending qi and inducing diuresis so that dampness is eliminated and fullness relieved. These five ingredients play the part of adjuvant drugs. As guiding drug, No. 9 can invigorate the spleen and regulate the middle-energizer as well as mediate drug properties. Fresh ginger and Chinese dates are meant to regulate the spleen and stomach so as to strengthen the effect of warming the middle-energizer and reinforcing the spleen.

This recipe and Zhenwu Tang both have the function of warming and invigorating the spleen and kidney yang to promote diuresis and used in treating edema due to yang deficiency. The latter focuses on warming the kidney yang, while the former on warming the spleen yang. The latter, besides the action of warming yang and inducing diuresis, can also relieve spasm and relax tendons, nourish the liver and relieve pain, which is fit for edema due to deficiency of the kidney yang concomitant with abdominal pain or twitching of skeletal muscles. The former, however, possesses a good effect of activating yang and

阳虚,不能运化水湿,泛溢肌肤而成,治宜温阳健脾,行气利水之法。方中附子善温肾阳,可助气化以行水;干姜专温脾阳,可助运化以制水,两者合用,温肾暖脾,扶阳抑阴,共为君药。茯苓健脾运湿,利水消肿,同为臣药。君臣配伍,温阳利水,标本兼治。木瓜化湿利水,协茯苓使水湿从小便而利;厚朴、木香、槟榔、草果下气导滞,化湿利水,使气行则湿化,气顺则胀消,均为佐药。炙甘草益脾和中,调和药性,为使药。煎加生姜、大枣调补脾胃,以助诸药温中补脾之效。

本方与真武汤均有温补脾肾,助阳利水的作用,可治疗阳虚水肿。真武汤偏于温肾,实脾散重在暖脾。真武汤温阳利水,兼能缓急舒筋,柔肝止痛,故适用于肾阳不足,水湿内停之水肿,兼有腹痛或身瞤动者;实脾散助阳散寒之力较胜,且能行气化滞,适用于脾阳不足,水湿内停之水肿,兼有胸腹胀满,大便溏

dispelling cold and can promote the flow of qi and remove stagnation. Thus it is suitable for edema due to deficiency of the spleen yang concomitant with chest and abdominal fullness, flatulence and loose stool.

Bixie Fenqing Yin
(*Decoction of Collett Yam*
for Clearing Turbid Urine)

Source: *Danxi Xinfa* (*Danxi's Experiential Therapy*).

Ingredients:

No.1 Chuanbixie (*Rhizoma Dioscoreae Hypoglaucae*) 9 g;

No.2 Wuyao (*Radix Linderae*) 9 g;

No.3 Yizhiren (*Fructus Alpiniae Oxyphyllae*) 9 g;

No.4 Shichangpu (*Rhizoma Acori Tatarinowii*) 9 g.

Administration: Grind the above drugs into powder; take 15 g each time and add to it a little salt before decocting in water for oral application.

Actions: Warming the kidney and promoting diuresis, separating the clear from the turbid.

Clinical Application: This recipe is indicated for turbid urine due to deficiency-cold, marked by frequency of urination with turbid urine as if rice gruel or cream, pale tongue with whitish fur, deep pulse. It is applicable to chyluria, chronic prostatitis and others, which pertain to deficiency-cold in the lower energizer. If concomitant with abdominal pain due to deficiency cold, add Rougui (*Cortex Cinnamomi*) and Xiaohuixiang (*Fructus Foeniculi*) to warm the middle-energizer and dispel cold. If concomitant with soreness of the waist and cold limbs, add Tusizi (*Semen Cuscutae*) and Duzhong (*Cortex Eucommiae*) to warm the kidney-yang. In case of qi deficiency as the result of long illness, add Huangqi (*Radix Astragali seu Hedysari*) and Baizhu (*Rhizoma Atractylodis Macrocephalae*) to supplement qi and eliminate dampness.

薄者。

萆薢分清饮

【方源】 《丹溪心法》。

【组成】 川萆薢、乌药、益智仁、石菖蒲各9g。

【用法】 共研粗末,每次15g,加食盐少许,水煎服。

【功用】 温肾利湿,分清化浊。

【临床应用】 适用于虚寒白浊。症见小便频数,白如米泔,凝如膏糊,舌淡苔白,脉沉。乳糜尿、慢性前列腺炎等属下焦虚寒者,可用本方治疗。若兼虚寒腹痛者,可加肉桂、小茴香以温中祛寒;若兼腰酸肢冷者,可加菟丝子、杜仲以温肾助阳;若久病气虚者,可加黄芪、白术以益气祛湿。

Elucidation: The syndrome results from kidney-yang deficiency, causing disturbance of qi activity, failure in separating the clear from the turbid, and downward flow of dampness and turbidity. It should be treated by warming the kidney-yang and inducing diuresis, separating the clear from the turbid. No. 1 is capable of inducing diuresis and eliminating the turbid and is the monarch drug for treating turbid urine. No. 3 functions as minister drug, which can warm the kidney-yang and arrest polyuria. With the function of eliminating dampness and turbid substances, No. 4 can help No. 1 separate the clear from the turbid and assist No. 3 in expelling deficiency-cold from the bladder. No. 2 has the effect of warming the kidney and bladder and can deal with frequent urination. Thus No. 4 and No. 2 act together as adjuvant drugs. Salt added before decocting the drugs is meant to cause other drugs to take effect directly in the lower energizer, which serves as guiding drug.

Cautions: This recipe is contraindicated for turbid urine with frequent and urgent painful urination, reddened tongue and greasy yellowish fur.

2.13.5 Prescriptions for Expelling Wind and Eliminating Dampness

Qianghuo Shengshi Tang
(*Decoction of Notoperygium for Expelling Dampness*)

Source: *Neiwaishang Bianhuo Lun* (*Differentiation on Endogenous and Exogenous Diseases*).

Ingredients:

No. 1 Qianghuo (*Rhizoma seu Radix Notopterygii*) 9 g;

No. 2 Duhuo (*Radix Angelicae Pubescentis*) 9 g;

No. 3 Gaoben (*Rhizoma et Ligustici*) 4.5 g;

【方解】 本方证由肾阳不足,气化失常,清浊不分,湿浊下注所致,治宜温肾利湿,分清化浊之法。方中萆薢利湿化浊,为治白浊要药,故为君药。益智仁温肾助阳,固摄缩尿,为臣药。石菖蒲除湿化浊,助萆薢分清化浊之力,助益智仁祛膀胱虚寒;乌药温肾元,暖膀胱,治小便频数,均为佐药。煎加食盐少许,取其咸以入肾,引药直达下焦,为使药。

【注意事项】 小便混浊而兼尿频急涩痛,舌红苔黄腻者,禁用本方。

第五节 祛风胜湿剂

羌活胜湿汤

【方源】 《内外伤辨惑论》。

【组成】 羌活、独活各9 g,藁本、防风、炙甘草、川芎各4.5 g,蔓荆子3 g。

No. 4 Fangfeng (*Radix Ledebouriellae*) 4.5 g;

No. 5 Zhigancao (*Radix Glycyrrhizae Praeparatae*) 4.5 g;

No. 6 Chuanxiong (*Rhizoma Ligustici Chuanxiong*) 4.5 g;

No. 7 Manjingzi (*Fructus Viticis*) 3 g.

Administration: Decoct the above drugs in water for oral application.

Actions: Expelling wind-dampness.

Clinical Application: This recipe is indicated for exogenous wind-dampness syndrome, marked by heaviness and pain of the head, waist and back, or general pain of the body with difficulty in turning round, whitish fur and superficial pulse. It is applicable to common cold, rheumatic arthritis, hemicrania, angioneurotic headache and others, which pertain to attack by exogenous wind-dampness on the superficies and upper body. In case of severe aversion to cold and heaviness of the body, add Zhichuanwu (*Radix Aconiti Praeparata*) and Zhicaowu (*Radix Aconiti Kusnezoffii Praeparata*) to enhance the effect of dispelling cold and relieving pain. In case of prevailing dampness with heaviness of the body and greasy fur, replace No. 4 with Fangji (*Radix Stephaniae Tetrandrae*) and add Cangzhu (*Rhizoma Atractylodis*) to strengthen the action of eliminating dampness.

Elucidation: The syndrome arises when exogenous wind and dampness attack and retain in the superficies, leading to disorder of qi and blood of the meridians and collaterals. It should be treated by eliminating wind and dampness, removing obstruction and relieving pain. No. 1 and No. 2 are effective in expelling wind and dampness respectively from the upper and lower body and used as monarch drugs, whose combination can eliminate wind and dampness from the body and relieve pain. No. 3 and No. 4 are minister drugs with the action of eliminating wind and dampness so as to relieve headache. No. 6 has

【用法】 水煎服。

【功用】 祛风胜湿。

【临床应用】 适用于外感风湿证。症见头痛头重,腰背重痛,或一身尽痛,难以转侧,苔白脉浮。感冒、风湿性关节炎、偏头痛、血管神经性头痛等属外感风湿,病位在表在上者,可用本方治疗。若恶寒身痛较甚者,可加制川乌、制草乌以加强散寒止痛之效;若湿邪较盛,身重苔腻者,可将防风改为防己,再加苍术以助祛湿之力。

【方解】 本方证由外感风湿,郁于肌表,经络气血失和所致,治宜祛风胜湿,通痹止痛之法。方中羌活善祛上部风湿,独活善祛下部风湿,两药相合,能散周身风湿,通痹止痛,共为君药。防风、藁本祛风胜湿而止头痛,同为臣药。川芎活血通络,祛风止痛;蔓荆子升散风湿,善止头痛,均为佐药。炙甘草益气和

the function of activating blood circulation, removing obstruction from meridians, dispelling wind and relieving pain, while No. 7 possesses the function of dispersing wind and dampness to relieve headache, both playing the role of adjuvant drugs. No. 5 serves as guiding drug, which can not only supplement qi and regulate the middle-energizer so as to prevent other drugs from consuming qi, but also mediate drug properties.

Both this recipe and Jiuwei Qianghuo Tang comprise Qianghuo (*Rhizoma seu Radix Notopterygii*), Fangfeng (*Radix Ledebouriellae*), Chuanxiong (*Rhizoma Ligustici Chuanxiong*) and Gancao (*Radix Glycyrrhizae*) with the effect of eliminating wind and dampness and relieving headache and general pain. But the latter includes also Cangzhu (*Rhizoma Atractylodis*), Baizhi (*Radix Angelicae Dahuricae*), Xixin (*Herba Asari*), Shengdihuang (*Radix Rehmanniae*) and Huangqin (*Radix Scutellariae*), thus has a stronger effect in relieving exterior syndrome and can also clear away heat from the interior. It is fit for cases with chief manifestations as aversion to cold and fever concomitant with bitter mouth and slight thirst. The former, however, consists also of Duhuo (*Radix Angelicae Pubescentis*), Manjingzi (*Fructus Viticis*) and Gaoben (*Rhizoma et Ligustici*), which are mainly for eliminating wind and dampness from the body with a milder action of relieving exterior syndrome. Therefore it is suitable for cases chiefly manifested as heaviness of the head and body with slight aversion to cold and fever.

Cautions: This recipe is contraindicated for headache caused by hyperactivity of liver-yang or deficiency of both qi and blood.

Duhuo Jisheng Tang
(*Decoction of Pubescent Angelica and Loranthus*)
Source: *Beiji Qianjin Yaofang* (*Valuable Pre-*

中,防诸药升散耗气,又可调和药性,为佐使药。

本方与九味羌活汤组成中都有羌活、防风、川芎、甘草,均可祛风除湿,止头身之痛。但九味羌活汤配有苍术、白芷、细辛、生地黄、黄芩,因而解表之力略胜,兼能清内热,适宜于以恶寒发热为主,兼口苦微渴者。本方则配有独活、蔓荆子、藁本,重在祛周身风湿,而解表之力较弱,适宜于头身重痛为主,恶寒发热之表证不著者。

【注意事项】 肝阳上扰或气血不足而致头痛者,禁用本方。

独活寄生汤

【方源】 《备急千金要

scriptions for Emergencies).

Ingredients：

No. 1 Duhuo（*Radix Angelicae Pubescentis*）9 g;

No. 2 Sangjisheng（*Ramulus Loranthi*）6 g;

No. 3 Duzhong（*Cortex Eucommiae*）6 g;

No. 4 Niuxi（*Radix Achyranthis Bidentatae*）6 g;

No. 5 Xixin（*Herba Asari*）6 g;

No. 6 Qinjiao（*Radix Gentianae Macrophyllae*）6 g;

No. 7 Fuling（*Poria*）6 g;

No. 8 Rouguixin（*Cortex Cinnamoni*）6 g;

No. 9 Fangfeng（*Radix Ledebouriellae*）6 g;

No. 10 Chuanxiong（*Rhizoma Ligustici Chuanxiong*）6 g;

No. 11 Renshen（*Radix Ginseng*）6 g;

No. 12 Gancao（*Radix Glycyrrhizae*）6 g;

No. 13 Danggui（*Radix Angelicae Sinensis*）6 g;

No. 14 Shaoyao（*Radix Paeoniae*）6 g;

No. 15 Gandihuang（*Radix Rehmanniae*）6 g.

Administration：Decoct the above drugs in water for oral application.

Actions：Eliminating wind and dampness, relieving arthralgia, reinforcing the liver and kidney, nourishing qi and blood.

Clinical Application：This recipe is indicated for chronic bi-syndrome with deficiency of both the liver and kidney and insufficient qi and blood, marked by pain of the waist and knees, limited movement or numbness of joints, aversion to cold with preference for warmth, palpitation and short breath, pale tongue with whitish fur, thready and weak pulse. It is applicable to chronic arthritis, lumbar muscle strain, hyperosteogeny, rheumatic sciatica and others, which have a long course of illness and manifest deficiency of the liver and kidney as well as insufficiency of qi and blood. In terms of Ingredient No. 14, Baishaoyao（*Radix Paeoniae Alba*）can be used for nourishing blood

方》。

【组成】 独活 9 g,桑寄生、杜仲、牛膝、细辛、秦艽、茯苓、肉桂心、防风、川芎、人参、甘草、当归、芍药、干地黄各 6 g。

【用法】 水煎服。

【功用】 祛风湿,止痹痛,益肝肾,补气血。

【临床应用】 适用于痹证日久,肝肾两虚,气血不足证。症见腰膝疼痛,肢节屈伸不利,或麻木不仁,畏寒喜温,心悸气短,舌淡苔白,脉细弱。慢性关节炎、腰肌劳损、骨质增生症、风湿性坐骨神经痛等病程较久,见有肝肾两虚,气血不足之象者,可用本方治疗。方中芍药,欲养血者选用白芍药,欲活血者选用赤芍药。若痹证疼痛较剧者,可加

and Chishaoyao (*Radix Paeoniae Rubra*) for promoting blood circulation. In case of sharp pain from arthralgia, add Zhichuanwu (*Radix Aconiti Praeparata*), Zhicaowu (*Radix Aconiti Kusnezoffii Praeparata*) and Baihuashe (*Agkistrodon Acutus*) to expel wind and remove obstruction from the collaterals, activate blood flow and relieve pain. In case of prevailing cold, add Fuzi (*Radix Aconiti*) and Ganjiang (*Rhizoma Zingiberis*) to warm yang and dispel cold. In case of prevailing dampness, subtract No. 15 and add Fangji (*Radix Stephaniae Tetrandrae*), Yiyiren (*Semen Coicis*) and Cangzhu (*Rhizoma Atractylodis*) to eliminate dampness and subduing swelling. In the absence of lowered body resistance, subtract No. 15 and No. 11.

Elucidation: The syndrome is caused by protracted bi-syndrome due to wind, cold and dampness, which lead to hepatic and spleni impairment as well as consumption and impairment of qi and blood. Ingredient No. 1 is capable of eliminating wind, cold and dampness from the lower-energizer and alleviating arthralgia and used as monarch drug. No. 6 and No. 9 function as minister drugs, which help the monarch drug in eliminating wind and dampness and relieving pain. No. 8 is warm in nature with the function of dispelling cold and activating blood circulation, while No. 5 is effective in relieving pain by expelling wind and cold. No. 2, No. 3 and No. 4 bear the action of reinforcing the liver and kidney and strengthening tendons and bones, while No. 13, No. 14, No. 15 and No. 10 possess the function of enriching blood and activating its circulation. No. 11, No. 7 and No. 12 are capable of supplementing qi and invigorating the spleen so as to build up body resistance. These twelve ingredients are all used as adjuvant drugs. No. 12 also serves as guiding drug, mediating the properties of other drugs.

制川乌、制草乌、白花蛇以助搜风通络,活血止痛之力;若寒邪偏盛者,可加附子、干姜以温阳散寒;若湿邪偏盛者,可去地黄,加防己、薏苡仁、苍术以祛湿消肿;若正虚不明显者,可去地黄、人参。

【方解】 本方治证由风寒湿痹日久不愈,以致损伤肝肾,耗伤气血所致。方中独活祛下焦风寒湿邪,蠲痹止痛,为君药。防风、秦艽助君药祛风胜湿,祛邪止痛,为臣药。肉桂心温散寒邪,通利血脉;细辛祛风散寒,善止疼痛;桑寄生、牛膝、杜仲补益肝肾,强壮筋骨;当归、芍药、干地黄、川芎养血活血;人参、茯苓、甘草补气健脾,扶助正气,均为佐药。甘草调和药性,兼作使药。

Cautions：This recipe should not be used for bi-syndrome without deficiency of healthy qi or with reddness, swelling and pain of the joints.

【注意事项】　痹证正气不虚或关节红肿疼痛者,不宜使用本方。

2.14 Prescriptions for Eliminating Phlegm

第十四章
祛痰剂

Precriptions that are made up of expectorants with the action of eliminating phlegm, and applied in the treatment of various phlegm syndromes are known as prescriptions for eliminating phlegm.

Phlegm syndromes, in the light of the pathogenic factors, are roughly divided into damp-phlegm syndrome, heat-phlegm syndrome, dryness-phlegm syndrome, cold-phlegm syndrome and wind-phlegm syndrome. Consequently prescriptions for eliminating phlegm are also classified correspondingly into prescriptions for drying dampness and eliminating phlegm, prescriptions for clearing away heat and eliminating phlegm, prescriptions for moistening dryness and eliminating phlegm, prescriptions for warming and eliminating cold and phlegm, and prescriptions for eliminating phlegm and subduing wind.

Prescriptions for drying dampness and eliminating phlegm are mainly composed of expectorant drugs with the actions of desiccating dampness, promoting the flow of qi and regulating the middle-energizer, which are indicated for phlegm syndrome generated from accumulation of dampness as the result of dysfunction of the spleen in transportation and transformation. Prescriptions for clearing away heat and eliminating phlegm mainly consist of heat-clearing and expectorant drugs, which have the actions of clearing away heat and eliminating phlegm as well as regulating the flow of qi and relieving cough and are indicated for phlegm syndrome caused by excessive heat

凡以祛痰药为主组成,具有消除痰饮作用,用于治疗各种痰病的方剂,统称祛痰剂。

痰病据其成因不同大致可分为湿痰、热痰、燥痰、寒痰与风痰五种,因而祛痰剂相应地分为燥湿化痰剂、清热化痰剂、润燥化痰剂、温化寒痰剂与化痰熄风剂五类。

燥湿化痰剂由燥湿化痰药为主组成,具有燥湿化痰,行气和中作用,适用于脾失健运,湿聚成痰之证。清热化痰剂由清热化痰药为主组成,具有清热化痰,理气止咳作用,适用于火热内盛,灼津为痰之证。润燥化痰剂以润肺化痰药为主组成,具有润肺清热,化痰止咳作用,适用于肺燥津亏,虚火烁液为痰之证。温化寒痰剂以温肺化痰药为主组

accumulation in the interior, leading to transformation of body fluid into phlegm. Prescriptions for moistening dryness and eliminating phlegm are chiefly composed of drugs that moisten the lung and eliminate phlegm, which possess the actions of moistening the lung and clearing away heat, removing phlegm and relieving cough, and are fit for phlegm syndrome due to lung-dryness and deficiency of body fluid, leading to phlegm transformed from fluid by deficiency-fire. Prescriptions for warming and eliminating cold and phlegm are mainly formed by drugs with the effect of warming the lung and reducing phlegm to stop cough and suitable for cold fluid-retention due to yang deficiency of the spleen and kidney or fluid-retention due to lung-cold. Prescriptions for eliminating phlegm and subduing wind include expectorants in combination with drugs that calm the liver and suppress pathogenic wind, which have the actions of resolving phlegm and suppressing endogenous wind. They are indicated for retention of turbid phlegm in the middle-energizer and upward disturbance of wind-phlegm due to stirring of liver-wind.

Phlegm is often generated from the accumulation of dampness and, because the spleen is in charge of the transportation and transformation of dampness, there goes the saying "The spleen is the source of phlegm". Phlegm is substantial pathogenic factor, and apt to disturb qi-function. Thus expectorant prescriptions often invole drugs with the action of reinforcing the spleen so as to deal with the root cause of phlegm and drugs with the action of regulating flow of qi to make the flow of qi smooth and remove phlegm. Prescriptions for drying dampness and eliminating phlegm are mostly warm and dry in nature and apt to stir blood, which should be used with caution for patients with hemoptysis.

成,具有温肺蠲饮,化痰止咳作用,适用于脾肾阳虚,寒饮内停或肺寒留饮之证。化痰熄风剂由化痰药配伍平肝熄风药为主组成,具有化痰熄风作用,适用于痰浊中阻,肝风内动,风痰上扰之证。

痰多由湿聚而生,脾主运化水湿,故有"脾为生痰之源"之说;痰为有形之邪,易于阻滞气机,因而祛痰剂中常配伍健脾药以治生痰之本,配伍理气药以使气顺痰消。燥湿化痰药性多温燥,易于动血,有咳血倾向者慎用。

2.14.1   Prescriptions for Drying Dampness and Eliminating Phlegm

Erchen Tang
(*Erchen Decoction*)

Source：*Taiping Huimin Hejiju Fang* (*Benevolent Prescriptions from Taiping Pharmaceutical Bureau*).

Ingredients：

No. 1 Banxia (*Rhizoma Pinelliae*) 15 g;

No. 2 Jupi (*Pericarpium Citri Reticulatae*) 15 g;

No. 3 Fuling (*Poria*) 9 g;

No. 4 Zhigancao (*Radix Glycyrrhizae Praeparatae*) 5 g.

Administration：Grind the above drugs into fine powder; decoct in water 12 g at one time after adding to it 7 slices of fresh ginger and 1 piece of Wumei (*Fructus Mume*).

Actions：Drying dampness, resolving phlegm, promoting the flow of qi and regulating the middle-energizer.

Clinical Application：This recipe is indicated for cough or vomiting due to phlegm-dampness, marked by cough with much whitish sputum which is easy to expectorate, fullness and choking sensation in the chest, nausea and vomiting, lassitude, or dizziness and palpitation, greasy whitish fur and smooth pulse. It is applicable to such diseases with much whitish sputum as chronic bronchitis, pulmonary emphysema, chronic gastritis, vomiting of pregnancy and neurotic vomiting, and others that are caused by phlegm-dampness. It is a basic recipe for treating phlegm syndrome and can be modified to treat various kinds of such syndrome. In case of heat-phlegm, add Huangqin (*Radix Scutellariae*) and Danxing (*Arisaema cum Bile*) to clear away heat and remove phlegm. In case

第一节　燥湿
化痰剂

二陈汤

【方源】 《太平惠民和剂局方》。

【组成】 半夏、橘皮各15 g,茯苓9 g,炙甘草5 g。

【用法】 共研粗末,每次12 g,加生姜7片,乌梅1个,水煎服。

【功用】 燥湿化痰,理气和中。

【临床应用】 适用于湿痰咳嗽或呕吐。症见咳嗽,痰多色白易咯,胸膈痞闷,恶心呕吐,肢体倦怠,或头眩心悸,舌苔白腻,脉滑。慢性支气管炎、肺气肿、慢性胃炎、妊娠呕吐、神经性呕吐等见有痰白量多,属湿痰为患者,可用本方治疗。本方又是治痰的基本方,可加减应用于多种痰证。若为热痰,可加黄芩、胆星以清热化痰;若为寒痰,可加干姜、细辛以温化寒痰;若为风痰,可加天南星、竹沥以熄风

of cold phlegm, add Ganjiang (*Rhizoma Zingiberis*) and Xixin (*Herba Asari*) to warm and dispel cold phlegm. In case of wind phlegm, add Tiannanxing (*Rhizoma Arisaematis*) and Zhuli (*Succus Phyllostachydis Henonis*) to subdue wind and remove phlegm. In case of phlegm from indigestion, add Laifuzi (*Semen Raphani*) and Shenqu (*Massa Fermentata Medicinalis*) to promote digestion and remove phlegm.

Elucidation: The syndrome is caused by dysfunction of the spleen in transportation and transformation and disorder of qi activity, leading to accumulation of dampness, which is then transformed into phlegm. This should be treated by drying dampness, resolving phlegm and regulating the circulation of qi and the middle-energizer. Pungent, warm and dry in nature, No. 1 acts as monarch drug, which is effective in stopping cough by drying dampness and eliminating phlegm, and capable of suppressing the adversely ascendant qi and regulating the stomach so as to relieve vomiting. Used as minister drug, No. 2 can promote the effect of No. 1 as well as promote the flow of qi to eliminate phlegm. No. 3 acts as adjuvant drug, and can reinforce the spleen and promote diuresis to root out "the source of producing phlegm", and achieve the effect of treating both the superficial symptoms and the root cause of the disease when in combination with the monarch and minister drugs. No. 4 serves as guiding drug, which bears the function of regulating the spleen and mediating drug properties. Fresh ginger is meant to assist No. 1 and No. 2 in their action of promoting the flow of qi, removing phlegm, regulating the stomach and relieving vomiting as well as to reduce the toxic effect of No. 1. Wumei (*Fructus Mume*) is supposed to preserve the lung-qi so that phlegm is removed without body resistance impaired. This compatibility focuses on eliminating damp-

化痰；若为食痰，可加莱菔子、神曲以消食化痰。

【方解】　本方证由脾失健运，湿邪内停，聚而成痰，气机失畅所致，治宜燥湿化痰，理气和中之法。方中半夏辛温性燥，善能燥湿化痰以止咳，并可降逆和胃以止呕，为君药。橘皮助半夏化痰与和胃之力，并可行气以使气顺痰消，为臣药。茯苓健脾渗湿，治生痰之源，与君、臣药相伍可收标本兼治之功，为佐药。炙甘草和中益脾，调和药性，为使药。煎药时加生姜，取其降逆化饮，助半夏、橘皮行气消痰，和胃止呕，并制半夏之毒；再用少许乌梅收敛肺气，与君、臣药相伍，散中有收，可使祛痰而不伤正。诸药合用，燥湿化痰为主而兼健脾理气，体现了治疗痰病的基本大法，故本方又为祛痰的通用方剂。方中半夏、橘皮宜选用较陈久者以减其燥散之性，故方以"二陈"为名。

ness and removing phlegm but has also the effect of reinforcing the spleen and regulating the flow of qi, which is a reflection of the basic principle in treating phlegm syndrome. That is why this recipe is universal for various kinds of such syndrome. It is advisable to use the old ones in the selection of No. 1 and No. 2 so as to reduce the dry and dispersive action of both.

Cautions: Warm and dry as this recipe is, it is contraindicated for dryness syndrome of the lung due to yin deficiency or hemoptysis.

【注意事项】 本方药性温燥,故阴虚肺燥及咯血者禁用。

Wendan Tang
(*Decoction for Clearing away Gallbladder Heat*)

温胆汤

Source: *Sanyin Jiyi Bingzheng Fanglun* (*Treatise on the Three Categories of Pathogenic Factors of Diseases*).

【方源】《三因极一病证方论》。

Ingredients:

No. 1 Banxia (*Rhizoma Pinelliae*) 6 g;

No. 2 Zhuru (*Caulis Bambusae in Taeniam*) 6 g;

No. 3 Zhishi (*Fructus Aurantii Imaturus*) 6 g;

No. 4 Jupi (*Pericarpium Citri Reticulatae*) 9 g;

No. 5 Zhigancao (*Radix Glycyrrhizae Praeparatae*) 3 g;

No. 6 Fuling (*Poria*) 5 g.

【组成】 半夏、竹茹、枳实各 6 g,橘皮 9 g,炙甘草 3 g,茯苓 5 g。

Administration: Grind the above drugs into fine powder; decoct in water 15g at one time after adding to it 5 slices of fresh ginger and 2 pieces of Dazao (*Fructus Ziziphi Jujubae*).

【用法】 共研粗末,每次 15 g,加生姜 5 片,大枣 2 枚,水煎服。

Actions: Regulating the flow of qi to remove phlegm, clearing away gallbladder-heat and regulating the stomach.

【功用】 理气化痰,清胆和胃。

Clinical Application: This recipe is indicated for disharmony between the gallbladder and stomach and attack of phlegm-heat in the interior, marked by susceptibility to fright, restlessness, insomnia and dreaminess, vomiting and hiccup, or epilepsy, greasy whitish and yel-

【临床应用】 适用于胆胃不和,痰热内扰证。症见胆怯易惊,虚烦不宁,失眠多梦,呕吐呃逆,或癫痫,舌苔白腻微黄,脉弦滑。神经官能症、

lowish fur, taut and smooth pulse. It is applicable to such
diseases with the above symptoms as neurosis, acute gastritis, chronic gastritis, chronic bronchitis, Meniere's
syndrome and vomiting of pregnancy. In case of vexation,
add Huanglian (*Rhizoma Coptidis*) and Maimendong
(*Radix Ophiopogonis*) to clear away heat and relieve
vexation. In case of dry mouth and tongue, subtract No. 1
and add Maimendong (*Radix Ophiopogonis*) and Tianhuafen (*Radix Trichosanthis*) to moisten dryness and
increase body fluid. In case of epilepsy with convulsion,
add Danxing (*Arisaema cum Bile*) and Gouteng (*Ramulus Uncariae cum Uncis*) to subdue wind and relieve
convulsion. In case of severe insomnia, add Shengmuli
(*Concha Ostreae Recens*) and Suanzaoren (*Semen Ziziphi Spinosae*) (baked) to tranquilize mind.

Elucidation: The syndrome is caused by attack of
phlegm-heat in the interior and disharmony between the
gallbladder and the stomach. It should be treated by regulating the flow of qi to remove phlegm, clearing away heat
from the gallbladder and regulating the stomach. No. 1 is
the monarch drug in the recipe, which can eliminate
dampness and phlegm as well as descend qi and regulate
the stomach. No. 2 functions as minister drug to clear a-
way heat from the gallbladder, regulate the stomach, arrest vomiting and relieve vexation. No. 3 and No. 4 possess the action of regulating the flow of qi so as to reduce
phlegm, while No. 6 has the function of reinforcing the
spleen and inducing diuresis so that phlegm is never to be
generated when dampness is eliminated, the three playing
the part of adjuvant drugs. No. 5 is used as guiding drug to
invigorate the spleen and mediate drug properties. Fresh
ginger and Dazao (*Fructus Ziziphi Jujubae*) can not only
enhance the effect of reinforcing the spleen and regulating
the stomach, but also reduce the toxic effect of No. 1.

急性胃炎、慢性胃炎、慢性支气管炎、梅尼埃综合征、妊娠呕吐等见有上述症状者,可用本方治疗。若心中烦热者,可加黄连、麦门冬以清热除烦;若口干舌燥者,可去半夏,加麦门冬、天花粉以润燥生津;若癫痫抽搐者,可加胆星、钩藤以熄风止痉;若失眠较甚者,可加生牡蛎、炒酸枣仁以宁心安神。

【方解】　本方证由痰浊化热内扰,胆胃失和所致,治宜理气化痰,清胆和胃。方中半夏燥湿化痰,降逆和胃,为君药。竹茹清胆和胃,止呕除烦,为臣药。枳实、橘皮理气化痰,使气顺痰消;茯苓健脾利湿,使湿去则痰不生,均为佐药。炙甘草益脾和中,调和药性,为使药。煎加生姜、大枣,既可增强补脾和胃之力,又可制半夏之毒。

Cautions：This recipe should not be used for verti-go, insomnia or palpitation due to deficiency of yin and in-sufficiency of blood.

【注意事项】 阴虚血少之眩晕、失眠、心悸者,不宜使用本方。

2.14.2 Prescriptions for Clearing away Heat and Eliminating Phlegm

第二节　清热化痰剂

Qingqi Huatan Wan
(*Pill for Clearing away Heat and Phlegm*)

清气化痰丸

Source：*Yifangkao* (*Textual Research on Pre-scriptions*).

【方源】 录自《医方考》。

Ingredients：

No. 1 Gualouren (*Semen Trichosanthis*) 30 g;

No. 2 Jupi (*Pericarpium Citri Reticulatae*) 30 g;

No. 3 Huangqin (*Radix Scutellariae*) 30 g;

No. 4 Xingren (*Semen Pruni Armentiacae*) 30 g;

No. 5 Zhishi (*Fructus Aurantii Immaturus*) 30 g;

No. 6 Fuling (*Poria*) 30 g;

No. 7 Danxing (*Arisaema cum Bile*) 45 g;

No. 8 Banxia (*Rhizoma Pinelliae*) 45 g.

【组成】 瓜蒌仁、橘皮、黄芩、杏仁、枳实、茯苓各30 g,胆星、半夏各45 g。

Administration：Grind the above drugs into fine powder and make into pillets with ginger juice; take orally 6 g each time with warm boiled water. Or decoct them with dosages in proportion to the original recipe.

【用法】 共研细末,加姜汁制成小丸,每次 6 g,温开水送下。亦可作汤剂,用量按原方比例酌定。

Actions：Clearing away heat and resolving phlegm, regulating the flow of qi and arresting cough.

【功用】 清热化痰,理气止咳。

Clinical Application：This recipe is indicated for cough due to phlegm-heat, marked by cough with difficult expectoration of thick yellowish sputum, fullness of the chest, or short breath and nausea if serious, reddened tongue with greasy yellowish fur, smooth and rapid pulse. It is applicable to such diseases with thick yellowish spu-tum as pneumonia, acute bronchitis or acute attack of chronic bronchitis and others, which pertain to phlegm-heat

【临床应用】 适用于痰热咳嗽。症见咳嗽,痰稠色黄,咯之不爽,胸膈痞闷,甚则气急呕恶,舌红苔黄腻,脉滑数。肺炎、急性支气管炎或慢性支气管炎急性发作等见有痰稠色黄,属痰热为患者,可用本方治疗。若肺热壅盛,身

syndrome. In case of excessive heat in the lung with feverish body and thirst, add Shigao (*Gypsum Fibrosum*) and Zhimu (*Rhizoma Anemarrhenae*) to clear away heat from the lung. In case of excessive phlegm, add Tianhuafen (*Radix Trichosanthis*) and Yuxingcao (*Herba Houttuyniae*) to enhance the action of clearing away heat and removing phlegm. In case of constipation due to heat accumulation, add Zhidahuang (*Radix et Rhizoma Rhei Praeparata*) to descend and purge away heat and relieve constipation.

Elucidation: The syndrome is caused by heat in the lung, which scorches and converts body fluid into phlegm and further leads to obstructed flow of qi and dysfunction of the lung. This should be treated by clearing away heat to remove phlegm, regulating the flow of qi and arresting cough. No. 7 is good at clearing away heat and removing phlegm and acts as monarch drug. No. 3 can purge away fire from the lung and No. 1 clear away heat from the lung and remove phlegm, which are used as minister drugs and promote the effect of the monarch drug in this respect. No. 5 and No. 2 bear the effect of regulating the flow of qi to relieve fullness and remove phlegm, while No. 6 possesses the function of reinforcing the spleen and inducing diuresis so that phlegm is never generated. No. 4 is capable of descending the adverse flow of qi to relieve cough, while No. 8 has the function of eliminating dampness and removing phlegm. These five ingredients play the role of adjuvant drugs. Ginger juice is meant to strengthen the effect of removing phlegm on the one hand, and to reduce the toxic effect of No. 8 on the other.

Cautions: Cold in nature, this recipe should be used with caution for debilitated patients with loose bowels due to spleen-deficiency.

热口渴者，可加石膏、知母以清泻肺热；若痰多者，可加天花粉、鱼腥草以加强清热化痰之力；若热结便秘者，宜加制大黄以泻热通腑，导热下行。

【方解】　本方证由肺热灼津，煎熬成痰，痰热互结，阻滞气机，肺失清肃所致，治宜清热化痰，理气止咳之法。方中胆星长于清热化痰，为君药。黄芩清肺泻火，瓜蒌仁清肺化痰，二者合用，泻肺火，化痰热，助胆星清热化痰之力，同为臣药。枳实、橘皮行气开痞，使气顺而痰消；茯苓健脾渗湿，使痰无所生；杏仁降气止咳以治肺气之逆，半夏燥湿化痰而助祛痰之功，俱为佐药。姜汁为丸亦取其可助本方化痰之力，并解半夏之毒。

【注意事项】　本方药性寒凉，素体脾虚便溏者慎用。

Xiao Xianxiong Tang
(*Minor Decoction for Relieving Stuffiness in the Chest*)

小陷胸汤

Source：*Shanghan Lun* (*Treatise on Exogenous Febrile Diseases*).

【方源】《伤寒论》。

Ingredients：

No. 1 Huanglian (*Rhizoma Coptidis*) 6 g;

No. 2 Banxia (*Rhizoma Pinelliae*) 12 g;

No. 3 Quangualou (*Fructus Trichosanthis*) 20 g (decocted first).

【组成】　黄连 6 g,半夏 12 g,全瓜蒌 20 g(先煎)。

Administration：Decoct the above drugs in water for oral use.

【用法】　水煎服。

Actions：Clearing away heat and resolving phlegm, relieving chest stuffiness and dispersing stagnation.

【功用】　清热化痰,宽胸散结。

Clinical Application：This recipe is indicated for retention of both phlegm and heat, marked by chest and epigastric fullness with pain when pressed, or expectoration with thick yellowish sputum, greasy yellowish fur, smooth and rapid pulse. It is applicable to acute or chronic gastritis, pleurisy, pleural adhesion, acute bronchitis, intercostal neuralgia and others, which are chiefly marked by chest and epigastric fullness and pain as well as greasy yellowish fur, and are ascribed to retention of both phlegm and heat. If concomitant with costal and hypochondriac pain, add Yujin (*Radix Curcumae*) and Chaihu (*Radix Bupleuri*) to disperse the obstructed liver-qi and alleviate pain. If concomitant with vomiting, add Zhuru (*Caulis Bambusae in Taeniam*) and Shengjiang (*Rhizoma Zingiberis Recens*) to regulate the stomach and relieve vomiting. In case of difficult expectoration of thick sputum, add Danxing (*Arisaema cum Bile*) and Chuanbeimu (*Bulbus Fritillariae Cirrhosae*) to strengthen the effect of removing phlegm.

【临床应用】　适用于痰热互结证。症见胸脘痞闷,按之则痛,或咳痰黄稠,舌苔黄腻,脉滑数。急性胃炎、慢性胃炎、胸膜炎、胸膜粘连、急性支气管炎、肋间神经痛等以胸脘闷痛,舌苔黄腻为主症,属痰热互结者,可用本方治疗。若兼肋胁疼痛者,可加郁金、柴胡以疏肝止痛;若兼呕吐者,可加竹茹、生姜以和胃止呕;若痰粘稠难咯者,可加胆星、川贝母以加强化痰之力。

Elucidation：The syndrome is caused by accumulation

【方解】　本方证由热邪

of phlegm and heat in the chest and epigastrium as the result of consumption of body fluid by heat. It should be treated by clearing away heat and removing phlegm to relieve fullness. No. 3 has the function of clearing away heat, removing phlegm, regulating the flow of qi to relieve chest fullness as well as relieving constipation and descending lung-heat, and is used as monarch drug. No. 1 is cold in nature and capable of clearing away heat, while No. 2 is pungent and warm in nature and capable of removing phlegm and relieving fullness as well as descending qi and regulating the stomach. Both are minister drugs and their combination can promote the function of No. 3 in clearing away heat, removing phlegm and relieving fullness. The three altogether achieve the purpose of clearing away heat and descending qi simultaneously because of their warm, bitter and pungent nature. This is a primary recipe for treating chest and epigastric fullness and pain due to accumulation of both phlegm and heat.

Guntan Wan
(*Pill for Eliminating Stubborn Phlegm*)

Source: *Danxi Xinfa Fuyu* (*A Supplementary to Danxi's Experiential Therapy*).

Ingredients:

No. 1 Dahuang (*Radix et Rhizoma Rhei*) (steamed with wine) 240 g;

No. 2 Huangqin (*Radix Scutellariae*) (washed with wine) 240 g;

No. 3 Mengshi (*Lapis Micae Aureus Usta*) (calcined with Nitrum) 30 g;

No. 4 Chenxiang (*Lignum Aquilariae Resinatum*) 15 g.

Administration: Grind the above drugs into fine powder and make them into pills with water; take 5 - 9 g at one time after meals with tea or warm boiled water and once or twice daily.

灼津成痰,痰热结于胸脘所致,治宜清热化痰,宽胸散结之法。方中全瓜蒌清热化痰,理气宽胸,并可润肠通便,导肺热下行,为君药。黄连寒凉,清热降火;半夏辛温,化痰散结,降逆和胃,两药合用,以助瓜蒌清热化痰开结之效,为臣药。三药配伍,温清并用,苦降辛开,为治疗痰热互结,胸脘痞痛之要方。

滚痰丸

【方源】　录自《丹溪心法附余》。

【组成】　大黄(酒蒸)、黄芩(酒洗)各 240 g,礞石 30 g(与硝石同煅),沉香 15 g。

【用法】　共研细末,水泛为丸,每次 5～9 g,饭后以清茶或温开水送下,每日 1～2 次。

Actions: Purging away fire and eliminating phlegm.

Clinical Application: This recipe is indicated for excess heat with pertinacious phlegm syndrome, marked by manic-depressive psychosis with pavor, or severe palpitation and coma, or cough and dyspnea with thick sputum, or fullness, or vertigo and tinnitus, or lymphoid tuberculosis, or involuntary movements of the mouth and eyes, insomnia or dream of things grotesque in shapes and appearance, or indescribable sudden pain of the joints, or chocking sensation and vexation, constiptation, greasy yellow fur, smooth rapid and forceful pulse. It is applicable to schizophrenia, epilepsy, neurosis and others, which pertain to internal blockage by phlegm-fire.

Elucidation: The syndrome is caused by long-term excess heat syndrome with pertinacious phlegm, which either obstructs the seven orificies or disturb mentality or retain in the lung or retain in the meridians and collaterals as well as joints. It should be treated by purging away intense heat and eliminating phlegm. No.3 has a dry nature with drastic effect and is good at eliminating the pertinacious phlegm. It acts as monarch drug, whose purgative action is further enhanced when calcined with Xiaoshi (*Nitrum*). Used as minister drug, No.1 is capable of eliminating excess heat and descending phlegm-fire. With a cold nature and purgative action, No.2 helps the monarch and minister drugs in clearing away heat. No.4 possesses the function of sending down the adverse flow of qi, promoting the functions of the monarch and minister drugs in purging away intense heat on the one hand, and ensuring a easy flow of qi to remove phlegm on the other. Both play the role of adjuvant drugs. The combination of all constitutes an effective result in purging away intense heat and eliminating phlegm so that the pertinacious phlegm will descend through the intestines. This is a

【功用】 泻火逐痰。

【临床应用】 适用于实热老痰证。症见癫狂惊悸，或怔忡昏迷，或咳喘痰稠，或痞闷，或眩晕耳鸣，或绕项结核，或口眼㖞动，或不寐，或梦寐奇怪之状，或骨节卒痛难以名状，或噫息烦闷，大便秘结，舌苔黄腻，脉滑数有力。精神分裂症、癫痫、神经官能症等属痰火内闭者，可用本方治疗。

【方解】 本方证由实热顽痰久积，或上蒙清窍，或扰动心神，或内壅于肺，或留于经络、关节所致，治宜泻火逐痰之法。方中礞石药性燥悍重坠，善于攻逐陈积伏匿之顽痰，与硝石同煅，其攻逐下行之性更增，为君药。大黄荡涤实热，导痰火下行，为臣药。黄芩寒凉泻火，助君、臣药清热之力；沉香降逆下气，既可助君、臣药下行之力，又使气顺以助痰消，均为佐药。诸药配伍，泻火逐痰之力较著，可使顽固久积之痰火自肠腑而下，为攻逐实热老痰之峻剂。

drastic recipe for treating excess heat with pertinacious phlegm.

Cautions：Since this recipe is drastic in its potency, it should be used with caution for debilitated patients with deficiency of the spleen and stomach or with yang deficiency of the spleen and kidney or for pregnant women. Diarrhea may occur for a short period after this recipe is taken. A handful of patients may have viscid sensation in the throat or slight abdominal pain and tenesmus, which are the normal responses when healthy qi removes pathogenic factors and will get relieved spontaneously.

2.14.3　Prescriptions for Moistening Dryness and Eliminating Phlegm

Beimu Gualou San
(*Power of Fritillary Bulb and Snakegourd*)

Source：*Yixue Xinwu* (*A Summary on Medicine from Clinical Practice*).

Ingredients：

No.1 Beimu (*Bulbus Fritillariae*) 5 g;

No.2 Gualou (*Fructus Trichosanthis*) 3 g;

No.3 Tianhuafen (*Radix Trichosanthis*) 2.5 g;

No.4 Fuling (*Poria*) 2.5 g;

No.5 Jupi (*Exocarpium Citri Grandis*) 2.5 g;

No.6 Jiegeng (*Radix Platycodi*) 2.5 g.

Administration：Decoct the above drugs in water for oral use.

Actions：Moistening the lung, clearing away heat, resolving phlegm and relieving cough.

Clinical Application：This recipe is indicated for cough due to dryness-phlegm, marked by cough, expectorating sputum with difficulty, dry mouth, lips and throat, thin whitish and dry fur, thready or thready rapid pulse.

【注意事项】　本方药力颇峻,若素体脾胃虚弱,或脾肾阳虚,或孕妇等,皆应慎用。服本方后可有短时间腹泻,少数患者会出现咽喉粘滞,壅塞不利,或轻微腹痛、里急后重等现象,此均为正气祛邪的正常反应,很快便会自行消失,不必过虑。

第三节　润燥化痰剂

贝母瓜蒌散

【方源】　《医学心悟》。

【组成】　贝母 5 g,瓜蒌3 g,天花粉、茯苓、橘皮、桔梗各 2.5 g。

【用法】　水煎服。

【功用】　润肺清热,化痰止咳。

【临床应用】　适用于燥痰咳嗽。症见咳嗽,咯痰不爽,口唇咽喉干燥,舌苔薄白而干,脉细或细数。肺结核、

It is applicable to tuberculosis, pneumonia and others, which have the above symptoms, and are induced by dryness-phlegm. In case of excessive dryness and heat with dry and painful throat, add Xuanshen (*Radix Scrophulariae*), Maimendong (*Radix Ophiopogonis*) and Zhimu (*Rhizoma Anemarrhenae*) to enhance the action of clearing away heat and nourishing the lung as well as nourishing yin and promoting the production of body fluid. If concomitant with attack by exogenous wind manifesting cough, itching throat and slight aversion to wind-cold, add Sangye (*Folium Mori*), Xingren (*Semen Armeniacae Amarum*) and Niubangzi (*Fructus Arctii*) to facilitate the flow of the lung-qi and relieve sore throat as well as to dispel pathogenic wind.

Elucidation: The syndrome is caused by lung-dryness and consumption of body fluid, leading to the generation of phlegm. It should be treated by nourishing the lung and clearing away heat as well as eliminating phlegm and relieving cough. The first two ingredients have the above function and are used as monarch drugs. No. 3 acts as minister drug with the function of moistening dryness and promoting the production of body fluid as well as clearing away heat and removing phlegm. No. 5 has the effect of regulating the flow of qi so as to remove phlegm. No. 4 can stop the generation of phlegm because it is capable of reinforcing the spleen and inducing diuresis. No. 6 possesses the effect of facilitating the flow of the lung-qi, which plays the role of adjuvant drug together with No. 4 and No. 5.

Cautions: This recipe is contraindicated for the hyperactivity of fire due to yin deficiency, concomitant with hectic fever, night sweating and dysphoria with feverish sensation in chest, palms and soles.

肺炎等见有上述症状,属燥痰为患者,可用本方治疗。若燥热较甚,咽干痛明显者,可加玄参、麦门冬、知母以加强清热润肺,养阴生津之功;若兼感风邪,咳嗽咽痒,微恶风寒者,可加桑叶、杏仁、牛蒡子以宣肺利咽,疏风散邪。

【方解】 本方证由肺燥津亏,虚火烁津炼液为痰所致,治宜润肺清热,化痰止咳之法。方中贝母、瓜蒌润肺清热,化痰止咳,共为君药。天花粉润燥生津,清热化痰,为臣药。橘皮理气化痰,使气顺痰消;茯苓健脾渗湿,以杜生痰之源;桔梗宣利肺气,令肺金宣降有权,均为佐药。

【注意事项】 若阴虚火扰,兼见潮热盗汗,五心烦热者,禁用本方。

2.14.4   Prescriptions for Warming and Eliminating Cold and Phlegm

Linggan Wuwei Jiangxin Tang
(*Decoction of Poria*, *Licorice*, *Schisandra*, *Fried Ginger and Asarum*)

第四节   温化寒痰剂

苓甘五味姜辛汤

Source: *Jingui Yaolue* (*Synopsis of Prescriptions of the Golden Cabinet*).

【方源】《金匮要略》。

Ingredients:

No.1 Fuling (*Poria*) 12 g;

No.2 Gancao (*Radix Glycyrrhizae*) 6 g;

No.3 Ganjiang (*Rhizoma Zingiberis*) 9 g;

No.4 Xixin (*Herba Asari*) 9 g;

No.5 Wuweizi (*Fructus Schisandrae*) 6 g.

【组成】 茯苓 12 g,甘草 6 g,干姜、细辛各 9 g,五味子 6 g。

Administration: Decoct the above drugs in water for oral use.

【用法】 水煎服。

Actions: Warming the lung to resolve phlegm.

【功用】 温肺化饮。

Clinical Application: This recipe is indicated for cough due to cold retention, marked by cough with much thin whitish sputum, fullness in the chest, glossy whitish fur and taut smooth pulse. It is applicable to chronic bronchitis and pulmonary emphysema, which are ascribed to cold retention in the interior with cough and thin clear sputum. In case of copious phlegm with nausea, add Banxia (*Rhizoma Pinelliae*) to reduce phlegm and relieve nausea. In case of qi ascending adversely, add Guizhi (*Ramulus Cinnamomi*) to descend the adverse rising qi. In case of severe cough with dyspnea, add Xingren (*Semen Armeniacae Amarum*) and Houpo (*Cortex Magnoliae Officinalis*) to send down qi and relieve dyspnea.

【临床应用】 适用于寒饮咳嗽。症见咳嗽痰多,清稀色白,胸膈痞闷,舌苔白滑,脉弦滑。慢性支气管炎、肺气肿属寒饮内停而咳痰清稀者,可用本方治疗。若痰多欲呕者,可加半夏以化痰止呕;若兼冲气上逆者,可加桂枝以降逆平冲;若咳甚而喘者,可加杏仁、厚朴以降气平喘。

Elucidation: The syndrome results from deficiency of the spleen-yang, leading to generation of endogenous cold and dysfunction of the spleen in transportation and

【方解】 本方证由脾阳不足,寒从中生,运化失司,湿聚成饮,上贮于肺而成,治宜

transformation, and retention of dampness in the lung. This should be treated by warming the lung and resolving phlegm-fluid. No. 3 functions as monarch drug to warm the lung and dispel cold so as to eliminate phlegm as well as to warm and activate the spleen-yang in order to eliminate dampness. No. 4 is capable of warming the lung and dispelling cold, while No. 1 bears the function of reinforcing the spleen and eliminating dampness. Both are used as minister drugs, which can not only remove phlegm but also prevent its generation. Used as adjuvant drug, No. 5 has the function of preserving the lung-qi so as to stop coughing and achieves both astringent and dispersive actions when in compatibility with No. 4 and No. 3, thus preventing the consumption of the lung-qi. No. 2, as the guiding drug, mediates drug properties and regulates the middle-energizer. This recipe is effective for warming cold-fluid retention and has both warming and dispersing effects.

Both this recipe and the Xiao Qinglong Tang comprise the four ingredients of No. 4, No. 3, No. 5 and No. 2 with the action of warming the lung and removing retention and are used for the treatment of cold-fluid retention in the interior, cough and dyspnea with thin sputum. This recipe has No. 3 as the monarch drug, and, in compatibility with No. 1 that may reinforce the spleen so as to prevent the regeneration of phlegm, is specially designed for yin excess due to yang deficiency with cold-fluid retaining in the lung. The latter, however, takes Mahuang (*Herba Ephedrae*) and Guizhi (*Ramulus Cinnamomi*) as monarch drugs, thus possesses the effect of both warming the lung and removing retention and relieving the exterior syndrome and dispelling cold. It has the effects of treating both the exterior and interior syndromes and is indicated for attack by wind-cold and retention of cold-fluid.

温肺化饮之法。方中干姜温肺散寒以化饮,温运脾阳以化湿,为君药。细辛温肺散寒,助干姜温化寒饮;茯苓健脾渗湿,既可化已成之痰,又可杜生痰之源,同为臣药。五味子敛肺气而止咳,与细辛、干姜配伍,散中有收,可防肺气之耗散,为佐药。甘草和中,调和药性,为使药。诸药配伍,温散并行,开合相济,为温化寒饮之良方。

本方与小青龙汤的组成药物均有细辛、干姜、五味子、甘草,皆可温肺化饮,治疗寒饮内停,咳喘痰稀。但本方以干姜为君药,配用茯苓健脾渗湿以除生痰之源,为治疗阳虚阴盛,肺寒留饮证候的专方;小青龙汤则以麻黄、桂枝为君药,故既可温肺化饮,又能解表散寒,有表里兼治之功,适用于风寒外束,寒饮内停证候。

Sanzi Yangqin Tang
(Decoction of Three Kinds of Seeds for the Aged)

三子养亲汤

Source：*Hanshi Yitong*（*Han's Book on Medicine*）.

【方源】《韩氏医通》。

Ingredients：

No. 1 Baijiezi（*Semen Sinapis Albae*）6 g；

No. 2 Suzi（*Fructus Perillae*）9 g；

No. 3 Laifuzi（*Semen Raphani*）9 g.

【组成】　白芥子 6 g,苏子 9 g,莱菔子 9 g。

Administration：Smash the above drugs and wrap with a piece of cloth before decocting in water；take orally the decoction frequently.

【用法】　三药捣碎,纱布包煎,煎汤频服。

Actions：Dissolving phlegm to facilitate the flow of qi，checking the adversely ascending qi and promoting digestion.

【功用】　化痰利气,降逆消食。

Clinical Application：This recipe is indicated for syndrome of qi stagnation due to excessive phlegm，marked by cough and dyspnea with much sputum, chest distress, poor appetite and dyspepsia, greasy whitish fur and smooth pulse. It is applicable to chronic bronchitis, which is caused by phlegm, adverse flow of qi and indigestion and chiefly manifested as much sputum and poor appetite. In case of excessive cold-phlegm retaining in the lung with much thin sputum, add Xixin（*Herba Asari*）and Banxia（*Rhizoma Pinelliae*）to strengthen the effect of eliminating cold-phlegm. In case of deficient spleen-yang with loose stool, add Fuling（*Poria*）and Ganjiang（*Rhizoma Zingiberis*）to activate the spleen-yang, induce diuresis and remove phlegm. If concomitant with nausea or vomiting, add Banxia（*Rhizoma Pinelliae*）and Shengjiang（*Rhizoma Zingiberis Recens*）to regulate the stomach and send down the adverse qi so as to relieve nausea or vomiting.

【临床应用】　适用于痰壅气滞证。症见咳嗽气喘,痰多胸闷,食少难消,舌苔白腻,脉滑。慢性支气管炎属痰、气、食交阻为患,以痰多食少为主症者,可用本方治疗。若寒痰壅肺,痰多清稀者,可加细辛、半夏以助温化寒痰之力;若脾阳不足,大便溏薄者,可加茯苓、干姜以温阳健脾,渗湿化痰;若兼恶心或呕吐者,可加半夏、生姜以和胃降逆止呕。

Elucidation：The syndrome is caused by deficiency

【方解】　本方证由年老

of qi in the middle-energizer and dysfunction in transportation and transformation in old people. Phlegm is generated from dampness as the result of indigestion and retains upward in the lung, further giving rise to excess phlegm and qi stagnation. This should be treated by removing phlegm, promoting digestion, and descending the adverse qi to relieve cough and dyspnea. No. 1 has the function of removing phlegm and promoting the flow of qi and acts as monarch drug. No. 2 functions as minister drug to send down the adversely ascendant qi and remove phlegm so as to promote the effect of the monarch drug in relieving cough and dyspnea. No. 3 serves as adjuvant drug, which is capable of promoting digestion and regulating the stomach as well as descending qi and removing phlegm. The combined application of the three ingredients is a very effective recipe for the treatment of cough and dyspnea with much sputum and poor appetite as seen in the senile.

Cautions：When effective result is obtained after administration, the cause of the disease should be dealt with because this recipe is sinking and descending in nature and supposed to treat secondary cause, regulating the flow of qi and removing phlegm.

中虚,运化失常,以致停食生湿,湿聚成痰,上贮于肺,痰壅气滞而成,治宜化痰消食,下气降逆,止咳平喘之法。方中白芥子化痰利气,为君药。苏子降气化痰,止咳平喘,助君药化痰止咳之力,为臣药。莱菔子消食和胃,降气祛痰,为佐药。三药均有化痰理气降逆之功,合而用之,可使气机畅而痰涎化,食积消而咳喘平,为治老人咳喘痰多食少之证的良方。

【注意事项】 本方药性沉降,为理气化痰治标之剂,若服后得效,即应转调其本。

2.14.5　Prescriptions for Eliminating Phlegm and Subduing Wind

Banxia Baizhu Tianma Tang
（**Decoction of Pinellia, Bighead Atractylodes and Gastrodia**）

Source：*Yixue Xinwu*（*A Summary on Medicine from Clinical Practice*）.

Ingredients：

No. 1 Banxia（*Rhizoma Pinelliae*）9 g;

No. 2 Tianma（*Rhizoma Gastrodiae*）6 g;

第五节　化痰

熄风剂

半夏白术天麻汤

【方源】 《医学心悟》。

【组成】 半夏 9 g,天麻 6 g,茯苓 9 g,橘皮 6 g,白术 9 g,甘草 3 g。

No. 3 Fuling (*Poria*) 9 g;

No. 4 Jupi (*Exocarpium Citri Grandis*) 6 g;

No. 5 Baizhu (*Rhizoma Atractylodis Macrocephalae*) 9 g;

No. 6 Gancao (*Radix Glycyrrhizae*) 3 g.

Administration: Decoct the above drugs in water for oral application after adding to it 2 slices of fresh ginger and 3 pieces of Chinese dates.

Actions: Drying dampness, resolving phlegm, calming the liver and subduing wind.

Clinical Application: This recipe is indicated for the syndrome of upward attack of wind-phlegm, marked by vertigo, headache, nausea, vomiting, chest fullness, greasy whitish fur, taut and smooth pulse. It is applicable to aural vertigo, neurotic vertigo, and others, which are chiefly manifested as vertigo, nausea and greasy whitish fur and ascribed to upward disturbance by wind-phlegm. In case of excessive dampness-phlegm with glossy whitish fur, add Zexie (*Rhizoma Alismatis*) and Guizhi (*Ramulus Cinnamomi*) to induce diuresis and remove phlegm. In case of dizziness and distending pain of the head due to hyperactivity of the liver-yang, add Gouteng (*Ramulus Uncariae cum Uncis*) and Daizheshi (*Ochra Haematitum*) to suppress the hyperactive yang and subdue the endogenous wind. If concomitant with weakness due to deficient qi, add Dangshen (*Radix Codonopsis Pilosulae*) and Huangqi (*Radix Astragali seu Hedysari*) to supplement qi and build up strength.

Elucidation: The syndrome is caused by dysfunction of the spleen in transportation and transformation, thus phlegm is formed from accumulated dampness and accompanied by internal stirring of liver wind and disturbance of wind-phlegm on the head. It should be treated by eliminating dampness and phlegm and subduing the liver-wind. No. 1 is capable of removing dampness and phlegm and

【用法】 加生姜 2 片、大枣 3 枚,水煎服。

【功用】 燥湿化痰,平肝熄风。

【临床应用】 适用于风痰上扰证。症见眩晕头痛,恶心呕吐、胸膈痞闷,舌苔白腻,脉弦滑。耳源性眩晕、神经性眩晕等以眩晕呕恶,舌苔白腻为主症,属风痰上扰者,可用本方治疗。若湿痰偏盛,舌苔白滑者,可加泽泻、桂枝以利湿化饮;若肝阳偏亢,头晕胀痛者,可加钩藤、代赭石以潜阳熄风;若兼气虚乏力者,可加党参、黄芪以益气补虚。

【方解】 本方证由脾失健运,聚湿生痰,肝风内动,挟痰上扰清空所致,治宜燥湿化痰,平肝熄风之法。方中半夏燥湿化痰,降逆止呕;天麻平肝熄风,止痛除眩,两药配伍,善治风痰眩晕头痛,共为君

descending qi to relieve vomiting, while No. 2 has the function of subduing the liver-wind and relieving pain and vertigo. Both are used as monarch drugs and effective in treating vertigo and headache due to wind-phlegm. No. 5 and No. 3 possess the action of reinforcing the spleen and eliminating dampness so as to prevent regeneration of phlegm and function as minister drugs, which can enhance the effect of removing phlegm and treat both the superficial symptoms and the root cause of the disease when combined with No. 1. Used as adjuvant drug, No. 4 can strengthen the effect of the monarch and minister drugs on the one hand, and promote the easy flow of qi and the elimination of phlegm and dampness on the other because it has the function of eliminating dampness and phlegm and regulating the flow of qi and the middle-energizer. No. 6 plays the role of guiding drug, which supplements qi and regulates the middle-energizer as well as mediates the drug properties. The fresh ginger and Chinese dates are meant to regulate the spleen and stomach, further enhancing the effect of this recipe in regulating the middle-energizer and removing phlegm.

Cautions：This recipe is contraindicated for vertigo and headache as the result of hyperactivity of the liver-yang due to yin deficiency of the liver and kidney.

Dingxian Wan
(*Pill for Relieving Epilepsy*)

Source：*Yixue Xinwu* (*A summary on Medicine from Clinical Practice*).

Ingredients：

No. 1 Tianma (*Rhizoma Gastrodiae*) 30 g;

No. 2 Chuanbeimu (*Bulbus Fritillariae Cirrhosae*) 30 g;

No. 3 Jiangbanxia (*Rhizoma Pinelliae prepared with ginger juice*) 30 g;

No. 4 Fuling (*Poria*) 30 g;

药。白术、茯苓健脾祛湿,以除生痰之源,合半夏标本兼治,可加强化痰之功,同为臣药。橘皮燥湿化痰,行气和中,既可增强君、臣药燥湿化痰之力,又可使气机畅达以助痰湿的消除,为佐药。甘草益气和中,调和药性,为使药。兼加生姜、大枣调和脾胃,以助本方和中化痰之效。

【注意事项】 肝肾阴虚,肝阳上亢所致的眩晕头痛,禁用本方。

定痫丸

【方源】《医学心悟》。

【组成】 天麻、川贝母、姜半夏、茯苓、茯神各 30 g,胆星、石菖蒲、全蝎、僵蚕、琥珀、灯心草各 15 g,橘皮、远志各21 g,丹参、麦门冬各 60 g,朱砂(水飞)9 g。

No. 5 Fushen (*Sclerotium Poriae Circum Radicem Pini*) 30 g;

No. 6 Danxing (*Arisaema cum Bile*) 15 g;

No. 7 Shichangpu (*Rhizoma Acori Tatarinowii*) 15 g;

No. 8 Quanxie (*Scorpio*) 15 g;

No. 9 Jiangcan (*Bombyx Batryticatus*) 15 g;

No. 10 Hupo (*Succinum*) 15 g;

No. 11 Dengxincao (*Medulla Junci*) 15 g;

No. 12 Jupi (*Exocarpium Citri Grandis*) 21 g;

No. 13 Yuanzhi (*Radix Polygalae*) 21 g;

No. 14 Danshen (*Radix Salviae Miltiorrhizae*) 60 g;

No. 15 Maimendong (*Radix Ophiopogonis*) 60 g;

No. 16 Zhusha (*Cinnabaris*) (refined with water) 9 g.

Administration：Grind the above drugs into fine powder; take a small bowl of Zhuli (*Succus Phyllostachydis Henonis*), a cup of ginger juice and 120 g of Gancao (*Radix Glycyrrhizae*) and make them into ointment; mix up the powder and the ointment and make it into pills coated with No. 16. Take orally 6 g each time and twice daily with warm boiled water.

Actions：Subduing wind, resolving phlegm, inducing resuscitation and tranquilizing mind.

Clinical Application：This recipe is indicated for epilepsy due to phlegm-heat, marked by sudden onset, faint and falling down to the ground, unconsciousness, or convulsion, wry eyes and mouth, slobbering, and crying if serious; or indicated in manic-depressive psychosis due to phlegm-heat. It is applicable to epilepsy, schizophrenia, and others, which are ascribed to blocking of the clear orifices by phlegm-heat.

Elucidation：The syndrome is caused by emotional disorder and stagnated liver-qi, leading to the generation of phlegm. It may also result from irregular diet, causing generation of phlegm due to spleen-dampness, which will

【用法】　共研细末，用竹沥1小碗，姜汁1杯，再用甘草120 g 熬膏，与药粉和匀为丸，朱砂为衣。每次 6 g，温开水送下，每日 2 次。

【功用】　熄风化痰，开窍安神。

【临床应用】　适用于痰热痫证。症见忽然发作，眩仆倒地，不省人事，甚则抽搐，目斜口歪，痰涎直流，叫喊作声，以及痰热癫狂。癫痫、精神分裂症等属痰热蒙蔽清窍者，可用本方治疗。

【方解】　本方证由情志失调，肝气不畅，郁结生痰；或饮食不节，脾湿生痰，一俟肝气失和，肝风挟痰随气上逆，

obstruct the meridians and orifices in combination with the liver-wind as the result of functional disorder of the liver-qi. Both may give rise to sudden onset of epilepsy, which should be treated by subduing the liver-wind and removing phlegm as well as inducing resuscitation and tranquilizing mind. Zhuli (*Succus Bambosae*) is very effective in clearing away heat and removing phlegm as well as calming mind and inducing resuscitation, whose effects are strengthened when in compatibility with ginger juice. No. 6 has the function of eliminating fire and phlegm, tranquilizing mind and relieving epilepsy. Both are used as monarch drugs. No. 1, No. 8 and No. 9 possess the function of subduing the liver-wind and relieving convulsion, while No. 3 and No. 12 have the function of eliminating dampness and phlegm and promoting the flow of qi. These five play the role of minister drugs, promoting the effect of the monarch drug in subduing wind and removing phlegm. No. 4 and No. 2 are capable of removing dampness and phlegm, while No. 14, No. 7 and No. 13 inducing resuscitation and calming the mind. No. 10, No. 16, No. 11 and No. 5 can tranquilize mind, while No. 15 can nourish and prevent the impairment of yin. These ten ingredients function as adjuvant drugs. Gancao (*Radix Glycyrrhizae*) serves as guiding drug with the function of mediating properties of other drugs.

Cautions：This recipe is contraindicated for patients with deficiency of healthy qi due to frequent and protracted epilepsy since it is potent in the effect of removing phlegm and subduing wind.

壅闭经络,阻塞清窍,以致突然发痫,治宜熄风化痰,开窍宁神之法。方中竹沥善清热涤痰,镇惊利窍,配姜汁之温则更助其化痰利窍;胆星清火化痰,镇惊定痫,共为君药。天麻、全蝎、僵蚕平肝熄风止痉,半夏、橘皮燥湿化痰行气,助君药熄风化痰,同为臣药。茯苓、川贝母祛湿化痰,丹参、石菖蒲、远志开窍宁心,琥珀、朱砂、灯心草、茯神镇惊安神,麦冬滋润以防伤阴,均为佐药。甘草调和药性,为使药。

【注意事项】 本方涤痰熄风力较强,若痫证屡发,日久不愈,正气虚弱者禁用。

2.15 Peptic Prescriptions

第十五章
消食剂

Peptic prescriptions are mainly composed of peptic drugs with the function of promoting digestion, removing stagnation, and regulating the spleen and stomach, which are applied for the treatment of dyspepsia and stagnancy of food.

Since indigestion is usually the result of intemperance in eating and drinking or failure of the spleen in transporting and transforming food, peptic prescriptions are accordingly subdivided into two categories: prescriptions for promoting digestion by resolving stagnancy and prescriptions for promoting digestion by reinforcing the spleen.

The former is mainly made up of digestives and drugs with the functions of regulating the circulation of qi, purging away heat, eliminating dampness and clearing away heat, which have peptic action and are used for food retention in the interior due to impairment of the stomach as the result of overeating. The latter also consists chiefly of digestives in combination with drugs that supplement qi and reinforce the spleen. This group of prescriptions possesses the actions of activating qi and replenishing the spleen as well as promoting digestion and regulating the stomach, and is applicable to food retention in the interior due to weakness of the spleen and stomach.

Food retention in the interior often leads to disorders of qi activity and is likely to generate dampness and heat. Therefore in formulating a peptic recipe, it is necessary to employ proper drugs in the light of the degree of food

凡以消食药为主组成,具有消食化滞,健脾和胃作用,用于治疗宿食不化,食积内停的方剂,统称消食剂。

由于食积常因暴饮暴食或脾虚不运而成,因而消食剂相应地分为消食化滞剂与健脾消食剂两类。

消食化滞剂由消食药为主组成,常配伍理气、泻下、祛湿、清热之品,具有消食导滞作用,适用于过食伤中,食积内停之证。健脾消食剂亦由消食药为主组成,常配伍补气健脾之品,具有益气健脾,消食和胃作用,适用于脾胃虚弱,食积内停之证。

食积内停,常常导致气机运行不畅,并且极易生湿化热。因而用消食剂在遣药组方时应注意辨清食、气、湿、热

stagnancy, qi stagnation, accumulation of dampness and heat. If food and dampness-heat are transformed into stagnancy and retain in the stomach and intestines, leading to abdominal pain and constipation or diarrhea, it is necessary to employ some purgatives to remove mass.

的程度,酌情配伍相应的药物。若食积与湿热阻于肠胃形成积滞,导致腹痛便秘或泄泻,则须酌配泻下药以化滞攻积。

2.15.1　Prescriptions for Promoting Digestion by Removing Stagnancy

Baohe Wan
（**Lenitive Pill**）

Source：*Danxi Xinfa* (*Danxi's Experimental Therapy*).

Ingredients：

No. 1 Shanzha (*Fructus Crataegi*) 180 g;

No. 2 Shenqu (*Massa Fermentata Medicinalis*) 60 g;

No. 3 Banxia (*Rhizoma Pinelliae*) 90 g;

No. 4 Fuling (*Poria*) 90 g;

No. 5 Chenpi (*Pericarpium Citri Reticulatae*) 30 g;

No. 6 Lianqiao (*Fructus Forsythiae*) 30 g;

No. 7 Laifuzi (*Semen Raphani*) 30 g.

Administration：Grind the above drugs into fine powder and prepare into boluses, take 9 g each time with warm boiled water or malt water for oral use, three times daily; or prepare the drugs directly as oral decoction, with dosages reduced proportionally.

Actions：Promoting digestion and regulating the stomach.

Clinical Application：This recipe is indicated for food stagnancy due to indigestion, marked by epigastric and abdominal stuffiness and pain, belching and regurgitation, poor appetite and vomiting, or diarrhea, thick greasy fur and smooth pulse. It is applicable to acute or chronic gastritis, acute or chronic enteritis, dyspepsia,

第一节　消食化滞剂

保和丸

【方源】《丹溪心法》。

【组成】 山楂 180 g,神曲 60 g,半夏、茯苓各 90 g,陈皮、连翘、莱菔子各 30 g。

【用法】 共研细末,炊饼为丸,每次 9 g,温开水或麦芽汤送下,每日 3 次。亦可作汤剂,用量按原方比例酌定。

【功用】 消食和胃。

【临床应用】 适用于食积停滞证。症见脘腹痞满胀痛,嗳腐吞酸,厌食呕吐,或大便泄泻,舌苔厚腻,脉滑。急性胃炎、慢性胃炎、急性肠炎、慢性肠炎、消化不良、婴儿腹

infant diarrhea and others with the above symptoms, which pertain to food stagnancy. This is a peptic recipe with mild effect. Therefore Zhishi (*Fructus Aurantii Immaturus*) and Binglang (*Semen Arecae*) should be added in case of excessive food stagnancy so as to enhance the peptic action. And Huangqin (*Radix Scutellariae*) and Huanglian (*Rhizoma Coptidis*) should be added to clear away heat in case of heat transformed from food stagnancy, manifested as thirst and desire for drinking, yellowish fur and rapid pulse. Baizhu (*Rhizoma Atractylodis Macrocephalae*) should be added to activate the spleen in its transporting and transforming function in case of constipation due to weakness of the spleen.

Elucidation：The syndrome is caused by improper diet or intemperate eating and drinking, leading to indigestion, obstruction of qi activity, disharmony between the spleen and stomach as well as the generation of dampness and heat. This should be treated by promoting digestion and regulating the stomach. No. 1 in large dosage is capable of removing food stagnancy of whatever kind, especially the stagnancy of meat or oily food, and functions as monarch drug. No. 2 can activate the spleen and digest those long-standing liquor or food, while No. 7 can descend qi and digest the stagnated grain or flour food, both acting as minister drugs. The combination of the monarch and minister drugs can remove stagnancy of whatever kind. No. 3 and No. 5 have the function of promoting the circulation of qi and promoting digestion as well as regulating the stomach and relieving vomiting. No. 4 possesses the effect of inducing diuresis and reinforcing the spleen as well as regulating the middle-energizer and stopping diarrhea. No. 6 is capable of clearing away heat and resolving mass. These four ingredients play the role of adjuvant drugs in the recipe.

泻等见有上述症状，属食积内停者，可用本方治疗。本方为消食轻剂，若食滞较重者，可加枳实、槟榔以增强消食导滞之力；若食积化热较甚，口渴欲饮，苔黄脉数者，可加黄芩、黄连以清热；若兼脾虚便溏者，可加白术以健脾助运。

【方解】 本方证由饮食失节，暴饮暴食，以致食积内停，气机阻滞，脾胃失和，生湿化热而成，治宜消食和胃为主。方中重用山楂，能消一切饮食积滞，尤善消肉食油腻之积，为君药。神曲消食健脾，善化酒食陈腐之积；莱菔子下气消食，长于消谷面之积，同为臣药。君臣相配，可消一切饮食积滞。半夏、陈皮行气化滞，和胃止呕；茯苓渗湿健脾，和中止泻；连翘清热散结，均为佐药。

Cautions: This recipe, mild in its efficacy and with the actions of promoting digestion and regulating the stomach, should not be used for patients with abdominal distending pain and constipation.

Zhishi Daozhi Wan
(*Pill of Immature Bitter Orange*
for Removing Stagnancy)

Source: *Neiwaishang Bianhuo Lun* (*Treatise on Differentiation of Internal and External Injuries*).

Ingredients:

No. 1 Dahuang (*Radix et Rhizoma Rhei*) 30 g;

No. 2 Zhishi (*Fructus Aurantii Immaturus*) 15 g;

No. 3 Shenqu (*Massa Fermentata Medicinalis*) 15 g;

No. 4 Fuling (*Poria*) 9 g;

No. 5 Huangqin (*Radix Scutellariae*) 9 g;

No. 6 Huanglian (*Rhizoma Coptidis*) 9 g;

No. 7 Baizhu (*Rhizoma Atractylodis Macrocephalae*) 9 g;

No. 8 Zexie (*Rhizoma Alismatis*) 6 g.

Administration: Grind the above drugs into fine powder; soak and steam it to make pills; take orally 6 – 9 g each time and twice or three times daily with warm boiled water. Or decoct the above drugs with dosages in proportion to the original recipe.

Actions: Promoting digestion, removing stagnated food, eliminating heat and dampness.

Clinical Application: This recipe is indicated for syndrome of food stagnancy with dampness-heat, marked by epigastric and abdominal fullness and pain, diarrhea or constipation, scanty dark urine, greasy yellowish and thick fur, deep rapid and forceful pulse. It is applicable to gastrointestinal dysfunction, chronic dysentery and others with chief manifestations as epigastric and abdominal fullness and pain, irregular defecation, and reddened tongue

【注意事项】 本方药性平和,以消食和胃为主,若腹胀痛、便秘者不宜使用。

枳实导滞丸

【方源】 《内外伤辨惑论》。

【组成】 大黄 30 g,枳实、神曲各 15 g,茯苓、黄芩、黄连、白术各 9 g,泽泻 6 g。

【用法】 共研细末,汤浸蒸饼为丸,每次 6～9 g,温开水送下,每日 2～3 次。亦可作汤剂,用量按原方比例酌定。

【功用】 消食导滞,清热祛湿。

【临床应用】 适用于食积湿热证。症见脘腹胀痛,泄泻或便秘,小便短赤,舌苔黄腻而厚,脉沉数有力。胃肠功能紊乱、慢性痢疾等以脘腹胀痛,大便失常,舌红苔黄腻为主症,属湿热食积壅滞肠胃者,可用本方治疗。若腹胀痛

with greasy yellowish fur, which are ascribed to dampness-heat and food stagnancy retaining in the stomach and intestines. In case of severe abdominal fullness and pain, diarrhea and tenesmus, add Muxiang (*Radix Aucklandiae*) and Binglang (*Semen Arecae*) to promote the flow of qi and remove stagnancy. In case of dysentery with excessive heat, high fever, pus and blood in the stool, add Baitouweng (*Radix Pulsatillae*) and Jinyinhua (*Flos Lonicerae*) to clear away heat from the intestines and remove heat and toxins from the blood.

Elucidation: The syndrome is caused by dampness-heat and food retaining in the stomach and intestines, leading to food stagnancy, dysfunction of qi activity and disturbance of transportation. It should be treated by promoting digestion, removing stagnancy and eliminating heat and dampness. No.3 with the function of promoting digestion and No.2 with the function of promoting the circulation of qi and removing stagnancy play the role of monarch drugs together, ensuring an easy flow of qi of the middle-energizer. No.1 is the minister drug, which can purge away heat, relax the bowels and lead the stagnated food and dampness-heat downward. No.5 and No.6 are capable of clearing away heat and eliminating dampness, No.4 and No.8 eliminating dampness by inducing diuresis, while No.7 has the function of reinforcing the spleen so as to remove stagnancy without impairing the vital-qi, all these five serving as adjuvant drugs.

Cautions: This recipe is drastic in its purgative effect, thus it should be used with great caution for patients with dysentery but not severe stagnancy or those with weakness of the spleen due to protracted dysentery. It is also contraindicated for pregnant women.

较甚，腹泻，里急后重者，可加木香、槟榔以行气导滞；若痢疾热毒较重，高热便脓血者，可加白头翁、金银花以清肠凉血解毒。

【方解】　本方证由湿热与食积交阻肠胃，积滞内停，气机壅塞，传导失司所致，治宜消食导滞，清热祛湿之法。方中神曲消食助运，枳实行气导滞，二药合用，消食化滞，行气畅中，共为君药。大黄泻下通腑，导积滞湿热下行，使邪有去路，为臣药。黄连、黄芩清热燥湿；茯苓、泽泻利水渗湿；白术健脾化湿，使攻积而不伤正，俱为佐药。

【注意事项】　本方泻下导滞之力较强，若泄痢而积滞不甚，或利久脾虚者慎用。孕妇禁用。

2.15.2   Prescriptions for Promoting Digestion by Activating the Spleen

Zhizhu Wan
(*Pill of Immature Bitter Orange and Bighead Atractylodes*)

Source：*Zhang Jiegu's recipe*，*excerpted from Neiwaishang Bianhuo Lun* (*Treatise on Differentiation of Internal and External Injuries*).

Ingredients：

No. 1 Zhishi (*Fructus Aurantii Immaturus*) 30 g;

No. 2 Baizhu (*Rhizoma Atractylodis Macrocephalae*) 60 g.

Administration：Grind the above drugs into fine powder and put it into boiled rice wrapped with lotus leaf (*Folium Nelumbinis*) and make them into pills. Take 5 -10 g each time for oral dose and twice or 3 times daily with warm boiled water.

Actions：Reinforcing the spleen and removing stagnated food.

Clinical Application：This recipe is indicated for food stagnancy due to weakness of the spleen, marked by chest and epigastric stuffiness, no appetite, dyspepsia, or abdominal fullness and diarrhea. It is applicable to chronic gastritis, chronic enteritis, dyspepsia and others, which pertain to indigestion due to weakness of the spleen. In case of excessive deficiency of the spleen-qi, add Dangshen (*Radix Codonopsis Pilosulae*), Fuling (*Poria*) and Zhigancao (*Radix Glycyrrhizae Praeparatae*) to supplement the spleen-qi. In case of much stagnancy, add Shanzha (*Fructus Crataegi*), Shenqu (*Massa Fermentata Medicinalis*) and Maiya (*Fructus Hordei Germinatus*) to strengthen the effect of promoting digestion and

第二节　健脾
消食剂

枳术丸

【方源】　张洁古方,录自《内外伤辨惑论》。

【组成】　枳实 30 g,白术 60 g。

【用法】　共研细末,荷叶裹烧饭为丸,每次 5～10 g,温开水送下,每日 2～3 次。

【功用】　健脾消积。

【临床应用】　适用于脾虚食积证。症见胸脘痞满,不思饮食,食则难消,或腹满泄泻。慢性胃炎、慢性肠炎、消化不良等属脾虚饮食不化者,可用本方治疗。若脾气虚弱较甚者,可加党参、茯苓、炙甘草以助健脾补气之力;若积滞较重者,可加山楂、神曲、麦芽以助消食化积之功。

removing stagnancy.

Elucidation: The syndrome is caused by indigestion and obstructed flow of qi due to weakness of the spleen and stomach. It should be treated by reinforcing the spleen to remove stagnated food. No. 2 with larger dosage is meant to activate the spleen and eliminate dampness and used as monarch drug. No. 1 is capable of promoting the circulation of qi, removing stagnancy and relieving fullness and functions as minister drug. Putting fine powder into boiled rice wrapped with lotus leaf and making them into pills after lotus leaf is removed can nourish the spleen and stomach and ascend lucid yang so as to help No. 2 to reinforce the spleen and invigorate the stomach, acting as the adjuvant drug. The application of both brings about the result of both removing stagnancy and reinforcing the spleen, with the latter prevailing over the former. Lotus leaf can lift up the lucid yang and No. 1 can descend turbid substances so that ascending and descending function of the spleen and stomach is restored.

Jianpi Wan
(*Pill of Invigorating the Spleen*)

Source: *Zhengzhi Zhunsheng* (*Standards of Diagnosis and Treatment*).

Ingredients:

No. 1 Chaobaizhu (*Rhizoma Atractylodis Macrocephalae*) (baked) 75 g;

No. 2 Muxiang (*Radix Aucklandiae*) 22.5 g;

No. 3 Huanglian (*Rhizoma Coptidis*) (parched with wine) 22.5 g;

No. 4 Gancao (*Radix Glycyrrhizae*) 22.5 g;

No. 5 Fuling (*Poria*) 60 g;

No. 6 Renshen (*Radix Ginseng*) 45 g;

No. 7 Chaoshenqu (*Massa Fermetata Medicinalis*) (baked) 30 g;

【方解】　本方证由脾胃虚弱,饮食不消,阻滞气机所致,治宜健脾消积之法。方中重用白术健脾祛湿,以助脾之运化,为君药。枳实行气化滞,消痞除满,为臣药。荷叶烧饭为丸,取其养脾胃而升清,助白术健脾益胃之功,为佐药。方中白术补脾,枳实化滞,消补兼施,以补为主;荷叶升清,枳实降浊,升降复常,则脾健胃和。

健脾丸

【方源】　《证治准绳》。

【组成】　炒白术 75 g,木香、黄连(酒炒)、甘草各 22.5 g,茯苓 60 g,人参 45 g,炒神曲、陈皮、砂仁、炒麦芽、山楂、山药、肉豆蔻各 30 g。

No. 8 Chenpi (*Pericarpium Citri Reticulatae*) 30 g;

No. 9 Sharen (*Fructus Amoni*) 30 g;

No. 10 Chaomaiya (*Fructus Hordei Germinatus*) (baked) 30 g;

No. 11 Shanzha (*Fructus Crataegi*) 30 g;

No. 12 Shanyao (*Rhizoma Dioscoreae*) 30 g;

No. 13 Roudoukou (*Semen Myristicae*) 30 g.

Administration: Grind the above drugs into fine powder before steaming and making it into pills. Take 9 g each time and twice or 3 times daily with warm boiled water or old rice gruel before meals. Or decoct them in water with dosages in proportion to the original recipe.

Actions: Reinforcing the spleen and regulating the stomach, promoting digestion and arresting diarrhea.

Clinical Application: This recipe is indicated for food stagnancy due to weakness of the spleen, marked by poor appetite and indigestion, epigastric and abdominal distention and fullness, loose stool, greasy yellowish fur, feeble pulse. It is applicable to chronic gastritis, chronic enteritis, dyspepsia and others, which pertain to indigestion due to weakness of the spleen and stomach. If concomitant with yang deficiency, cold sensation and pain of the epigastrium, aversion to cold and preference for warmth, subtract No. 3 and add Ganjiang (*Rhizoma Zingiberis*) to warm the middle-energizer and dispel cold. In case of dampness syndrome with diarrhea and thick greasy fur, add Cheqianzi (*Semen Plantaginis*) and Zexie (*Rhizoma Alismatis*) to eliminate dampness by inducing diuresis and arresting diarrhea.

Elucidation: The syndrome is caused by usual weakness of the spleen and stomach, leading to their hypofunction in transporting and digesting food so that dampness and heat are generated when food gets stagnated. This should be treated by reinforcing the spleen and

【用法】 共研细末,蒸饼为丸。每次 9 g,饭前以温开水或陈米汤送下,每日 2～3 次。亦可作汤剂,用量按原方比例酌定。

【功用】 健脾和胃,消食止泻。

【临床应用】 适用于脾虚食积证。症见食少难消,脘腹痞闷,大便溏薄,苔腻微黄,脉象虚弱。慢性胃炎、慢性肠炎、消化不良等属脾胃虚弱,饮食不消者,可用本方治疗。若兼阳虚,脘腹冷痛,喜温畏寒者,可去黄连,加干姜以温中祛寒;若湿象较甚,泄泻,舌苔厚腻者,可加车前子、泽泻以利水渗湿止泻。

【方解】 本方证由素体脾胃虚弱,运化乏力,食入难消,停滞成积,生湿化热所致,治宜健脾和胃,消食止泻之法。方中山楂、神曲、麦芽消

regulating the stomach as well as promoting digestion and arresting diarrhea. No. 11, No. 7 and No. 10 are monarch drugs with the function of promoting digestion, removing stagnancy and regulating the stomach. No. 6, No. 1, No. 5 and No. 4 together, namely the Sijunzi Tang, have the function of supplementing qi and reinforcing the spleen and are used as minister drugs, of which No. 1 and No. 5 with larger dosage are meant to activate the spleen and eliminate dampness so as to relieve diarrhea. No. 12 and No. 13 have a tonic and astringent effect respectively on the spleen and intestines and promote the function of the minister drugs. No. 2, No. 9 and No. 8 possess the function of regulating the flow of qi and the stomach, promoting the effect of transportation and transformation and relieving fullness. No. 3 can clear away heat and eliminate dampness generated from stagnated food. The above six ingredients act together as adjuvant drugs. No. 4 also serves as guiding drug to mediate drug properties. All are together used for elimination and reinforcement in combination with the latter prevailing over the former, thus making the spleen invigorated, stomach regulated, dampness eliminated, heat cleared away and all symptoms relieved.

Both this recipe and Zhizhu Wan possess dispersive and tonic action simultaneously and are applied in the treatment of indigestion due to weakness of the spleen. But the former has a better effect than the latter in supplementing qi and activating the spleen as well as relieving dyspepsia, and can also eliminate dampness to arrest diarrhea. The latter, however, focuses on activating the spleen and promoting the flow of qi so as to relieve fullness. The former is fit for indigestion due to weakness of the spleen with chief manifestations as poor appetitie, loose stool and greasy yellowish fur, while the latter suit-

食化滞和胃以治食积之标,为君药。人参、白术、茯苓、甘草,即四君子汤,益气健脾助运以培脾虚之本,其中白术、茯苓用量偏重,意在健脾渗湿以止泻,为臣药。山药、肉豆蔻补脾涩肠,助四君子健脾止泻;木香、砂仁、陈皮理气和胃,助运化而消痞满;黄连清热燥湿以除食积酿生之湿热,俱为佐药。甘草调和药性,兼作使药。诸药配伍,消补兼施,补重于消,使脾健胃和,湿祛热清,诸证自除。

本方与枳术丸均有消补兼施之功,同治脾虚食积之证,但本方益气健脾与消食化滞之力均胜于枳术丸,并可化湿止泻;枳术丸则重在健脾行气,消痞除满。健脾丸适宜于脾虚食积以食少便溏,苔腻微黄为主症者;枳术丸则适宜于脾虚食积以气机阻滞,脘腹痞满较甚为主症者。

able for that mainly characterized by obstructed flow of qi and severe fullness sensation in the epigastrium.

Caution：This recipe is contraindicated for weakness of the spleen with poor appetite but without stagnancy.

【注意事项】 脾虚食少，内无积滞者禁用本方。

2.16 Prescriptions for Treating Carbuncles

Those that possess detoxicating action and effect of removing swelling and can promote the evacuation of pus and regeneration of tissues for the treatment of carbuncle, cellulites, sores and furuncles are known as prescriptions for treating carbuncles.

Carbuncles, cellulites, sores and furuncles may appear on the surface of the body (briefed as external carbuncle) or occur inside the body (briefed as internal carbuncle). Therefore this group of prescriptions is classified accordingly into two categories, namely the prescriptions for external carbuncles and those for internal carbuncles.

External carbuncles with local redness, swelling, pyrexia and pain, are known as yang syndrome and those with local diffuse swelling, hardness or softness, unchanged skin color in a scattered way are known as yin syndrome. Treatment of external carbuncles comprises external and internal therapies. Discussed in this chapter are only prescriptions of the latter therapy. In the application of internal therapy, resolving method, expulsion method and tonic method should be employed respectively in the light of the three stages of carbuncle development (i. e. initial stage, pus formation and post ulceration stage). Resolving method is used at the initial stage of non-suppuration to eliminate toxins and subdue swelling. In case of yang syndrome, prescriptions should be aimed at clearing away heat and toxins, while in case of yin syndrome, aimed at dispelling cold and removing phlegm.

第十六章 治痈剂

凡具有解毒消肿、排脓生肌等作用,用于治疗痈疽疮疡的方剂,统称治痈剂。

由于痈疽疮疡有发生于体表者(简称外痈),亦有发生于体内者(简称内痈),因而治痈剂相应地分为治疗外痈剂与治疗内痈剂两类。

发生于体表的痈疡,若局部红、肿、热、痛明显者称为阳证,而局部漫肿、坚硬或绵软、皮色不变、范围松散者称为阴证。体表痈疡的治疗有外治法与内治法两类,本章主要介绍内治的部分方剂。外痈的内治方法,一般是按照痈疡发展过程的三个阶段(初起、脓成、溃后),分别使用消、托、补三法。消法,用于痈疡尚未成脓的初期,可使毒散肿消,若阳证者治以清热解毒为主,阴证者治以散寒化痰为主。托法,用于痈疡中期正虚邪陷,脓成难溃之证,通过扶正透脓

Expulsion method is employed at the intermediate stage of carbuncles when pus is formed but difficult to be expelled due to deficiency of vital-qi and retaining of pathogenic factors. This method can cause the internal toxins to shift to the superficies of the body, and make pus easy to fester and the wound to heal soon. Tonic method is often applied at the later stage of carbuncles manifested as deficiency of both qi and blood, thin clear watery pus and unhealed vent. The tonic drugs can replenish qi and promote the production of blood and tissue regeneration.

Prescriptions for internal carbuncles mainly consist of drugs with the function of clearing away heat and toxins, removing stasis and draining pus, which can clear away heat from the vescera, remove stasis and evacuate pus as well as resolve mass and promote wound healing.

It is the first priority to differentiate the location, nature and different stages of carbuncles in the application of these prescriptions so that corresponding prescriptions could be employed properly. It is necessary to adopt tonic method at the later stage of carbuncles with deficiency of vital-qi, but not too early or exclusively so as to prevent the unremoved toxins from lingering on.

可促使疮毒移深就浅,易溃、易敛。补法,用于疮疡后期气血皆虚,脓液清稀,疮口久溃不敛之证,通过补益方药的治疗,可使气充血实,促进溃处生肌收口。

治疗内痈剂由清热解毒,逐瘀排脓药为主组成,具有清解脏腑热毒,祛腐逐瘀排脓,散结消肿敛疮作用。

使用治痈剂时首先应当辨明疮疡发生的部位、性质和阶段,以酌情选用有针对性的方剂。痈疡后期正气不足者固应温补,但切忌用补过早或纯补,以防余毒未尽,邪气流连不去。

2.16.1 Prescriptions for External Carbuncles

Xianfang Huoming Yin
(*Fairy Decoction for Treating Cutaneous Infections*)

Source: *Jiaozhu Furen Liangfang* (*The Revised Complete Effective Prescriptions for Diseases of Women*).

Ingredients:

No. 1 Baizhi (*Radix Angelicae Dahuricae*) 3 g;

第一节　治疗外痈剂

仙方活命饮

【方源】《校注妇人良方》。

【组成】　白芷、贝母、防风、赤芍药、当归尾、甘草、炒

No. 2 Beimu (*Bulbus Fritillariae*) 3 g;

No. 3 Fangfeng (*Radix Ledebouriellae*) 3 g;

No. 4 Chishaoyao (*Radix Paeoniae Rubra*) 3 g;

No. 5 Dangguiwei (*tail of Radix Angelicae Sinensis*) 3 g;

No. 6 Gancao (*Radix Glycyrrhizae*) 3 g;

No. 7 Chaozaojiaoci (*Spina Gleditsiae*) (parched) 3 g;

No. 8 Zhichuanshanjia (*Squama Manitis Praeparatae*)3 g;

No. 9 Tianhuafen (*Radix Trichosanthis*) 3 g;

No. 10 Ruxiang (*Olibanum*) 3 g;

No. 11 Moyao (*Myrrha*) 3 g;

No. 12 Jinyinhua (*Flos Lonicerae*) 9 g;

No. 13 Jupi (*Pericarpium Citri Reticulatae*) 9 g.

Administration: Decoct the above drugs in water or in the mixture of water and wine with equal amount for oral application. The residue can be smashed for external application.

Actions: Clearing away heat and toxins, subduing swelling and disintegrating mass, promoting the circulation of blood and relieving pain.

Clinical Application: This recipe is indicated for carbuncles in the early stage, marked by local redness, swelling, pyrexia and pain, pus being not yet formed or formed already, or feverish body with slight aversion to cold, thin whitish or thin yellowish fur, rapid and forceful pulse. It is applicable to such diseases with purulent inflammations as phlegmon, suppurative tonsillitis, mastadenitis, impetigo herpetifomis, furuncle, deep abscess, and others, which pertain to yang syndrome and excess syndrome. In case of severe heat-toxin and local redness and swelling, add Pugongying (*Herba Taraxaci*), Lianqiao (*Fructus Forsythiae*), Zihuadiding (*Herba Violae*) and Yejuhua (*Flos Chrysanthemi Indici*) to strengthen the effect of clearing away heat and removing toxins. In case of constipation, add Dahuang (*Radix et Rhizoma*

皂角刺、炙穿山甲、天花粉、乳香、没药各 3 g,金银花、橘皮各 9 g。

【用法】 水煎或水酒各半煎服。药渣亦可捣烂外敷。

【功用】 清热解毒,消肿溃坚,活血止痛。

【临床应用】 适用于痈疡肿毒初起。症见局部红肿热痛,脓未成或已成,或身热微恶寒,舌苔薄白或薄黄,脉数有力。蜂窝织炎、化脓性扁桃体炎、乳腺炎、脓疱疮、疖肿、深部脓肿等化脓性炎症属阳证实证者,可用本方治疗。若热毒较著,局部红肿痛甚者,可加蒲公英、连翘、紫花地丁、野菊花以加强清热解毒之力;若便秘者,可加大黄以泻火通腑,导热下行。此外还可根据疮疡肿毒所在部位的不同,适当加入引经药,以使药

Rhei) to purge away fire and relax bowels as well as to lead heat downward. In addition, guiding herbs could be added in accordance with the location of carbuncles so as to cause the drugs to take effect directly at the affected part.

Elucidation: The syndrome is caused by excessive accumulation of heat and toxins inside, leading to qi stagnation, blood stasis and stagnation of phlegm. This should be treated by clearing away heat and toxins, subduing swelling and resolving mass, promoting blood circulation and relieving pain. Because of the effect of eliminating heat and toxins as well as subduing swelling, No. 12 was thus named holy herb for carbuncles by our forefathers and functions as monarch drug in this recipe. No. 5, No. 4, No. 10, No. 11 and No. 13 have the function of promoting the flow of qi, removing obstruction from the meridians, promoting blood circulation and resolving stasis so as to subdue swelling, all playing the role of minister drugs. No. 1 and No. 3 can expel wind and heat, No. 8 and No. 7 can ensure smooth flow of qi in the meridians and collaterals, promote pus discharge and resolve mass. No. 9 and No. 2 possess the function of clearing away heat, removing phlegm, resolving mass and subduing swelling so that pus is resolved before it can be formed. These six ingredients act as adjuvant drugs together. No. 6 is the guiding drug with the action of clearing away heat and toxins as well as mediating drug properties. The wine is meant to enhance the potency of the recipe so that all ingredients will quickly take effect at the affected part because wine can ensure smooth circulation of blood in the vessels.

Cautions: Cold in nature and drastic in the effect of expelling pathogenic factors, this recipe should be contraindicated for patients with healed carbuncles. It should also be used with caution for those with usual weakness of the spleen and stomach as well as deficiency of both qi and blood.

力直达病所。

【方解】 本方证由热毒内壅,气滞血瘀痰结所致,治宜清热解毒,消肿溃坚,活血止痛之法。方中金银花清热解毒,消散痈肿,前人誉之谓疮疡圣药,故为君药。当归尾、赤芍药、乳香、没药、橘皮行气通络,活血散瘀,使气畅血行而瘀去肿消,同为臣药。白芷、防风疏风散邪,使热毒从外透解;穿山甲、皂角刺通行经络,透脓溃坚,使脓已成者即溃;天花粉、贝母清热化痰,散结消肿,使脓未成者消散,均为佐药。生甘草清热解毒,调和药性,为使药。煎药时加酒,可利用其通调血脉之性以助药势,使诸药速达病所。

【注意事项】 本方药性寒凉,通透之力较著,故疮疡已溃者禁用;素体脾胃虚弱,气血不足者慎用。

Tounong San
(*Powder for Promoting Pus Discharge*)

Source: *Waike Zhengzong* (*Orthodix Treatis on surgical Diseases*).

Ingredients:

No. 1 Shenghuangqi (*Radix Astragali seu Hedysari*) 12 g;

No. 2 Danggui (*Radix Angelicae Sinensis*) 6 g;

No. 3 Chaochuanshanjia (*Squama Manitis*) (parched) 3 g;

No. 4 Zaojiaoci (*Spina Gleditsiae*) 5 g;

No. 5 Chuanxiong (*Rhizoma Ligustici Chuanxiong*) 9 g.

Administration: Decoct the above drugs in water for oral application.

Actions: Expelling toxin and promoting pus discharge.

Clinical Application: This recipe is indicated for swelling and pain from carbuncles and inability to drain pus because of deficiency of vital-qi, marked by pus inside which can hardly break, diffuse swelling, or soreness, distending sensation, pyrexia and pain. It is applicable to various purulent inflammations occurring on the surface of body, which are manifested as unrelieved carbuncle and swelling, not easy to form pus and unfit for being cut open. In case of severe local redness and swelling, add Jinyinhua (*Flos Lonicerae*) and Liangqiao (*Fructus Forsythiae*) to clear away heat and toxins so as to relieve carbuncle. In case of hardness of carbuncle when pressed with severe pain, add Ruxiang (*Olibanum*) and Moyao (*Myrrha*) to promote blood circulation, subdue swelling and relieve pain.

Elucidation: The syndrome is caused by unexpelled toxic substances due to deficiency of vital-qi, leading to formation of pus, which is hard to break. This should be

【方源】《外科正宗》。

【组成】 生黄芪 12 g,当归 6 g,炒穿山甲 3 g,皂角刺 5 g,川芎 9 g。

【用法】 水煎服。

【功用】 托毒溃脓。

【临床应用】 适用于痈疡肿痛,正虚不能托毒。症见痈疡内已成脓,外不易溃,漫肿无头,或酸胀热痛。体表各种化脓性炎症见有痈肿不消,成脓不易,切开又不适宜者,可用本方治疗。若局部红肿较甚者,可加金银花、连翘以清热解毒消痈;若痈肿按之较硬,疼痛较甚者,可加乳香、没药以活血消肿止痛。

【方解】 本方证由正虚不能托毒外透,以致脓成难溃,毒亦难泄,治宜托毒溃脓

treated by promoting pus discharge. No. 1 is capable of replenishing qi and expelling toxins, while No. 3 promoting pus discharge and resolving mass, both acting as monarch drugs. No. 2 and No. 5 possess the function of enriching and promoting the circulation of blood, which not only promote No. 1 in its effect of building up vital-qi but also relieve swelling and pain, both used as minister drugs. No. 4 functions as adjuvant drug, which is capable of subsiding swelling to dissipate indurated mass and expelling toxin and helps No. 3 in resolving mass and draining pus. All ingredients together involve expelling pathogenic factors and building up healthy qi simultaneously so that toxins are removed with pus and tissue regeneration follows.

Cautions：This recipe belongs to those for promoting pus discharge and thus it is contraindicated for the initial stage of carbuncles without formation of pus.

之法。方中黄芪益气托毒,穿山甲透脓溃坚,共为君药。当归、川芎养血活血,既助黄芪扶正补虚之力,又有消肿止痛之功,同为臣药。皂角刺消散通透,助穿山甲软坚溃脓,为佐药。诸药配伍,祛邪之中兼以扶正,使毒随脓泄,腐去新生。

【注意事项】 本方属于托法之剂,痈疡初起脓未成者禁用。

Yanghe Tang
(Yang-activiting Decoction)

Source：*Waike Quanshengji* (*Treatise on Diagnosis and Treatment of Surgical Diseases*).

Ingredients：

No. 1 Shudihuang (*Radix Rehmanniae Praeparatae*) 30 g;

No. 2 Rougui (*Cortex Cinnamomi*) 3 g;

No. 3 Mahuang (*Herba Ephedrae*) 2 g;

No. 4 Lujiaojiao (*Colla Cornus Cervi*) 9 g;

No. 5 Baijiezi (*Semen Sinapis Albae*) 6 g;

No. 6 Paojiang (*Rhizoma Zingiberis Praeparatae*) 2 g;

No. 7 Shenggancao (*Radix Glycyrrhizae*) 3 g.

Administration：Decoct the above drugs in water for oral application.

Actions：Warming yang and enriching blood, dispelling cold and removing obstruction.

阳和汤

【方源】 《外科全生集》。

【组成】 熟地黄 30 g,肉桂 3 g,麻黄 2 g,鹿角胶 9 g,白芥子 6 g,炮姜 2 g,生甘草 3 g。

【用法】 水煎服。

【功用】 温阳补血,散寒通滞。

Clinical Application：This recipe is indicated for yin-type carbuncle, marked by local diffuse swelling, unchanged skin color, soreness without pyrexia, absence of thirst, pale tongue with whitish fur, deep thready or slow thready pulse. It is applicable to bone tuberculosis, peritoneal tuberculosis, chronic osteomyelitis, periostitis, chronic lymphnoditis, rheumatoid arthritis, thromboangiitis obliterans, deep abscess, and others, which are ascribed to syndrome of cold accumulation due to insufficient blood.

Elucidation：The syndrome is caused by insufficient blood due to usual deficiency of yang and attack by exogenous cold, leading to accumulation of cold and phlegm, which retain in the tissues, tendons, blood vessels and joints. This should be treated by warming yang and enriching blood, dispelling cold and removing phlegm so as to remove stagnation and subdue swelling. With a larger dosage, No. 1 is meant to nourish blood. No. 4 is supposed to replenish essence, activate the kidney-yang and strengthen tendons and bones. Both can deal with the root cause of the disease by nourishing blood and yang and function as monarch drugs. No. 6 and No. 2 possess the function of warming the interior to dispel cold as well as ensuring smooth circulation of blood, playing the role of minister drugs. Used as adjuvant drugs, No. 3 and No. 5 can promote the flow of blood and qi on the one hand, and bring about the tonic action of No. 1 and No. 4 and prevent stagnation on the other because No. 3 is capable of removing obstruction from meridians and collaterals and No. 5 eliminating stagnation of phlegm from the muscular striae, tendons and vessles. No. 7 is the guiding drug in the recipe, which can remove toxin and mediate drug properties.

Caution：This recipe is contraindicated for patients with yang syndrome of external carbuncle.

【临床应用】　适用于阴疽。症见局部漫肿无头，皮色不变，酸痛无热，口中不渴，舌淡苔白，脉沉细或迟细。骨结核、腹膜结核、慢性骨髓炎、骨膜炎、慢性淋巴结炎、类风湿关节炎、血栓闭塞性脉管炎、肌肉深部脓疡等属血虚寒凝者，可用本方治疗。

【方解】　本方证由素体阳虚血少，外受寒邪，寒凝痰滞，痹阻于肌肉、筋骨、血脉、关节所致，治宜温阳补血，散寒化痰，通滞消肿之法。方中重用熟地黄温补营血，配以鹿角胶血肉有情之品填精益髓，补肾助阳，强壮筋骨，两药配伍，养血助阳以治本，共为君药。炮姜、肉桂温里散寒，通达血脉，同为臣药。麻黄宣通经络，开腠理以达表，白芥子善祛肌腠筋脉之痰滞，两药既能使血气宣通，又可令熟地黄、鹿角胶补而不滞，均为佐药。甘草解毒而调和药性，为使药。

【注意事项】　外痈阳证禁用本方。

2.16.2   Prescriptions for Internal Carbuncles

Weijing Tang
(*Reed Stem Decoction*)

Source: *Beiji Qianjin Yaofang* (*Valuable Prescriptions for Emergency*).

Ingredients:

No. 1 Weijing (*Rhizoma Phragmitis*) 60 g;

No. 2 Yiyiren (*Semen Coicis*) 15 g;

No. 3 Dongguazi (*Semen Benincasae*) 15 g;

No. 4 Taoren (*Semen Persicae*) 9 g.

Administration: Decoct No. 1 first in water to get the decoction, in which the rest ingredients are decocted. Remove residue from the decoction, which is to be taken separately.

Actions: Clearing away heat from the lung and resolving phlegm, removing stasis and promoting pus discharge.

Clinical Application: This recipe is indicated for pulmonary abscess, marked by expectoration of yellowish stench sputum with blood and pus and stinking smell, vague pain in the chest which aggravates while coughing, reddened tongue with greasy yellowish fur, smooth and rapid pulse. It is applicable to pulmonary abscess, lobar pneumonia, bronchitis, pertussis, and others, which have chief manifestations as chest pain, cough, expectoration of sputum with stinking smell or pus and blood, reddened tongue with greasy yellowish fur and pertain to accumulation of heat and phlegm in the lung. If pus is not yet formed, add Jinyinhua (*Flos Lonicerae*) and Yuxingcao (*Herba Houttuyniae*) to strengthen the effect of eliminating heat and toxin. If pus is already formed, add

第二节   治疗

内痈剂

苇茎汤

【方源】 《备急千金要方》。

【组成】 苇茎 60 g,薏苡仁 15 g,冬瓜子 15 g,桃仁 9 g。

【用法】 以水先煎苇茎取汁,再以苇茎汁煎余药,汤成去滓分服。

【功用】 清肺化痰,逐瘀排脓。

【临床应用】 适用于肺痈。症见咳吐腥臭黄痰脓血,胸中隐隐作痛,咳时尤甚,舌红苔黄腻,脉滑数。肺化脓症、大叶性肺炎、支气管炎、百日咳等以胸痛咳嗽、吐腥臭痰或脓血,舌红苔黄腻为主证,属肺热痰瘀互结者,可用本方治疗。若肺痈未成脓者,可加金银花、鱼腥草以增强清热解毒之功;若脓已成者,可加桔梗、甘草、贝母以增强化痰排脓之效。

Jiegeng (*Radix Platycodi*), Gancao (*Radix Glycyrrhizae*) and Beimu (*Bulbus Fritillariae*) to promote the effect of removing phlegm and discharge pus.

Elucidation: The syndrome is caused by excessive heat in the lung, complicated with phlegm accumulation. It should be treated by clearing away heat from the lung and removing phlegm so as to promote pus discharge. No. 1 has the function of clearing and purging away heat from the lung and is considered the primary drug for treating carbuncles, which functions as monarch drug in this recipe. No. 3 is capable of eliminating heat and phlegm in order to discharge pus, while No. 2 clearing away heat and inducing diuresis to promote pus discharge. Both are minister drugs. No. 4 possesses the function of promoting blood circulation and removing stasis as well as moistening the lung and loosening bowels and plays the role of adjuvant drug, which can direct the accumulated phlegm downward when combined with No. 3 so that phlegm is removed and carbuncle subdued.

Dahuang Mudan Tang
(*Decoction of Rhubarb Root and Moutan Bark*)

Source: *Jingui Yaolue* (*Synopsis of Prescriptions of the Golden Cabinet*).

Ingredients:

No. 1 Dahuang (*Radix et Rhizoma Rhei*) 12 g;

No. 2 Mudanpi (*Cortex Moutan Radicis*) 9 g;

No. 3 Taoren (*Semen Persicae*) 12 g;

No. 4 Dongguazi (*Semen Benincasae*) 30 g;

No. 5 Mangxiao (*Natrii Sulphas*) 9 g.

Administration: Decoct the first four ingredients in water; then remove the residue from the decoction and dissolve No. 5 in it. The decoction is to be taken separately.

Actions: Purging away heat and removing blood stasis, dispersing pathogenic accumulation and subduing

【方解】　本方证由热毒壅肺,痰瘀互结,蕴蓄成痈所致,治宜清肺化痰,逐瘀排脓之法。方中苇茎清肺泄热,乃治肺痈要药,为君药。冬瓜子清热化痰排脓,薏苡仁清热利湿排脓,同为臣药。桃仁活血祛瘀,且润燥滑肠,与冬瓜子相伍,可导痰瘀下行,使邪去而痈消,为佐药。

大黄牡丹汤

【方源】　《金匮要略》。

【组成】　大黄 12 g,牡丹皮 9 g,桃仁 12 g,冬瓜子 30 g,芒消 9 g。

【用法】　前四药水煎,汤成去滓,溶入芒消分服。

【功用】　泻热破瘀,散结消肿。

swelling.

Clinical Application：This recipe is indicated for intestinal abscess in the early stage, marked by pain and tenderness in the right lower abdomen, or limitation of the right foot to stretch and aggravating pain when stretched, or constant fever, spontaneous perspiration with aversion to cold, thin yellowish and greasy fur, slow and tense or smooth and rapid pulse. It is applicable to acute simple appendicitis that is ascribed to accumulation of dampness-heat, as well as acute pelvic inflammation, infection after ligation of oviduct, and others, which pertain to heat accumulation in *xuefen*. In case of excessive heat with high fever, thirst and sharp abdominal pain, add Pugongying (*Herba Taraxaci*), Jinyinhua (*Flos Lonicerae*) and Baijiangcao (*Herba Patriniae*) to enhance the effect of clearing away heat and toxin. In case of dysentery-like stool with difficulty in defecation, reddened tongue and thready rapid pulse, which are suggestive of yin impairment, it is advisable to subtract No. 5 to reduce the purgative effect and add Xuanshen (*Radix Scrophulariae*) and Shengdihuang (*Radix Rehmanniae*) to nourish yin and clear away heat.

Elucidation：The syndrome arises when dampness-heat and toxic substances retain in the intestines and lead to stagnation of qi and blood, giving rise to carbuncles. This should be treated by purging away heat and removing blood stasis, dispersing pathogenic accumulation and subduing swelling. No. 1 has the function of purging away intense heat, toxin and dampness-heat from the intestines, while No. 3 possesses the function of promoting blood flow and removing blood stasis, both acting as monarch drugs. No. 5 is capable of purging away heat and pathogenic accumulation and, when in combination with No. 1, can remove heat of excess type from the intestines. No. 2 is

【临床应用】 适用于肠痈初起。症见右下腹疼痛拒按，或右足屈而不伸，伸则痛甚，或时时发热，自汗恶寒，舌苔薄黄而腻，脉迟紧或滑数。急性单纯性阑尾炎属湿热瘀滞者，以及妇科急性盆腔炎、输卵管结扎后感染等属血分瘀热者，均可用本方治疗。若热毒较重，高热口渴，腹痛较剧者，可加蒲公英、金银花、败酱草以加强清热解毒之力；若大便似痢不爽，舌质红，脉细数者，为阴伤之象，宜去芒消以减缓泻下之力，并加玄参、生地黄以养阴清热。

【方解】 本方证由湿热毒邪结于肠中，气血凝聚，蕴蓄成痈所致，治宜泻热破瘀，散结消肿之法。方中大黄泻火解毒，攻下肠中湿热瘀滞；桃仁活血破瘀，两药合用以攻逐肠中湿热瘀毒，共为君药。芒消泻热导滞，软坚散结，与大黄合用以荡涤肠中实热；牡丹皮凉血化瘀，消肿散结，与桃仁配伍以助其活血破瘀之功，同为臣药。冬瓜子清肠利

capable of clearing away heat from blood and removing blood stasis, and can promote the function of No. 3. Therefore No. 5 and No. 2 function together as minister drugs. No. 4 is the adjuvant drug in the recipe, which has the function of clearing away heat from the intestines, inducing diuresis and promoting pus discharge.

Cautions: This recipe should be contraindicated for patients after degeneration, the aged, pregnant women and women after delivery. Besides, it should not be used for severe case of acute suppurative or gangrenous appendicitis, appendicitis complicated with peritonitis, and acute infantile appendicitis.

湿,排脓消痈,为佐药。

【**注意事项**】 肠痈溃后, 或老人、孕妇、产后患者禁用 本方。重型急性化脓性或坏 疽性阑尾炎、阑尾炎合并腹膜 炎、婴儿急性阑尾炎等,亦不 宜使用本方。

3 Appendix 附 录

I. Commonly Used Chinese Patent Medicines 一、常用中成药

Chart I   Medicines for Inducing Diaphoresis, Relieving Cough and Asthma

Name of the Recipe	Ingredients	Functions	Indications	Directions & Dosage	Specifications
Wushicha Chongji	Old Folium Gemmae Camelliae Sinensis, Fructus Forsythiae, Rhizoma Atractylodis, Radix Bupleuri, Radix Ledebouriellae, Fructus Aurantii Immaturus, Radix Peucedani, Radix Platycodi, Fructus Crataegi, Rhizoma Ligustici Chuanxiong, Rhizoma seu Radix Notopterygii, Pericarpium Citri Reticulatae, Herba Agastachis, Folium Perillae, Massa Fermentata Medicinalis, Cortex Magnoliae Officinalis, Radix Glycyrrhizae, Fructus Hordei Germinatus, Radix Angelicae Dahuricae	Relieving exterior syndrome, regulating the middle-energizer, promoting digestion, removing phlegm	Attack by wind-cold and indigestion, alternating chills and fever, cough, poor appetitie, abdominal pain, vomiting, diarrhea	Take warmly one piece at each time after it is decocted in water, once or twice daily; or drink as tea after it is soaked in boiling water	9 g each
Tongxuan Lifei Wan	Folium Perillae, Radix Scutellariae, Fructus Aurantii, Radix Glycyrrhizae, Pericarpium Citri Reticulatae, Radix Platycodi, Poria, Semen Armeniacae Amarum, Radix Peucedani, Herba Ephedrae, Rhizoma Pinelliae	Relieving exterior syndrome to dispel cold, facilitating the flow of the lung-qi to stop coughing	Cough due to exogenous pathogenic factors, fever with aversion to cold, headache without perspiration, soreness of the limbs, clear nasal discharge	2 pills orally at one time and twice or 3 times daily	6 g each.
Lingqiao Jiedu Wan	Cornu Saigae Tattaricae, Flos Lonicerae, Fructus Forsythiae, Herba Menthae, Herba Schizonepetae, Semen Sojae Praeparatum, Fructus Arctii, Radix Platycodi, Herba Lophatheri, Radix Glycyrrhizae	Relieving superficial syndrome with drugs of pungent flavor and cool nature, Clearing away heat and toxin	Common cold due to wind-heat with fever, headache, cough, dry mouth, and sore throat	One pill orally at one time and twice or 3 times daily	3 g each

Name of the Recipe	Ingredients	Functions	Indications	Directions & Dosage	Specifications
Xiao'er Jind-an Pian	Rhizoma seu Radix Notopterygii, Radix Ledebouriellae, Radix Puerariae, Spica Schizonepetae, Cacumen Tamaricis, Cornu Bubali, Cornu Saigae Tattaricae, Folium Isatidis, Radix Rehmanniae, Radix Paeoniae Rubra, Borneolum, Field Mint, Caulis Akebiae, Radix Scrophulariae, Bulbus Fritillariae, Exocarpium Citri Rubrum, Arisaema cum Bile, Radix Peucedani, Fructus Aurantii, Fructus Arctii, Radix Platycodi, Rhizoma Pinelliae, Cinnabaris, Ramulus Uncariae cum Uncis, Rhizoma Gastrodiae, Radix Glycyrrhizae	Dispelling wind, Clearing away heat, promoting eruption, eliminating phlegm, arresting cough, removing heat from the liver and subduing endogenous wind	Common cold due to wind-heat, cough and asthma due to phlegm-heat, convulsion due to phlegm-heat, as well as failure of urticaria in eruption, mumps in children	Two tablets for children over one year old; and appropriately reduced dose for children under one year; twice daily	0.3 g each
Qingxuan Wan	Rhizoma Ligustici Chuanxiong, Radix Angelicae Dahuricae, Gypsum Fibrosum, Herba Menthae, Spica Schizonepetae	Dispelling wind and Clearing away heat to alleviate pain	Attack by wind-heat manifested as headache and dizziness, or nasal obstruction with thick discharge, or red swelling gum	30 - 45 pills each time orally and once or twice daily	Weighing 1 g every five pills
Jinyi Qushu Wan	Herba Agastachis, Herba Elsholtziae seu Moslae, Folium Perillae, Fructus Chaenomelis, Poria, Flos Syzygii Aromatici, Lignum Santali, Radix Glycyrrhizae	Expelling cold from the superficies, eliminating summer-heat and dampness	Attack by wind-cold in combination with dampness accumulation due to internal injury in summer time, characterized by aversion to cold, fever, headache, chest distress, epigastric and abdominal pain, vomiting and diarrhea	2 pills each time orally and twice daily	7.5 g each
Shedan Chen-pi San	Snake bile, Pericarpium Citri Reticulatae	Regulating the flow of qi and removing phlegm, dispelling wind and reinforcing the stomach	Cough due to wind-cold with much sputum and nausea	0.3 - 0.6 g each time orally and twice or 3 times daily	0.3 g per bottle

(**Following table**)

Name of the Recipe	Ingredients	Functions	Indications	Directions & Dosage	Specif- ications
Shedan Chua- nbei San	*Snake bile, Bulbus Frit- illariae Cirrhosae*	Clearing away heat from the lung and remo- ving phlegm to arrest coug- hing	Cough due to heat in the lung with much expectoration	0.3 – 0.6 g each time orally and twice or 3 times daily	0.3 g per bottle
Chuanbei Pipa Tangjiang	*Liquid extract of Bulbus Fritillariae Cirrhosae, Folium Eriobotryae, Menthol, Radix Platyco- di*	Clearing away heat from the lung, stopping cough and re- moving phlegm	Attack by wind- heat, functional disorder of the lung, cough with profuse sputum	10 ml each time orally and 3 times daily	
Fufang Chua- nbeijing Pian	*Bulbus Fritillariae Cir- rhosae, Herba Ephedrae, Pericarpium Citri Retic- ulatae, Rhizoma Pinelli- ae, Radix Polygalae, Ra- dix Platycodi, Fructus Schisandrae, Radix Gly- cyrrhizae*	Promoting the flow of lung-qi and removing phlegm, stop- ping cough and asthma	Excessive phlegm re- taining in the lung and functional disor- der of the lung-qi marked by cough and asthma, chest dis- tress with much ex- pectoration of thin whitish sputum	3 – 6 tablets each time orally and 3 times daily	0.5 g per tablet
Fufang Yux- ingcao Pian	*Herba Houttuyniae, Ra- dix Isatidis, Radix Scute- llariae, Flos Lonicerae, Fructus Forsythiae*	Relieving su- perficial syn- drome with drugs of pun- gent flavor and cool nature, purging away heat from the lung	Excessive heat in the lung due to at- tack by wind-heat manifested as fe- ver, cough, diffi- cult expectoration of thick yellowish sputum, and sore throat; or pulmona- ry abscess marked be cough and spu- tum complicated with pus	4 – 6 tablets each time orally and 3 times daily	0.25 g per tablet
Jizhi Tangjiang	*Rhizoma Fagopyri Cymo- si, Folium Ilicis Chinen- sis, Herba Houttuyniae, Radix Peucedani, etc.*	Clearing away heat and toxin, removing phlegm and stopping cough	Attack by wind-heat or phlegm-heat re- taining in the lung manifested as fe- ver, flushed face, cough with yellow- ish sputum, chest distress, or blood streak in sputum, or expectoration with pus and blood in severe case	20 – 30 ml each time orally and 3 – 4 times daily	100 ml per bottle

（**Following table**）

Name of the Recipe	Ingredients	Functions	Indications	Directions & Dosage	Specif- ications
Daige San	*Indigo Naturalis, Concha Meretricis seu Cyclinae*	Clearing away heat and removing phlegm to arrest cough	Accumulated heat in the lung and liver and internal accumulation of phlegm-heat manifested as dizziness, tinnitus, cough and sputum with blood, uncomfortable throat	3 g each time orally and twice daily	30 g per packet
Ermu Ningsou Wan	*Bulbus Fritillariae Thunbergii, Rhizoma Anemarrhenae, Gypsum Fibrosum, Radix Scutellariae, Fructus Gardeniae, Cortex Mori Radicis, Semen Trichosanthis, Pericarpium Citri Reticulatae, Fructus Schisandrae, Poria, Fructus Aurantii Immaturus, Radix Glycyrrhizae*	Clearing away heat and moistening the lung, removing phlegm and arresting cough	Yin impairment due to dryness in the lung manifested as cough with less thick yellowish sputum and difficulty in expectoration, or husky cough without sputum, dry mouth and throat or husky voice and sore throat, reddened tongue with little fur, thready and rapid pulse	1 pill each time orally and twice daily	9 g per pill
Qiuli Gao	*Fructus Pyrus Ussuriensis, Bulbus Fritillariae Thunbergii, Radix Ophiopogonis, radish, fresh lotus root*	Nourishing yin and moistening the lung, arresting cough and removing phlegm	Deficiency of the lung-yin due to long standing cough manifested as husky cough, short breath, less but thick sputum, or sputum with blood streak, dry mouth and throat, slim figure, even afternoon fever and dysphoria with feverish sensation in chest, palms and soles if serious	15 g each time orally and twice daily	60 g per big bottle and 30 g per small one
Jinguo Yin	*Radix Rehmanniae, Radix Scrophulariae, Radix Hordei Germinatus, Radix Adenophorae, Xiqingguo, Periostracum Cicadae, Semen Sterculiae Scaphigerae, Radix Pseudostellariae, Pericarpium Citri Reticulatae, Oleum Menthae*	Nourishing yin and moistening the lung, Clearing away heat and relieving sore throat	Flaming-up of deficiency fire due to insufficient lung-yin manifested as dry, itching and sore throat, cough with less but thick sputum, difficult expectoration	10 ml each time orally and 3 times daily	10 ml per vial

（Following table）

Name of the Recipe	Ingredients	Functions	Indications	Directions & Dosage	Specifications
Gejie Ding-chuan Wan	*Gecko, Semen Trichosanthis, Radix Asteris, Herba Ephedrae, Carapax Trionycis, Radix Scutellariae, Radix Glycyrrhizae, Radix Ophiopogonis, Rhizoma Coptidis, Bulbus Lilii, Fructus Perillae, Gypsum Fibrosum, Semen Armeniaccae Amarum*	Reinforcing the kidney and moistening the lung, Clearing away heat and removing phlegm, stopping cough and asthma	Yin deficiency of the lung and kidney manifested as cough and asthma, which is aggravated on slight exertion, afternoon fever, soreness of the waist and knees, mental fatigue and lassitude	1 pill each time orally and twice daily	9 g per pill
Bushen Fang-chuan Pian	*Slices of Radix Aconiti Lateralis Praeparata, Fructus Psoraleae, Herba Epimedii, Radix Rehmanniae Praeparata, Rhizoma Dioscoreae Pericarpium Citri Reticulatae, etc.*	Warming and promoting the function of the kidney, consolidating the body resistance and preventing asthma	Deficiency of the kidney-yang manifested as protracted cough and asthma, short breath and lassitude, which are aggravated on slight exertion, cold limbs, soreness of the waist and knees, spontaneous perspiration and mental fatigue	4 – 6 g each time orally and 3 times daily	0.25 g per tablet

（一）解表止咳平喘类

方　名	组　成	功　用	主　治	用法与用量	规　格
午时茶冲剂	陈茶叶,连翘,苍术,柴胡,防风,枳实,前胡,桔梗,山楂,川芎,羌活,陈皮,藿香,苏叶,神曲,厚朴,甘草,麦芽,白芷。	解表和中,消食化痰。	感冒风寒,内停食积,寒热咳嗽,不思饮食,腹痛吐泻。	口服:每次1块,水煎热服,每日1~2次,或开水浸泡代茶饮用。	每块重9 g。
通宣理肺丸	苏叶,黄芩,枳壳,甘草,陈皮,桔梗,茯苓,杏仁,前胡,麻黄,法半夏。	解表散寒,宣肺止咳。	外感咳嗽,发热恶寒,头痛无汗,肢体酸楚,鼻流清涕。	口服:每次2丸,每日2~3次。	每丸重6 g。
羚翘解毒丸	羚羊角,金银花,连翘,薄荷,荆芥,淡豆豉,牛蒡子,桔梗,淡竹叶,甘草。	辛凉透表,清热解毒。	风热感冒,发热头痛,咳嗽口干,咽喉疼痛。	口服:每次1丸,每日2~3次。	每丸重3 g。

方　名	组　　成	功　用	主　　治	用法与用量	规　格
小儿金丹片	羌活,防风,葛根,荆芥穗,桎柳,水牛角,羚羊角,大青叶,生地黄,赤芍药,冰片,薄荷冰,木通,玄参,川贝母,橘红,胆星,前胡,枳壳,牛蒡子,桔梗,半夏,朱砂,钩藤,天麻,甘草。	疏风清热,透疹解毒,化痰止咳,凉肝熄风。	小儿风热感冒,热痰咳喘,痰热惊风,以及里热郁闭,隐疹不出,痄腮。	口服:周岁以上每次2片,周岁以内酌减,每日2次。	每片重0.3 g。
清眩丸	川芎,白芷,石膏,薄荷,荆芥穗。	散风清热止痛。	外感风热,头痛目眩,或鼻塞流浊涕,或牙龈红肿疼痛。	口服:每次30～45粒,每日1～2次。	每5粒重1 g。
金衣祛暑丸	藿香,香薷,苏叶,木瓜,茯苓,丁香,檀香,甘草。	解表散寒,祛暑化湿。	暑月外感风寒,内伤湿滞,恶寒发热,头痛胸闷,脘腹疼痛,呕吐泄泻。	口服:每次2丸,每日2次。	每丸重7.5 g。
蛇胆陈皮散	蛇胆汁,陈皮。	理气化痰,祛风健胃。	风寒咳嗽,痰多呕逆。	口服:每次0.3 g～0.6 g,每日2～3次。	每瓶重0.3 g。
蛇胆川贝散	蛇胆汁,川贝母。	清肺化痰止咳。	肺热咳嗽,痰多。	口服:每次0.3～0.6 g,每日2～3次。	每瓶重0.3 g。
川贝枇杷糖浆	川贝母流浸膏,枇杷叶,薄荷脑,桔梗。	清热肃肺,止咳化痰。	外感风热,肺失清肃,咳嗽痰多。	口服:每次10 ml,每日3次	
复方川贝精片	川贝母,麻黄,陈皮,半夏,远志,桔梗,五味子,甘草。	宣肺化痰,止咳平喘。	痰浊壅肺,肺失宣降,咳嗽气喘,胸闷痰多,色白质稀。	口服:每次3～6片,每日3次。	每片重0.5 g。
复方鱼腥草片	鱼腥草,板蓝根,黄芩,金银花,连翘等。	辛凉透表,清泄肺热。	风热袭肺,肺热壅盛,发热咳嗽,痰黄粘稠难咯,咽喉肿痛,或肺痈咳吐脓痰。	口服:每次4～6片,每日3次。	每片重0.25 g。
急支糖浆	金荞麦,四季青,鱼腥草,前胡等。	清热解毒,化痰止咳。	风热袭肺,或痰热蕴肺,发热面赤,咳嗽痰黄,胸闷,甚或咳痰带血,或咳吐脓血。	口服:每次20～30 ml,每日3～4次。	每瓶100 ml。
黛蛤散	青黛,蛤壳。	清热化痰止咳。	肺肝郁热,痰火内蕴,头晕耳鸣,咳痰带血,咽喉不利。	口服:每次3 g,每日2次。	每袋装30 g。

续表

方　名	组　成	功　用	主　治	用法与用量	规　格
二母宁嗽丸	象贝母,知母,石膏,黄芩,栀子,桑白皮,瓜蒌仁,陈皮,五味子,茯苓,枳实,甘草。	清热润肺,化痰止咳。	肺燥阴伤,咳嗽,痰黄粘稠量少,不易咳出,或干咳无痰,咽干口燥或声哑喉痛,舌红少苔,脉细数。	口服:每次1丸,每日2次。	每丸重9 g。
秋梨膏	秋子梨,象贝母,麦门冬,青萝卜,鲜藕。	养阴润肺,止咳化痰。	久咳伤肺,肺阴不足,干咳短气,痰少而稠,或咳痰带血,口干咽燥,形体消瘦,甚则午后潮热,五心烦热。	口服:每次15 g,每日2次。	大瓶装60 g,小瓶装30 g。
金果饮	生地黄,玄参,麦门冬,南沙参,西青果,蝉蜕,胖大海,太子参,陈皮,薄荷油。	养阴润肺,清热利咽。	肺阴不足,虚火上炎,咽痒燥痛,咳嗽痰少而粘,不易咯出。	口服:每次10 ml,每日3次。	每支10 ml。
蛤蚧定喘丸	蛤蚧,瓜蒌仁,紫菀,麻黄,鳖甲,黄芩,甘草,麦门冬,黄连,百合,苏子,石膏,杏仁。	益肾润肺,清热化痰,止咳定喘。	肺肾阴虚,咳嗽气喘,动则尤甚,午后潮热,腰膝酸软,神疲乏力。	口服:每次1丸,每日2次。	每丸重9 g。
补肾防喘片	附片,补骨脂,淫羊藿,熟地黄,山药,陈皮等。	温肾纳气,固本防喘。	肾阳不足,气失摄纳,咳喘日久,短气乏力,动则尤甚,形寒肢冷,腰膝酸软,自汗神疲。	口服:每次4～6 g,每日3次。	每片重0.25 g。

Chart Two　Medicines for Clearing away Heat，Purging Fire and Eliminating Toxin

Name of the Recipe	Ingredients	Functions	Indications	Directions & Dosage	Specifications
Niuhuang Qingre San	*Calculus Bovis*, *Rhizoma Coptidis*, *Calcitum*, *Carapax Eretmochelydis*, *Borneolum*, etc.	Clearing away heat and toxin, subduing endogenous wind to relieve convulsion	Lingering high fever, restlessness, thirst, convulsion, even coma and delirium, reddened tongue with yellowish fur, slippery and rapid pulse	1.5 g each time orally and 2 - 4 times daily in light of the condition	3 g per bottle

Name of the Recipe	Ingredients	Functions	Indications	Directions & Dosage	Specifications
Niuhuang Shangqing Wan	Calculus Bovis, Rhizoma Coptidis, Radix Scutellariae, Cortex Phellodendri, Fructus Gardeniae, Radix et Rhizoma Rhei, Gypsum Fibrosum, Fructus Forsythiae, Flos Chrysanthemi, Herba Menthae, Herba Schizonepetae, Radix Angelicae Dahuricae, Rhizoma Ligustici Chuanxiong, Radix Angelicae Sinensis, Radix Paeoniae Rubra, Radix Rehmanniae, Radix Platycodi, Radix Glycyrrhizae, Borneolum	Clearing away heat and dispelling wind, purging fire and relieving constipation	Headache, vertigo, epidemic hemorrhagic conjunctivitis, oral ulcers, sore throat, swelling pain of gums	1 pill each time orally and twice daily	6 g per pill
Niuhuang Jiedu Wan	Calculus Bovis, Borneolum, Realgar, Radix Platycodi, Radix Scutellariae, Radix Glycyrrhizae, Radix et Rhizoma Rhei, Gypsum Fibrosum	Clearing away heat and toxin	Sore throat, toothache, swelling gums, oral ulcers, redness and swelling pain of the eyes	1 pill each time orally and twice or 3 times daily	3 g per pill
Liushen Wan	Calculus Bovis, Moschus, Borneolum, Venenum Bufonis, Margarita, Realgar	Clearing away heat and toxin, relieving swelling pain	Laryngopharyngitis, acute tonsillitis, sore throat and carbuncles and furuncles due to heat and toxin	Orally: Keep in the mouth till it dissolves fully; 3 - 5 pills for 3 - 10 year old and 5 -10 pills for adults and twice daily. Externally: Dissolve 10 pills in a little amount of boiled water or rice vinegar till it looks like paste and then place it on the affected part several times daily. It's contraindicated in pregnant women	0.3 g per 10 pills and 30 pills contained in one bottle
Pianzaihuang	Omitted	Clearing away heat and toxins, relieving swelling pain	Upward invasion of wind-fire manifested as redness and swelling pain of the eyes, gums and throat, tinnitus, otalgia; or hypochondriac pain and jaundice as seen in internal accumulation of dampness-heat	0.15-0.3 g for children between 1 and 8 years, and 0.6 g for children over it each time and adults; twice or 3 times daily	3 g per piece and 0.6 per bag

(**Following table**)

Name of the Recipe	Ingredients	Functions	Indications	Directions & Dosage	Specifications
Meihua Dianshe Dan	*Venenum Bufonis Praeparata*, *Calculus Bovis*, *Borneolum*, *Margarita*, *Fel Ursi*, *Resina Draconis*, *Olibanum*, *Resina Commiphoraee Myrrhae*, *Moschus*, *Lignum Aquilariae Resinatum*, *Borax*, *Realgar*, *Cinnabaris*, *Semen Lepiddii seu Descurainiae*, *Baimeihua*, *Concha Haliotidis*	Clearing away heat and toxins, promoting blood circulation, relieving swelling, promoting tissue regeneration and relieving pain	Initial stage of skin eruptions, or swelling pain of the throat and gums, or oral ulcers and various unknown swelling	Orally: First drink a mouthful of warm boiled water, put 3 pills on the tongue till it gets numb and then swallow them down with warm millet wine or warm boiled water. Externally: Place it on the affected part after dissolving it in vinegar	1 g per 10 pills
Jinyinhua Lu	*Flos Lonicerae*	Clearing away heat and toxin	Thirst due to summer-heat, sudamina and sores	60–120 g each time orally and twice or 3 times daily	30 g available composition contained in 500 g liquid.
Xianglian Wan	*Rhizoma Coptidis* (*prepared with Fructus Erodiae*), *Radix Aucklandiae*	Clearing away heat and dampness, promoting the flow of qi and removing stagnancy	Dysentery due to dampness-heat, abdominal pain, rectal tenesmus, stool with pus and blood	3–6 g each time orally and twice or 3 times daily	18 g per bag
Xiakucao Gao	*Spica Prunellae*	Purging liver-fire, resolving phlegm and removing mass	Upward invasion of liver-fire manifested as headache, conjunctival congestion, vertigo and tinnitus; or scrofula and goiter as seen in accumulation of phlegm-heat	15 g each time orally and twice daily	60 g per big bottle and 30 g per small one
Bingpeng San	*Borneolum*, *Borax*, *Natrii Sulfa Exsiccatus*, *Cinnabaris*	Clearing away heat and toxin, relieving swelling pain	Sore throat, swelling pain of gums, and oral ulcers	Externally: Take a proper amount of the powder and blow it into the affected part several times daily	3 g per bottle
Xilei San	*Indigo Naturalis*, *Calculus Bovis*, *Borneolum*, *Uroctea*, *Margarita*, *ivory bits*, *human nails*	Clearing away heat and toxins, promoting tissue regeneration	Erosion and swelling pain of the throat, mouth and tongue, and gums	Externally: Take a proper amount of the powder and blow it into the affected part several times daily	0.3 g per bottle

（二）清热泻火解毒类

方　名	组　成	功　用	主　治	用法与用量	规　格
牛黄清热散	牛黄,黄连,寒水石,玳瑁,冰片等。	清热解毒,熄风定惊。	高热不退,烦躁口渴,惊厥抽搐,甚则神昏谵语,舌红苔黄,脉滑数。	口服:每次 1.5 g,根据病情每日服2～4次。	每瓶装3 g。
牛黄上清丸	牛黄,黄连,黄芩,黄柏,栀子,大黄,石膏,连翘,菊花,薄荷,荆芥,白芷,川芎,当归,赤芍药,地黄,桔梗,甘草,冰片。	清热散风,泻火通便。	头痛眩晕,暴发火眼,口舌生疮,咽喉肿痛,牙龈肿痛。	口服:每次 1 丸,每日 2 次。	每丸重6 g。
牛黄解毒丸	牛黄,冰片,雄黄,桔梗,黄芩,甘草,大黄,生石膏。	清热解毒。	咽喉肿痛,牙痛龈肿,口舌生疮,目赤肿痛。	口服:每次 1 丸,每日 2～3 次。	每丸重3 g。
六 神 丸	牛黄,麝香,冰片,蟾酥,珍珠,雄黄。	清热解毒,消肿止痛。	咽喉炎,急性扁桃体炎,咽喉肿痛及热毒痈疮疖疔等。	含化:3～10 岁每次3～5 粒,成人每次5～10 粒,每日 2 次。外用:取 10 粒用开水或米醋少许溶成糊状,每日数次敷搽。孕妇忌服。	每瓶装30 粒,每10 粒重0.3 g。
片仔癀	略。	清热解毒,消肿止痛。	风火上攻,目赤肿痛,牙龈肿痛,耳鸣耳聋,咽喉红肿疼痛,或湿热内蕴,胁痛黄疸。	口服:1～8 岁儿童每次 0.15～0.3 g,8 岁以上及成人每次 0.6 g,每日 2～3 次。	每块重3 g,每包重0.6 g。
梅花点舌丹	制蟾酥,牛黄,冰片,珍珠,熊胆,血竭,乳香,没药,麝香,沉香,硼砂,雄黄,朱砂,葶苈子,白梅花,石决明。	清热解毒,活血消肿,生肌定痛。	疔疮痈肿初起,或咽喉牙龈肿痛,或口舌生疮,以及各种无名肿毒。	口服:每次 3 粒,先饮温开水一口,将药放在舌上,以口麻为度,再用温黄酒或温开水送下。外用:以醋化开,敷于患处。	每 10 粒重1 g。
金银花露	金银花。	清热解毒。	暑热口渴,痱子疮疖等。	口服:每次 60～120 g,每日 2～3 次。	每 500 g相当于金银花30 g。
香连丸	黄连(吴茱萸制),木香。	清热燥湿,行气化滞。	湿热痢疾,腹痛,里急后重,大便脓血。	口服:每次 3～6 g,每日 2～3 次。	每袋重18 g。

方　名	组　　成	功　用	主　治	用法与用量	规　格
夏枯草膏	夏枯草。	清泻肝火，化痰散结。	肝火上炎，头痛目赤，眩晕耳鸣；或痰火郁结，瘰疬、瘿瘤等。	口服：每次 15 g，每日 2 次。	大瓶装 60 g，小瓶装30 g。
冰硼散	冰片，硼砂，玄明粉，朱砂。	清热解毒，消肿止痛。	咽喉疼痛，牙龈肿痛，口舌生疮。	外用：取药粉适量，吹敷患处，每日数次。	每瓶装 3 g。
锡类散	青黛，牛黄，冰片，壁钱炭，珍珠，象牙屑，人指甲。	清热解毒，化腐生新。	咽喉、口舌、牙龈糜烂肿痛。	外用：取药粉适量，吹敷患处，每日数次。	每瓶装 0.3 g。

Chart Three Medicines for Purgation，Relaxing Bowels and Removing Stagnancy

Name of the Recipe	Ingredients	Functions	Indications	Directions & Dosage	Specifications
Qingning Wan	Radix et Rhizoma Rhei, Semen Phaseoli Radiatus, Herba Plantaginis, Rhizoma Atractylodis Macrocephalae, Rhizoma Pinelliae, Semen Sojae, Rhizoma Cyperi, Ramulus Mori, Ramulus Sophorae, Cortex Magnoliae Officinalis, Fructus Hordei Germinatus Pericarpium Citri Reticulatae, Radix Scutellariae	Clearing away heat and purging fire, loosening bowels to relieve constipation	Accumulated heat in zang-fu organs manifested as sore throat, oral ulcers, conjunctival congestion and pain, abdominal fullness and constipation	1 pill each time orally and twice daily	9 g per pill
Jiuzhi Dahuang Wan	Radix et Rhizoma Rhei	Relieving constipation and eliminating dryness, promoting digestion and removing stagnancy	Stagnancy in stomach and intestines manifested as constipation, or dysentery due to dampness-heat, vexation, thirst and yellowish urine	6 g each time daily	6 g per bag
Gengyi Wan	Aloe, Cinnabaris	Purging fire to relieve constipation	Hyperactivity of fire in the heart and liver as well as heat accumulation in intestines and stomach manifested as constipation, vexation and irritability, restless sleep at night, bitter mouth and conjunctival congestion	3 g each time orally and once or twice daily	3 g per 25 pills

(Following table)

Name of the Recipe	Ingredients	Functions	Indications	Directions & Dosage	Specif- ications
Banliu Wan	*Rhizoma Pinelliae，Sulfur*	Warming the kidney and dispelling cold, activating yang and purging turbid substances	Deficiency of kidney-yang and excess of yin due to old age manifested as dyschesia, distending sensation or pain in abdomen, pale complexion, and cold extremities	1. 5 – 3 g each time orally and once or twice daily	1 g per 15 pills
Maren Runchang Wan	*Fructus Cannabis，Radix et Rhizoma Rhei，Pericarpium Citri Reticulatae，Radix Aucklandiae，Semen Armeniacae Amarum，Radix Paeoniae Alba*	Loosening the bowels and purging heat, promoting the flow of qi and relieving constipation	Dryness-heat in the intestines and stomach manifested as constipation, abdominal fullness, dry mouth and reddened tongue	1 pill each time orally and 3 times daily	6 g per pill
Wuren Runchang Wan	*Semen Perisicae，Fructus Cannabis，Semen Pruni，Semen Biotae，Semen Pini Koraiensis，Radix Rehmanniae，Pericarpium Citri Reticulatae，Radix et Rhizoma Rhei，Radix Angelicae Sinensis，Herba Cistanchis*	Nourishing yin and blood, loosening the bowels to relieve constipation	Deficiency of yin and fluid as well as constipation as the result of old age, weak constitution, long course of illness, delivery or operation	1 pill each time orally and twice daily	9 g per pill
Fangfeng Tongsheng Wan	*Radix Ledebouriellae，Herba Schizonepetae，Fructus Forsythiae，Herba Ephedrae，Herba Menthae，Rhizoma Ligustici Chuanxiong，Radix Angelicae sinensis Radix Paeoniae Alba，Fructus Gardeniae，Radix et Rhizoma Rhei（prepared with wine），Natrii Sulfas，Gypsum Fibrosum，Radix Scutellariae，Radix Platycodi，Radix Glycyrrhizae，Talcum，Rhizoma Atractylodis Macrocephalae*	Relieving superficial symptoms by dispelling wind, purging heat to relax the bowels	Excess syndrome of both the interior and exterior due to attack by wind and internal accumulation of heat manifested as aversion to cold, high fever, headache, dry throat, constipation, dark yellowish urine, initial stage of carbuncles and furuncles, eczema and pruritus	6 g each time orally and once or twice daily	18 g per bag

（三）泻下通便逐邪类

方　名	组　成	功　用	主　治	用法与用量	规　格
清宁丸	大黄,绿豆,车前草,白术,法半夏,黑豆,香附,桑枝,槐枝,厚朴,大麦,陈皮,黄芩。	清热泻火,润肠通便。	脏腑积热,咽喉肿痛,口舌生疮,目赤肿痛,腹胀便秘。	口服:每次1丸,每日2次。	每丸重9g。
九制大黄丸	大黄。	通便润燥,消食化滞。	胃肠积滞,大便秘结,或湿热下痢,心胸烦热,口渴尿黄。	口服:每次6g,每日1次。	每袋重6g。
更衣丸	芦荟,朱砂。	泻火通便。	心肝火盛,肠胃热结,大便不通,心烦易怒,夜寐不安,口苦目赤。	口服:每次3g,每日1～2次。	每25粒重3g。
半硫丸	半夏,硫黄。	温肾逐寒,通阳泄浊。	老人肾阳不足,阴气凝结,大便艰涩,腹中气攻或疼痛,面色无华,四肢不温。	口服:每次1.5～3g,每日1～2次。	每15粒重1g。
麻仁润肠丸	火麻仁,大黄,陈皮,木香,杏仁,白芍药。	润肠泄热,行气通便。	肠胃燥热,大便干结,脘腹胀满,口干舌红。	口服:每次1丸,每日3次。	每丸重6g。
五仁润肠丸	桃仁,火麻仁,郁李仁,柏子仁,松子仁,生地黄,陈皮,大黄,当归,肉苁蓉。	滋阴养血,润肠通便。	年老体弱,久病、产后、术后阴虚津枯,大便干燥。	口服:每次1丸,每日2次。	每丸重9g。
防风通圣丸	防风,荆芥,连翘,麻黄,薄荷,川芎,当归,白芍药,栀子,酒制大黄,芒硝,石膏,黄芩,桔梗,甘草,滑石,白术。	疏风解表,泻热通便。	外感风邪,内有蕴热,表里俱实。恶寒壮热,头痛咽干,大便秘结,小便黄赤,疮疡初起,湿疹瘙痒。	口服:每次6g,每日1～2次。	每袋重18g。

Chart Four　Medicines for Nourishing, Building up Body Resistance and Preserving Life

Name of the Recipe	Ingredients	Functions	Indications	Directions & Dosage	Specifications
Renshen Yangrong Wan	*Radix Ginseng, Rhizoma Atractylodis Macrocephalae, Poria, Radix Glycyrrhizae Praeparata, Radix Angelicae Sinensis, Radix*	Replenishing qi and enriching blood, tranquilizing mind	Deficiency of the heart and spleen as well as qi and blood manifested as slim physique, mental	1 pill each time orally and once or twice daily	9 g per pill

Name of the Recipe	Ingredients	Functions	Indications	Directions & Dosage	Specifications
	Rehmanniae Praeparata, Radix Paeoniae Alba, Radix Astragali seu Hedysari, Pericarpium Citri Reticulatae, Radix Polygalae, Cortex Cinnamomi, Fructus Schisandrae		fatigue, poor appetite, loose stool, palpitation, amnesia, spontaneous perspiration, short breath, dry throat and lips, and weak constitution after illness		
Shenqi Gao	Radix Codonopsis Pilosulae, Radix Astragali seu Hedysari, crystal sugar	Invigorating the spleen and replenishing qi, lifting yang and strengthening body resistance	Qi deficiency of the spleen and stomach manifested as lassitude, mental fatigue, unwillingness to speak, spontaneous perspiration with aversion to wind, loose stool, or fever, aggravated by strain	15 g each time orally and 3 times daily	200 g per bottle
Yiqi Congming Wan	Rhizoma Cimicifugae, Radix Puerariae, Cortex Phellodendri, Radix Paeoniae Alba, Fructus Viticis, Radix Codonopsis Pilosulae, Radix astragali seu Hedysari, Radix Glycyrrhizae Praeparata	Replenishing qi and lifting yang, improving hearing and eyesight	Qi deficiency of the spleen and stomah and failure of lucid yang in lifting manifested as blurring of vision, vertigo, tinnitus, insomnia, amnesia, lassitude	6 g each time orally and twice or 3 time daily.	1 g per 12 pills
Shihu Yeguang Wan	Herba Dendrobii, Radix Asparagi, Radix Ginseng, Poria, Radix Ophiopogonis, Radix Rehmanniae Praeparata, Radix Rehmanniae Recens, Semen Cuscutae, Flos Chrysanthemi, Semen Cassiae, Semen Armeniacae Amarum, Rhizoma Dioscoreae, Fructus Lycii, Radix Achyranthis Bidentatae, Fructus Schisandrae, Fructus Tribuli, Herba Cistanchis, Rhizoma Ligustici Chuanxiong, Radix Glycyrrhizae Praeparata, Fructus Aurantii, Semen Celosiae, Radix Ledebouriellae, Rhizoma Coptidis, Cornu Bubali, Cornu Antelopis	Subduing liver-wind, nourishing yin and improving acuity of vision	Deficiency of the liver and kidney and hyperactivity of fire due to yin deficiency manifested as catarct, dim eyesight, blurring of vision	1 pill each time orally in the morning and evening	9 g per pill

(**Following table**)

Name of the Recipe	Ingredients	Functions	Indications	Directions & Dosage	Specifications
Erzhi Wan	*Fructus Ligustri Lucidi*, *Herba Ecliptae*	Reinforcing the liver and kidney, nourishing yin and blood	Yin deficiency of the liver and kidney manifested as vertigo, insomnia, dreaminess, flaccid lower limbs, white beard and hair at an earlier age	1 pill each time orally twice daily	15 g per pill
Sangma Wan	*Folium Mori*, *black sesame*	Reinforcing the liver and kidney, dispelling wind and improving acuity of vision	Deficiency of the liver and kidney manifested as vertigo, blurred vision, epiphora induced by wind	6 g each time orally and 3 times daily	1 g per 20 pills
Huanshao Wan	*Rhizoma Dioscoreae*, *Radix Polygalae*, *Rhizoma Acori Tatarinowii*, *Radix Morindae Officinalis*, *Herba Cistanchis*, *Fructus Lycii*, *Radix Rehmanniae Praeparata*, *Radix Achyranthis Bidentatae*, *Fructus Corni*, *Cortex Eucommiae*, *Poria*, *Fructus Broussonetiae*, *Fructus Schisandrae*, *Fructus Ziziphi Jujubae*	Reinforcing the kidney and spleen, strengthening yang and essence	Deficiency of the spleen and kidney manifested as slim physique and weak constitution, soreness of waist and knees, vertigo and tinnitus, sexual impotence, emission, amnesia and severe palpitation	9 g each time orally taken with light salty water and twice daily	9 g per pill
Banlong Wan	*Cornu Cervi Degelatinatum*, *Colla Cornus Cervi*, *Semen Cuscutae*, *Radix Rehmanniae Praeparata*, *Poria*, *Fructus Psoraleae*, *Semen Biotae*	Reinforcing the kidney, enriching essence and strengthening yang	Deficiency of kidney essence manifested as soreness of waist and knees, sexual impotence, prospermia, dizziness, tinnitus, thin leukorrhea, frequent urination at night	1 pill each time orally taken with light salty water and twice daily	9 g per pill
Heche Dazao Wan	*Placenta Hominis*, *Radix Rehmanniae Praeparata*, *Radix Asparagi*, *Radix Ophiopogonis*, *Cortex Eucommiae*, *Radix Achyranthis Bidentatae*, *Cortex Phellodendri*, *Plastrum Testudinis*	Reinforcing the lung and kidney, nourishing yin and Clearing away heat	Yin deficiency of the lung and kidney manifested as hectic fever, cough, night sweat, emission, weakness of waist and knees	6 g each time orally for, hydro-honeyed bolus, 9 g for small honeyed pills and 1 for large ones; twice daily	9 g per large honeyed pill

(Following table)

Name of the Recipe	Ingredients	Functions	Indications	Directions & Dosage	Specifications
Quanlu Wan	Fresh deer meat, Colla Cornus Cervi, Cornu Cervi Pantotrichum, deer kidney, deer tail, Radix Ginseng, Radix Astragali seu Hedysari, Rhizoma Atractylodis Macrocephalae (parched), Poria, Radix Glycyrrhizae, Rhizoma Dioscoreae, Radix Rehmanniae Praeparata, Radix Rehmanniae, Radix Angelicae Sinensis, Rhizoma Ligustici Chuanxiong, Fructus Lycii, Semen Cuscutae, Fructus Broussonetiae, Fructus Rubi, Semen Trigonellae, Cortex Eucommiae, Radix Dipsaci, Radix Achyranthis Bidentatae, Fructus Psoraleae, Radix Morindae Officinalis, Herba Cistanchis, Herba Cynomorii, Halitum, Qiushi (made from human urine sediment and salt), Radix Asparagi, Radix Ophiopogonis, Fructus Foeniculi, Pericarpium Zanthoxyli, Lignum Aquilariae Resinatum, Pericarpium Citri Reticulatae, Semen Euryales, Fructus Schisandrae	Strengthening yang and nourishing yin, replenishing qi and enriching blood	Deficiency of yin and yang manifested as weak constitution, dizziness, tinnitus, nocturnal emission, spermatorrhea, soreness of waist and knees, poor appetite, lassitude, spontaneous perspiration, night sweating, metrorrhagia and metrostaxis, leukorrhagia, etc.	1 pill each time orally and twice daily	9 g per pill
Shenrong Wan	Radix Ginseng, Cornu Cervi Pantotrichum, Radix Rehmanniae Praeparata, Radix Morindae Officinalis, Radix Salviae Miltiorrhizae, Radix Codonopsis Pilosulae, Fructus Lycii, Herba Cistanchis, Fructus Mediae Toosendan (Fructus Meliae Toosendan, Semen Euryales, Arillus Longan, Radix Polygalae, Rhizoma Dioscoreae, etc	Replenishing qi and strengthening yang, enriching blood and essence	Deficiency of both yin and yang manifested as mental fatigue, short breath, tinnitus, palpitation, emission, prospermia, soreness of waist and weakness of legs, metrorrhagia and metrostaxis, leukorrhagia	1 pill each time orally and twice daily	9 g per pill

(**Following table**)

Name of the Recipe	Ingredients	Functions	Indications	Directions & Dosage	Specifications
Guiling Ji	*Cornu Cervi Pantotrichum, Radix Ginseng, Radix Rehmanniae Recens, Radix Rehmanniae Praeparata, Hippocampus, Cortex Eucommiae, Herba Cistanchis, Herba Cynomorii, Fructus Psoraleae, Semen Cuscutae, Fructus Lycii, Radix Asparagi, Radix Aconiti Lateralis Praeparata, sparrow brains Maquemao, silk moth, dragonfly, Flos Syzygii Aromatici, Radix Glycyrrhizae, Herba Epimedii, Halitum, Herba Asari, Fossilia Spiriferis, Fructus Amomi, Semen Impatientis, Squama Manitis, Cortex Lycii Radicis, Cinnabaris, Radix Achyranthis Bidentatae, etc*	Reinforcing the kidney and strengthening yang	Insufficient kidney-yang manifested as sexual impotence, emission, short breath, dyspnea, cough, cold sensation in waist and knees, contracture of the lower abdomen, dizziness, tinnitus, poor memory, metrorrhagia and metrostaxis, leukorrhagia with pus and blood, morning diarrhea	0.3 g each time orally and once daily	3 g per bottle
Jingang Wan	*Herba Cistanchis, Cortex Eucommiae, Semen Cuscutae, Rhizoma Dioscoreae Hypoglaucae, pig kidney*	Reinforcing kidney and replenishing essence, strengthening muscles and tendons	Deficiency of the liver and kidney, malnutrition in channels and collaterals manifested as flaccid muscles and tendons in flaccidity syndrome, or soreness and weakness of waist and legs in arthralgia syndrome, or sexual impotence, prospermia and soreness of waist and knees	1 pill each time orally and twice daily	9 g per pill
Wubi Shanyao Wan	*Rhizoma Dioscoreae, Radix Rehmanniae, Halloysitum Rubrum, Radix Morindae Officinalis, Poria, Radix Achyranthis Bidentatae, Fructus Corni, Rhizoma Alismatis, Fructus Schisandrae, Herba Cistanchis, Semen Cuscutae, Cortex Eucommiae*	Enriching essence and reinforcing the kidney, nourishing yin and yang moderately	Weakness of the kidney manifested as soreness of waist and legs, emission, frequent urination, vertigo, dizziness, slim physique, poor appetite	1 pill each time orally taken with warmed wine or thin rice gruel before meals; twice daily	9 g per pill

（**Following table**）

Name of the Recipe	Ingredients	Functions	Indications	Directions & Dosage	Specifications
Wuzi Yanzong Wan	*Fructus Lycii*, *Fructus Rubi*, *Fructus Schisandrae*, *Semen Plantaginis*, *Semen Cuscutae*	Reinforcing the kidney and enriching essence	Soreness of waist due to deficiency of kidney, dribbling urination	6 g each time orally for hydro- honeyed bolus, 9 g for small honeyed pills and 1 pill for large ones; twice daily	1 g every 10 g hydro-honeyed bolus, every 5 small honeyed pills and 9 g per large one
Wuji Baifeng Wan	*Pullus cum Osse Nigro*, *Radix Ginseng*, *Colla Cornus Cervi*, *Concha Ostreae*, *Radix Paeoniae Alba*, *Radix Angelicae Sinensis*, *Radix Astragali seu Hedysari*, *Carapax Trionycis*, *Ootheca Mantidis*, *Radix Rehmanniae Recens*, *Radix Rehmanniae Praeparata*, *Rhizoma ligustici Chuanxiong*, *Radix Glycyrrhizae*, *Radix Salviae Miltiorrhizae*, *Semen Euryales*, *Rhizoma Dioscoreae*, *Radix Stellariae*, *Cornu Cervi Degelatinatum*, *Radix Asparagi*, *Rhizoma Cyperi*	Replenishing qi and enriching blood, regulating menstruation and leukorrhea	Insufficient qi and blood manifested as slim physique, soreness of the waist and knees, irregular menstruation, metrorrhagia and metrostaxis, leukorrhagia	1 pill each time orally and twice daily	9 g per pill
Erlong Zuoci Wan	*Magnetitum* (calcined), *Radix Rehmanniae Praeparatae*, *Fructus Corni*, *Rhizoma Dioscoreae*, *Poria*, *Rhizoma Alismatis*, *Cortex Moutan Radicis*, *bamboo leaves*, *Radix Bupleuri*	Reinforcing the kidney and subduing liver-wind	Yin deficiency of the liver and kidney manifested as tinnitus, deafness, and vertigo	6 g each time orally for hydro- honeyed bolus, 9 g for small honeyed pills and 1 pill for large ones; twice daily	9 g per large honeyed pill

（四）滋补强身延年类

方　名	组　成	功　用	主　治	用法与用量	规　格
人参养荣丸	人参，白术，茯苓，炙甘草，当归，熟地黄，白芍药，炙黄芪，陈皮，远志，肉桂，五味子。	温补气血，养心安神。	心脾不足，气血两虚，形瘦神疲，食少便溏，惊悸健忘，自汗短气，咽干唇燥及病后体弱。	口服：每次1丸，每日1～2次。	每丸重9g。

续表

方　名	组　成	功　用	主　治	用法与用量	规　格
参芪膏	党参,黄芪,冰糖。	补中益气,升阳固表。	脾胃气虚,倦怠乏力,神疲懒言,自汗恶风,大便溏泻,或发热,劳则加重。	口服:每次15 g,每日3次。	每瓶重200 g。
益气聪明丸	升麻,葛根,黄柏,白芍药,蔓荆子,党参,黄芪,炙甘草。	益气升阳,聪耳明目。	脾胃气虚,清阳不升,视物昏花,眩晕耳鸣,失眠健忘,怠惰乏力。	口服:每次6 g,每日2~3次。	每12粒重1 g。
石斛夜光丸	石斛,天冬,人参,茯苓,麦门冬,熟地黄,生地黄,菟丝子,菊花,决明子,杏仁,山药,枸杞子,牛膝,五味子,白蒺藜,肉苁蓉,川芎,炙甘草,枳壳,青葙子,防风,黄连,水牛角,羚羊角。	平肝熄风,滋阴明目。	肝肾两亏,阴虚火旺,内障目暗,视物昏花。	口服:每次1丸,早晚各1次。	每丸重9 g。
二至丸	女贞子,旱莲草。	补肝肾,养阴血。	肝肾阴虚,头目眩晕,失眠多梦,下肢痿软,须发早白。	口服:每次1丸,每日2次。	每丸重15 g。
桑麻丸	桑叶,黑芝麻。	滋养肝肾,祛风明目。	肝肾不足,头晕眼花,迎风流泪。	口服:每次6 g,每日3次。	每20粒重1 g。
还少丸	山药,远志,石菖蒲,巴戟天,肉苁蓉,枸杞子,熟地黄,怀牛膝,山茱萸,杜仲炭,茯苓,楮实子,五味子,红枣。	益肾补脾,壮阳固精。	脾肾两虚,形瘦体弱,腰膝酸软,头晕耳鸣,阳痿遗精,健忘征忡等。	口服:每次9 g,淡盐水送下,每日2次。	每丸重9 g。
斑龙丸	鹿角霜,鹿角胶,菟丝子,熟地黄,茯苓,补骨脂,柏子仁。	补肾填精壮阳。	肾虚精亏,腰膝酸软,阳痿早泄,头晕耳鸣,带下清稀,夜尿频多。	口服:每次1丸,淡盐水送下,每日2次。	每丸重9 g。
河车大造丸	紫河车,熟地黄,天门冬,麦门冬,杜仲,牛膝,黄柏,龟版。	补肺益肾,滋阴清热。	肺肾阴虚,潮热咳嗽,盗汗遗精,腰膝无力。	口服:水蜜丸每次6 g,小蜜丸每次9 g,大蜜丸每次1丸,每日2次。	大蜜丸每丸重9 g。

方　名	组　成	功　用	主　治	用法与用量	规　格
全鹿丸	鲜鹿肉,鹿角胶,鹿茸,鹿肾,鹿尾,人参,黄芪,炒白术,茯苓,甘草,山药,熟地黄,干地黄,当归,川芎,枸杞子,菟丝子,楮实子,覆盆子,胡芦巴,杜仲,续断,牛膝,补骨脂,巴戟天,肉苁蓉,锁阳,大青盐,秋石,天门冬,麦门冬,小茴香,花椒,沉香,陈皮,芡实,五味子。	壮阳益阴,补气养血。	阴阳两虚,身体虚弱,头晕耳鸣,梦遗滑精,腰膝酸痛,食少乏力,自汗盗汗,妇女崩漏带下等。	口服:每次1丸,每日2次。	每丸重9g。
参茸丸	人参,鹿茸,熟地,巴戟天,丹参,党参,枸杞子,肉苁蓉,莲子,芡实,龙眼肉,远志,山药等。	补气壮阳,养血生精。	阴阳两虚,神疲气短,耳鸣,心悸,遗精早泄,腰酸腿软,妇女崩漏带下。	口服:每次1丸,每日2次。	每丸重9g。
龟龄集	鹿茸,人参,生地黄,熟地黄,海马,杜仲炭,肉苁蓉,锁阳,补骨脂,菟丝子,枸杞子,天门冬,黑附子,麻雀脑,蚕蛾,蜻蜓,丁香,甘草,淫羊藿,大青盐,细辛,石燕,砂仁,急性子,穿山甲,地骨皮,朱砂,牛膝等。	补肾壮阳。	肾阳虚弱,阳痿遗精,气短喘嗽,腰膝冷痛,小腹拘急,头晕耳鸣,记忆减退,妇女崩漏,带下赤白,五更泄泻。	口服:每次0.3g,每日1次。	每瓶装3g。
金刚丸	肉苁蓉,杜仲,菟丝子,草薢,猪肾。	补肾益精,强壮筋骨。	肝肾亏虚,经脉失养,痿证筋骨痿软,或痹证腰腿酸痛无力,或阳痿、早泄,腰膝酸软等。	口服:每次1丸,每日2次。	每丸重9g。
无比山药丸	山药,干地黄,赤石脂,巴戟天,茯苓,牛膝,山茱萸,泽泻,五味子,肉苁蓉,菟丝子,杜仲。	填精固肾,平补阴阳。	肾虚腰痛腿软,遗精尿多,头晕目眩,形瘦纳差。	口服:每次1丸,食前以温酒或米汤送下,每日2次。	每丸重9g。
五子衍宗丸	枸杞子,覆盆子,五味子,车前子,菟丝子。	补肾益精。	肾亏腰疼,溺后余沥。	口服:水蜜丸每次6g;小蜜丸每次9g;大蜜丸每次1丸,均日服2次。	水蜜丸每10粒重1g;小蜜丸每5粒重1g;大蜜丸每丸重9g。

方 名	组 成	功 用	主 治	用法与用量	规 格
乌鸡白凤丸	乌鸡,人参,鹿角胶,牡蛎,白芍药,当归,黄芪,鳖甲,桑螵蛸,生地黄,熟地黄,川芎,甘草,丹参,芡实,山药,银柴胡,鹿角霜,天冬,香附。	补气养血,调经止带。	气血亏损而致身体瘦弱,腰膝酸痛,月经不调,崩漏带下。	口服:每次1丸,每日2次。	每 丸 重 9 g。
耳聋左慈丸	煅磁石,熟地黄,山茱萸,山药,茯苓,泽泻,牡丹皮,竹叶,柴胡。	滋肾平肝。	肝肾阴虚,耳鸣耳聋,头晕目眩。	口服:水蜜丸每次6 g,小蜜丸每次9 g,大蜜丸每次1丸,每日2次。	大蜜丸,每 丸 重 9 g。

Chart Five　Medicines for Tranquilization and Resuscitation

Name of the Recipe	Ingredients	Functions	Indications	Directions & Dosage	Specifications
Zhenzhong Wan	*Plastrum Testudinis*, *Os Draconis*, *Rhizoma Acori Tatarinowii*, *Radix Polygalae*	Reinforcing the kidney and tranquilizing mind	Deficiency of the heart and kidney manifested as palpitation, amnesia, insomnia, dreaminess, dizziness, tinnitus, soreness of the waist and knees, nocturnal emission	1 pill each time orally and twice or 3 times daily	9 g per pill
Jiaotai Wan	*Rhizoma Coptidis*, *Cortex Cinnamomi*	Restoring the coordination between the heart and kidney, and tranquilizing mind	Breakdown of the normal physiological coordination between the heart and kidney manifested as vexation, insomnia, palpitation, amnesia, dysphoria with feverish sensation in chest, palms and soles, soreness of the waist, loose stool, frequent urination or enuresis, emission	2 - 3 g each time orally taken half hour before going to bed	30 g every 500 pills

Name of the Recipe	Ingredients	Functions	Indications	Directions & Dosage	Specifications
Zhenheling Pian	*Margarita Powder, Ganoderma Lucidum seu Japonicum, Radix Glycyrrhizae*	Exerting a tonic effect on the heart and tranquilizing mind, subduing the liver-wind and Clearing away heat	Hyperactivity of liver-yang due to insufficient heart-yin manifested as palpitation, short breath, dreaminess, amnesia, dizziness, lassitude, tinnitus, taut, thready and rapid pulse	3 - 4 tablets each time orally and 3 times daily	0.35 g per tablet
Qingkailing Zhusheye	*Cholic acid, Cornu Bubali, baicalin, Margarita cengfen, Fructus Gardeniae, Radix Isatidis, extract of Flos Lonicerae, etc.*	Clearing away heat and inducing resuscitation, relieving convulsion and tranquilizing mind	Heat retaining in the heart meridian manifested as high fever, flushed face, coma and delirium, or macular eruptions, tic of limbs, reddened tongue, slippery and rapid pulse	IM: 1 - 2 vials each time and twice or 3 times daily. IV: 1 - 2 vials with 500 ml 5% glucose injection added to it	2 ml per vial
Niuhuang Qingxin Wan	*Calculus Bovis, Cornu Rhinoceri, Cornu Antelopis, Radix Scutellariae, Radix Ampelopsis, Radix Platycodi, Semen Armeniaccae Amarum, Cortex Cinnamomi, Pollen Typhae, Radix Bupleuri, Radix Ledebouriellae, Radix Ginseng, Poria, Rhizoma Atractylodis Macrocephalae, Radix Glycyrrhizae, Rhizoma Zingiberis, Fructus Ziziphi Jujubae, Rhizoma Dioscoreae, Radix Angelicae Sinensis, Radix Paeoniae Alba, Rhizoma Ligustici Chuanxiong, Radix Ophiopogonis, Colla Corii Asini, Massa Dermentata Medicinalis, Semen Sojae Germinatum, Moschus, Realgar, Borneolum, Cinnabaris*	Clearing away heat from the heart to restore consciousness, removing phlegm and obstruction in meridians, replenishing qi and enriching blood	Deficiency of qi and blood, stagnation of phlegm-heat manifested either as hemiparalysis, alternating consciousness and unconsciousness, rale, dysphasia, or as vertigo, vexation, irritability, numbness of the extremities, or as palpitation, restlessness, insomnia and dreaminess	One pill each time orally and 2 pills in severe case; twice daily. Those with rale may take it with the decoction of Succus Bambosae	3 g per pill

(Following table)

Name of the Recipe	Ingredients	Functions	Indications	Directions & Dosage	Specifications
Niuhuang Baolong Wan	Calculus Bovis, Concretio Silicea Bambusae, Arisaema cum Bile, Scorpio, Bombyx Batryticatus, Cinnabaris, Succinum, Realgar, Moschus, Poria	Clearing away heat and relieving convulsion, removing phlegm and subduing wind	Infantile convulsion due to phlegm-heat manifested as high fever, coma, flushed face, excessive phlegm and saliva, short breath, clonic convulsion and trismus	1 pill each time orally and twice or 3 times daily taken with the decoction of Herba Menthae or warm boiled water; reduce the dosage appropriately for children below 12 months	1.5 g per pill
Houzao San	Calculus Macacae, Calculus Bovis, Moschus, Margarita, Succinum, etc	Removing phlegm, relieving convulsion and inducing resuscitation	Excessive phlegm and saliva in children manifested as cough and asthma, infantile convulsion with fever	Half bottle for children under one year and one bottle for those over; taken after dissolved in hot boiled water	0.3 g per bottle
Shixiang Fansheng Dan	Lignum Aquilariae Resinatum, Bombyx Batryticatus, Flos Syzygii Aromatici, Radix Curcumae, Lignum Santali, Plumula Nelumbinis, Radix Aristolochiae, Semen Trichosanthis, Lapis Micae Aureus, Fructus Chebulae, Rhizoma Cyperi, Herba Agastachis, Lignum Dalbergiae Odoriferae, Olibanum, Rhizoma Gastrodiae, Radix Glycyrrhizae, Succinum, Calculus Bovis, Borneolum, Cinnabaris, Resina Liquidambaris Orientalis, Benzomum, Moschus, etc.	Warming the channels and inducing resuscitation, removing phlegm and relieving convulsion	Obstruction of the heart channel by phlegm manifested as coma, unconsciousness, trismus, cold extremities, excessive sputum or saliva, dark complexion	1 pill each time orally and once or twice daily	6 g per pill
Guanxin Suhe Wan	Resina Liquidambaris Orientalis, Borneolum, Lignum Santali, Radix Aristolochiae, Olibanum, Cinnabaris	Warming the channels and inducing resuscitation, regulating the circulation of qi and blood to relieve pain	Angina pectoris of coronary heart disease with sudden chest pain, spontaneous perspiration of cold sweat, cold extremities, whitish fur and slow pulse	1 pill each time orally and 3 times daily	0.9 g per pill

(Following table)

Name of the Recipe	Ingredients	Functions	Indications	Directions & Dosage	Specifications
Subingdi Wan	*Styrax-zhi*, *Borneolum*, etc.	Acitivating yang, inducing resuscitation and relieving pain	Obstruction of chest-yang and heart channel manifested as chest distress and pain, palpitation and severe palpitation	2 - 4 pills each time orally and 3 times daily, kept in the mouth or swallowed down	100 pills in one bottle
Shayao	*Venenum Bufonis*, *Realgar*, *Cinnabaris*, *Moschus*, *Borneolum*, *Radix et Rhizoma Rhei*, *Herba Ephedrae*, *Flos Syzygii Aromatici*, *Rhizoma Atractylodis*, *Rhizoma Gastrodiae*, *Radix Glycyrrhizae*	Inducing resuscitation, removing turbid substances, eliminating summer-heat and toxin	Attack by summer-heat and turbid factors in summer time manifested as abdominal pain, vomiting, diarrhea, trismus, coldness of extremities, even faint	Orally: 0.75 g each time kept in the mouth for a while before swallow down. Externally: Grind into fine powder and blow a proper amount of the powder into the nose to have the patient sneeze; or dissolve it in vinegar and apply it over the furuncles and bites by insects	1 g every 33 pills; 3 g per pack and 1 g per bottle
Baijin Wan	*Radix Curcumae*, *Alumen*	Removing phlegm to induce resuscitation	Excessive phlegm and obstruction of heart channel manifested as mania, restlessness, or epilepsy and coma	1.5 g each time orally and twice daily	3 g every 40 pills
Zhuli Datan Wan	*Radix et Rhizoma Rhei*, *Radix Scutellariae*, *Pericarpium Citri Reticulatae*, *Lapis Chloriti* (*calcined with Yanxiao*), *Lignum Aquilariae Resinatum*, *Rhizoma Pinelliae*, *Succus Bambosae*	Purging heat and fire, removing phlegm and obstruction	Obstruction of heart channel due to intense heat and thick sputum manifested as mania, epilepsy induced by terror, cough, asthma with much sputum, fullness in chest, constipation, greasy yellowish fur, slippery and rapid pulse	6 g each time orally and twice daily	18 g per bag

(五) 宁心安神开窍类

方 名	组 成	功 用	主 治	用法与用量	规 格
枕 中 丸	龟版,龙骨,石菖蒲,远志。	补肾宁心,益智安神。	心肾不足,心悸健忘,失眠多梦,头晕耳鸣,腰膝酸软,梦寐遗精。	口服:每次 1 丸,每日 2~3 次。	每 丸 重 9 g。
交 泰 丸	黄连,肉桂。	交通心肾,宁心安神。	心肾不交,水火失济,心烦失眠,心悸健忘,五心烦热,腰酸便溏,尿频或遗溺、遗精。	口服:每次 2~3 g,临睡前半小时服。	每 500 粒重 30 g。
珍合灵片	珍珠层粉,灵芝,甘草。	补心安神,平肝清热。	心阴不足,肝阳偏亢,心悸气短,多梦健忘,头晕乏力,耳鸣,脉弦细数。	口服:每次 3~4 片,每日 3 次。	每 片 重 0.35 g。
清开灵注射液	胆酸,水牛角,黄芩甙,珍珠层粉,栀子,板蓝根,金银花提取物等。	清热开窍,镇惊安神。	热陷心包,高热面赤,神昏谵语,或发斑疹,四肢抽搐,舌质红绛,脉滑数。	肌肉注射:每次 1~2 支,每日 2~3次。静脉注射:1~2 支加入 5% 葡萄糖注射液 500 ml 中静脉滴注。	每支 2 ml。
牛黄清心丸	牛黄,犀角,羚羊角,黄芩,白蔹,桔梗,杏仁,肉桂,蒲黄,柴胡,防风,人参,茯苓,白术,甘草,干姜,红枣,山药,当归,白芍药,川芎,麦门冬,阿胶,神曲,大豆卷,麝香,雄黄,冰片,朱砂。	清心开窍,豁痰通络,益气养血。	气血不足,痰热闭阻,或半身不遂,神志时清时昧,喉中痰鸣,言语不利,或头晕目眩,心烦易怒,手足麻木;或心悸烦躁,失眠多梦。	口服:每次 1 丸,重者 2 丸,每日 2 次。喉中痰鸣者,可用竹沥水送下。	每 丸 重 3 g。
牛黄抱龙丸	牛黄,天竺黄,胆星,全蝎,僵蚕,朱砂,琥珀,雄黄,麝香,茯苓。	清热镇惊,涤痰熄风。	小儿痰热惊风,高热神昏,面色红赤,痰涎壅盛,呼吸气促,抽搐痉厥,牙关紧闭。	口服:每次 1 丸,每日 2~3 次,薄荷煎汤或温开水送服。周岁以内酌减。	每 丸 重 1.5 g。
猴 枣 散	猴枣,牛黄,麝香,珍珠,琥珀等。	除痰镇惊通窍。	小儿痰涎壅盛,咳嗽气喘,惊风发热。	1 岁以下,每服半瓶,1 岁以上,每服 1 瓶,滚开水调服。	每 瓶 装 0.3 g。

方　名	组　成	功　用	主　治	用法与用量	规　格
十香返生丹	沉香,僵蚕,丁香,郁金,檀香,莲子心,青木香,瓜蒌仁,青礞石,诃子,香附,藿香,降香,乳香,天麻,甘草,琥珀粉,牛黄,冰片,朱砂粉,苏合香,安息香,麝香等。	温通开窍,豁痰定惊。	痰浊蒙蔽心窍,神志昏迷,不省人事,牙关紧闭,四肢不温,痰涎壅盛,面色灰滞。	口服:每次1丸,每日1~2次。	每丸重6 g。
冠心苏合丸	苏合香,冰片,檀香,青木香,乳香,朱砂。	温通开窍,理气活血止痛。	冠心病心绞痛,突然胸痛,冷汗自出,四肢厥逆,苔白脉迟。	口服:每次1粒,每日3次。	每丸重0.9 g。
苏冰滴丸	苏合香酯,冰片等。	通阳宣窍止痛。	胸阳闭阻,心脉不通,胸闷胸痛,心悸怔忡。	口服:每次2~4粒,每日3次,含服或吞服。	每瓶装100粒。
痧　药	蟾酥,雄黄,朱砂,麝香,冰片,大黄,麻黄,丁香,苍术,天麻,甘草。	开窍辟秽,祛暑解毒。	夏令感受暑温秽浊之气,腹痛吐泻,牙关紧闭,四肢逆冷,甚则昏厥。	口服:每次0.75 g,噙少刻咽下。外用:研细末,取适量吹鼻取嚏。亦可以醋化开调涂治疗各种疔毒及虫蝎咬伤。	每33丸重1 g。每袋装3 g,每瓶装1 g。
白金丸	郁金,白矾。	豁痰开窍。	痰涎壅盛,心窍闭阻,癫狂烦躁,或癫痫昏仆。	口服:每次1.5 g,每日2次。	每40粒重3 g。
竹沥达痰丸	大黄,黄芩,陈皮,青礞石(与焰硝同煅),沉香,半夏,竹沥。	泻热降火,逐痰开郁。	实热老痰,蒙蔽心窍,癫狂惊痫,咳喘痰多,胸膈痞闷,大便秘结,舌苔黄腻,脉滑数。	口服:每次6 g,每日2次。	每袋装18 g。

Chart Six　Medicines for Regulating Qi, Promoting Blood Circulation and Relieving Pain

Name of the Recipe	Ingredients	Functions	Indications	Directions & Dosage	Specifications
Qizhi Weitong Chongji	*Radix Bupleuri, Fructus Aurantii, Radix Paeoniae Alba, Radix Glycyrrhizae, Rhizoma Cyperi, Rhizoma Corydalis, etc*	Dispersing stagnated liver-qi to relieve pain	Stagnated liver-qi manifested as fullness and pain in abdomen, hypochondrium and costae,	1 bag each time orally and twice daily	10 g per bag

Name of the Recipe	Ingredients	Functions	Indications	Directions & Dosage	Specifications
			which are aggravated on depression and anger, poor appetite, or irregular menstruation and fullness and pain in abdomen, hypochonrium and breasts before menstruation		
Jiuqi Niantong Wan	*Rhizoma Cyperi, Radix Aucklandiae, Rhizoma Alpiniae Officinarum, Pericarpium Citri Reticulatae, Radix Curcumae, Rhizoma Zedoariae, Rhizoma Corydalis, Semen Arecae, Radix Glycyrrhizae, Faeces Trogopterorum (baked)*	Regulating qi and promoting blood circulation, removing mass and relieving pain	Stomachache, hypochondriac fullness, abdominal mass	6 - 9 g each time orally and twice daily	1 g every 20 pills
Shixiang Zhitong Wan	*Lignum Aquilariae Resinatum, Radix Aucklandiae, Semen Litchi, Fructus Gleditsiae Abnormalis, Flos Syzygii Aromatici, Fructus Foeniculi, Rhizoma cyperi, Pericarpium Citri Reticulatae, Radix Linderae, Rhizoma Alismatis*	Promoting flow of qi and removing stasis, dispelling cold and relieving pain	Abdominal pain due to qi stagnation, distending pai due to various hernia, dysmenorrhea	1 pill each time orally and twice daily	6 g per pill
Fufang Danshen Pian	*Radix Salviae Miltiorrhizae, Radix Notoginseng, Borneolum*	Promoting blood circulation and removing blood stasis, removing obstruction in channels and relieving pain	Obstruction of qi in heart channel, stagnation of qi and blood, chest distress and heat pain, palpitation and short breath	4 tablets each time orally and 3 times daily	60 tablets contained in one bottle
Yuanhu Zhitong Pian	*Rhizoma Corydalis, Radix Angelicae Dahuricae*	Promoting the circulation of qi and blood to relieve pain	Obstruction of qi and blood stasis manifested as headache, stomachache, hypochondriac pain, obstruction of qi in the chest, dysmenorrhea, etc	4 - 6 tablets each time orally and 3 times daily	0.3 g per tablet

（Following table）

Name of the Recipe	Ingredients	Functions	Indications	Directions & Dosage	Specifications
Shixiao San	*Pollen Typhae*, *Faeces Trogopterorum*	Promoting blood circulation and removing blood stasis to relieve pain	Dysmenorrhea due to blood stasis, amenia, obstruction of heart-qi due to blood stasis, abdominal pain	6 g each time orally taken with millet wine and twice daily	6 g per bottle
Fuke Tiaojing Pian	*Rhizoma Cyperi*, *Rhizoma Corydalis*, *Radix Angelicae Sinensis*, *Radix Rehmanniae Praeparatae*, *Rhizoma Ligustici Chuanxiong*, *Radix Paeoniae Rubra*, *Radix Paeoniae Alba*, *Rhizoma Atractylodis Macrocephalae*, *Fructus Ziziphi Jujubae*, *Radix Glycyrrhizae*	Promoting circulation of qi and blood, regulating menstruation and relieving pain	Obstructed flow of liver-qi due to blood deficiency and blood stasis due to qi stagnation manifested as irregular menstruation, dysmenorrhea, pain in the lower abdomen, distending pain in breast and chest distress	4 tablets each time orally and 3 times daily	0.3 g per tablet
Dahuang Zhechong Wan	*Radix et Rhizoma Rhei*, *Eupolyphaga seu Steleophaga*, *Hirudo*, *Semen Perisicae*, *Jicao*, *Tabanus Bivittatus*, *Ganqi*, *Semen Armeniacae Amarum*, *Radix Scutellariae*, *Radix Rehmanniae Recens*, *Radix Paeoniae Alba*, *Radix Glycyrrhizae*	Removing blood stasis and promoting blood regeneration	Internal accumulation of blood stasis, amenia, slimness, squamous and dry skin, or abdominal mass	1 pill each time orally and 3 times daily	3 g per pill
Yimucao Gao	*Fresh Herba Leonuri*, *Radix Angelicaee Sinensis*, *Rhizoma Ligustici Chuanxiong*, *Radix Paeoniae Alba*, *Radix Rehmanniae Praeparatae*, *Flos Carthami*	Promoting blood circulation, removing blood stasis and relieving pain	Blood stasis in uterus, irregular menstruation, scanty menstruation or amenia, soreness of the waist and abdominal pain, or blood stasis and abdominal pain after delivery	15 g each time orally and twice daily	60 g per big bottle and 30 g per small bottle
Qili San	*Resina Draconis*, *Moschus*, *Borneolum*, *Resina Olibani*, *Resina Commiphorae Myrrhae*, *Flos Carthami*, *Cinnabaris*, *Catechu*	Promoting blood circulation and removing blood stasis, relieving pain and arresting bleeding	Blood stasis, swelling and pain due to trauma or broken tendons or fracture; or bleeding from wounds. Also indicated in unknown swelling, sores, burns or scalds	0.2 - 0.9 g each time orally taken with millet wine or warm boiled water. Or applied externally on the affected parts after mixed with spirit	3 g per bottle

Name of the Recipe	Ingredients	Functions	Indications	Directions & Dosage	Specifications
Baiyao	Omitted	Relieving pain and arresting bleeding, removing blood stasis and promoting blood regeneration	Trauma and wounds, long-standing blood stasis, and internal injury due to overstrain manifested as hemoptysis, hematemesis, swelling and pain of joints, numbness due to wind-dampness, abdominal pain due to indigestion, abdominal pain after delivery	For oral use: 0.2 – 0.3 g or no more than 0.5 g each time for adults and each time every 4 hours. 0.03 g each time for children over 2 years old and 0.06 g each time for children over 5 years. For severe trauma, the patient need first to take orally one pill of Baoxianzi (granule for emergency) with wine (only one pill daily). Sour and cold food, broad bean, fish and shrimps should be avoided after taking this medicine. Pregnant women should not take this medicine. For bleeding wounds, it can be applied externally; for swelling and pain of tendons and joints as well as blood stasis due to trauma, applied externally after mixed with liquor	4 g per bottle with one pill of Baoxianzi pill for emergency inside

(六) 理气活血止痛类

方　名	组　　成	功　用	主　治	用法与用量	规　格
气滞胃痛冲剂	柴胡,枳壳,白芍药,甘草,香附,延胡索等。	疏肝止痛。	肝郁气滞,脘腹胁肋胀满疼痛,郁怒则加重,纳差,妇女月经不调,经前腹胁乳房胀痛。	口服:每次1袋,每日2次。	每袋重10 g。

方　名	组　　成	功　用	主　治	用法与用量	规　格
九气拈痛丸	香附,木香,高良姜,陈皮,郁金,莪术,延胡索,槟榔,甘草,炒五灵脂。	理气活血,消癥止痛。	胃脘疼痛,两胁胀满,癥瘕积聚。	口服:每次6~9g,每日2次。	每20粒重1g。
十香止痛丸	沉香,木香,荔枝核,猪牙皂,丁香,小茴香,香附,陈皮,乌药,泽泻。	行气散结,祛寒止痛。	气滞腹痛,诸疝胀痛,妇女痛经。	口服:每次1丸,每日2次。	每丸重6g。
复方丹参片	丹参,参三七,冰片。	活血化瘀,通脉止痛。	心脉瘀阻,气血凝滞,胸闷心痛,心悸气短。	口服:每次4片,每日3次。	每瓶装60片。
元胡止痛片	延胡索,白芷。	行气活血止痛。	气滞血瘀,头痛,胃脘痛,胁痛,胸痹,痛经等。	口服:每次4~6片,每日3次。	每片重0.3g。
失笑散	蒲黄,五灵脂。	活血化瘀止痛。	瘀滞痛经、闭经,血瘀心痹、脘腹疼痛。	口服:每次6g,以黄酒调下,每日2次。	每瓶装6g。
妇科调经片	香附,延胡索,当归,熟地黄,川芎,赤芍药,白芍药,白术,红枣,甘草。	行气活血,调经止痛。	血虚肝郁,气滞血瘀,月经不调,经行不畅,少腹疼痛,乳胀胸闷。	口服:每次4片,每日3次。	每片重0.3g。
大黄䗪虫丸	大黄,土鳖虫,水蛭,桃仁,蛴螬,虻虫,干漆,杏仁,黄芩,生地黄,白芍药,甘草。	祛瘀生新。	干血内结,经闭不行,身体羸瘦,肌肤甲错,或腹中癥积痞块。	口服:每次1丸,每日3次。	每丸重3g。
益母草膏	鲜益母草,当归,川芎,白芍药,熟地黄,红花。	活血调经,散瘀止痛。	瘀阻胞宫,月经不调,量少或经闭,腰酸腹痛,产后瘀血腹痛。	口服:每次15g,每日2次。	每大瓶60g,每小瓶30g。
七厘散	血竭,麝香,冰片,乳香,没药,红花,朱砂,儿茶。	活血祛瘀,定痛止血。	跌打损伤,筋断骨折之瘀血肿痛,或刀伤出血。亦治无名肿毒、烧伤烫伤等。	口服每次0.2~0.9g,以黄酒或温开水送服。外用以烧酒调药适量敷伤处。	每瓶装3g。
白　药	略。	止痛止血,祛瘀生新。	跌打刀伤,陈年瘀患,劳积内伤,咳血吐血,筋骨肿痛,风湿麻木,心胃积痛,产后腹痛。	口服:成人每次服0.2~0.3g,最多不超过0.5g,每4小时服1次。小儿2岁以上每次服	每瓶4g,内装保险子1粒。

方 名	组　成	功　用	主　治	用法与用量	规 格
				0.03 g,5 岁以上每次服 0.06 g。跌损较重者先用酒送服保险子 1 粒(每日只能用 1 粒)。服药后忌食酸冷食物、蚕豆、鱼虾。孕妇忌服。刀伤见血者,兼用外敷;跌打损伤筋骨肿痛瘀积者,用白酒调和外搽。	

Chart Seven Medicines for Dispelling Wind，Relaxing Muscles and Tendons，and Removing Obstruction in Channels

Name of the Recipe	Ingredients	Functions	Indications	Directions & Dosage	Specifications
Xitong Wan	*Herba Siegesbeckiae*, *Folium Clerodendri*	Dispelling wind and removing obstruction in meridians subduing liver-wind and relieving dizziness	Arthralgia-syndrome due to wind-dampness manifested as numbness and pain of the limbs, limited movement; or up-stirring of the liver-wind manifested as vertigo and dizziness, numbness of the extremities, soreness and weakness of the waist and knees	10 pills each time orally and twice daily	120 pills per bottle
Tianma Wan	*Rhizoma Gastrodiae*, *Rhizoma seu Radix Notopterygii*, *Radix Angelicae Pubescentis*, *Rhizoma Dioscoreae Hypoglaucae*, *Cortex Eucommiae*, *Radix Achyranthis Bidentatae*, *Radix Aconiti Praeparata*, *Radix Rehmanniae*, *Radix Scrophulariae*, *Radix Angelicae Sinensis*	Expelling wind and eliminating dampness, relaxing the muscles and tendons, removing obstruction in meridians, activating blood circulation and relieving pain	Arthralgia due to wind-dampness manifested as spasm of the limbs, numbness of the extremities, soreness of the waist and knees	6 g each time orally for hydro-honeyed bolus and 1 pill for large honyed bolus; twice or 3 times daily	9 g per large honyed bolus

(Following table)

Name of the Recipe	Ingredients	Functions	Indications	Directions & Dosage	Specifications
Mugua Wan	*Fructus Chaenomelis, Radix Angelicae Sinensis, Rhizoma Ligustici Chuanxiong, Radix Angelicae Dahuricae, Radix Clematidis, Rhizoma Cibotii, Radix Achyranthis Bidentatae, Caulis Spatholobi, Caulis Piperis Futokadsurae, Radix Ginseng, Radix Aconiti, Radix Aconiti Kusnezoffii*	Expelling wind-cold, removing obstruction in channels and relieving pain	Arthralgia-syndrome due to wind-cold-dampness manifested as numbness of the limbs, general pain, weakness of the waist and knees, difficulty in walking	50 pills each time orally and twice daily	1.8 g per 10 pills
Shujin Huoluo Wan	*Cortex Acanthopanacis Radicis, Arisaema cum Bile, Rhizoma Ligustici Chuanxiong, Herba Siegesbeckiae, Ramulus Cinnamomi, Cortex Lycii Radicis, Radix Angelicae Pubescentis, Radix Achyranthis Bidentatae, Radix Angelicae Siensis, Fructus Chaenomelis, Radix Clematidis, Rhizoma seu Radix Notopterygii*	Dispelling wind and eliminating dampness, relaxing the muscles and tendons, and removing obstruction in channels	Arthralgia-syndrome due to wind-dampness manifested as painful joints, spasm of the muscles and tendons, numbness of the extremities, soreness and weakness of the waist and knees	1 pill each time orally and twice daily	6 g per pill
Wangbi Chongji	*Radix Rehmanniae Recens, Radix Rehmanniae Praeparata, Radix Aconiti Praeparata, Rhizoma Drynariae, Herba Epimedii, Radix Angelicae Pubescentis, Ramulus Cinnamomi, Radix Ledebouriellae, Scolopendra, Rhizoma Anemarrhenae, Spina Gleditsiae, sheep tibia, Radix Paeoniae Alba, Flos Carthami, Radix Clematidis, Herba Lycopodii, Fructus Psoraleae,* etc.	Reinforcing the liver and kidney, strengthening the tendons and bones, removing obstruction in channels to relieve pain	Retaining of pathogenic factors in the tendons and bone due to weakness of the liver and kidney manifested as swelling, pain, distortion and limited movement of the joints, even ankylosis, soreness and weakness of the waist and knees, aversion to cold and preference for warmth	1 bag each time orally and twice or 3 times daily; double the dosage in severe case	10 g per bag

Name of the Recipe	Ingredients	Functions	Indications	Directions & Dosage	Specifications
Renshen Zaizao Wan	*Agkistrodon Acutus*, *Herba Agastachis*, *Flos Caryophylli*, *Herba Asari*, *Radix Scrophulariae*, *Rhizoma Cyperi*, *Lumbricus*, *Radix Rehmanniae Praeparata*, *Lignum Santali*, *Radix Notoginseng*, *Olibanum*, *Pericarpium Citri Reticulatae Viride*, *Semen Myristicae*, *Radix Ledebouriellae*, *Radix Polygoni Multiflori*, *Rhizoma Ligustici Chuanxiong*, *Pianjianghuang*, *Radix Scutellariae*, *Radix Glycyrrhizae*, *Ramulus Loranthi*, *Poria*, *Radix Paeoniae Rubra*, *Rhizoma Coptidis*, *Radix et Rhizoma Rhei*, *Radix Puerariae*, *Herba Ephedrae*, *Scorpio*, *Radix Aconiti Praeparata*, *Fructus Piperis Longi*, *Plastrum Testudinis*, *Lignum Aquilariae Resinatum*, *Rhizoma Zingiberis Recens*, *Bombyx Batryticatus*, *Succinum*, *Rhizoma Atractylodis Macrocephalae*, *Rhizoma Gastrodiae*, *Cortex Cinnamomi*, *Radix Angelicae Sinensis*, *Radix Angelicae Dahuricae*, *Semen Alpiniae Katsumadai*, *Resina Commiphorae Myrrhae*, *Radix Clematidis*, *Radix Linderae*, *Rhizoma seu Radix Notopterygii*, *Radix Ginseng Rubra*, *Massa Fermentata Medicinalis*, *Exocarpium Citri Grandis*, *Resina Draconis*, *Concretio Silicea Bambusae*, *Cinnabaris*, *Calculus Bovis*, *Borneolum*, *Moschus*, *Cornu Bubali*	Replenishing qi and enriching blood, dispelling wind and removing phlegm, promoting blood circulation and removing obstruction in the channels	Insufficient qi and blood in the liver and kidney, obstructed flow of qi in channels due to phlegm manifested as hemiparalysis, distortion of the mouth and eyes, spasm and numbness of the limbs, painful joints. It can prevent stroke in the middle or old aged people who are in the state of deficiency of qi and blood in the liver and kidney in combination with excess of phlegm and dampness	1 pill each time orally and twice daily	7.5 g per pill

Name of the Recipe	Ingredients	Functions	Indications	Directions & Dosage	Specif- ications
Huatuo Zaizao Wan	*Radix Angelicae Sinensis, Rhizoma Ligustici Chuanxiong, Radix Paeoniae Alba, Flos Carthami, Radix Ginseng Rubra, Fructus Schisandrae, Semen Strychni, Rhizoma Arisaematis, Borneolum, etc*	Activating blood circulation to remove blood stasis, removing phlegm and promoting the flow of qi to relieve pain	Stroke and hemiparalysis manifested as distortion of the mouth and eyes, numbness and spasm of the extremities; obstruction of qi in the chest manifested as chest pain and palpitation; arthralgia-syndrome due to wind-cold-dampness manifested as painful joints, numbness and limited movement of the limbs	8 g each time orally and twice or 3 times daily	8 g or 80 g per bottle
Shenrong Mugua Yaojiu	*Herba Ephedrae, Ramulus Loranthi, Radix Ginseng, Rhizoma Cibotii, Radix Angelicae Pubescentis, Radix Aconiti Praeparata, Rhizoma seu Radix Notopterygii, Semen Persicae, Radix Glycyrrhizae, Radix Gentianae Macrophyllae, Cornu Cervi Pantotrichum, Radix Angelicae Sinensis, Radix Dipsaci, Fructus Chaenomelis, Rhizoma Atractylodis, Cortex Acanthopanacis Radicis, Radix Aconiti Kusnezoffii Praeparata, Radix Clematidis, Zaocys, Caulis Sinomenii, Radix Paeoniae Rubra, Radix Ledebouriellae, Herba Erodii seu Geranii, Lumbricus, Ramulus Cinnamomi, Radix Achyranthis Bidentatae, Flos Carthami, Caulis Piperis Futokadsurae, Rhizoma Ligustici Chuanxiong, Radix Angelicae Dahuricae, Herba Asari, white sugar, liquor*	Dispelling wind-cold, relaxing muscles and tendons to promote blood circulation, removing obstruction in the collaterals to relieve pain	Numbness or pain of the limbs, joints, waist and back, limited movement of the joints, aversion to cold and preference for warmth	10 – 15 ml each time orally and 3 times daily	450 ml per bottle

(Following table)

Name of the Recipe	Ingredients	Functions	Indications	Directions & Dosage	Specifications
Qishe Yaojiu	*Agkistrodon, Rhizoma seu Radix Notopterygii, Flos Carthami, Radix Ledebouriellae, rhizoma Gastrodiae, Radix Gentianae Macrophyllae, Cortex acanthopanacis Radicis, Radix Anelicae Sinensis, white sugar*	Dispelling wind-cold, eliminating dampness and removing obstruction in the collaterals	Arthralgia-syndrome due to wind-cold-dampness manifested as painful joints and limited movements	30 ml each time orally and twice daily	500 ml per bottle
Shiguogong Yaojiu	*Radix Glycyrrhizae, Rhizoma seu Radix Notopterygii, Rhizoma Ligustici Chuanxiong, Radix Angelicae Sinensis, Radix Angelicae Pubescentis, Radix Dipsaci, Excrementa Bombycum, Fructus Chaenomelis, Radix Achyranthis Bidentatae, Radix Ledebouriellae, Rhizoma Polygonati Odorati, Ramulus Loranthi, Rhizoma Atractylodis Macrocephalae, Flos Carthami, Colla Cornus Cervi, Colla Carapax Trionycis, Massa Dermentata Medicinalis, liquor*	Dispelling wind and eliminating dampness, nourishing blood and removing obstruction in the collaterals	Arthralgia-syndrome due to wind, cold and dampness manifested as numbness of limbs and painful joints	15 –20 ml each time warmly and orally and twice or 3 times daily	250 ml or 500 ml per bottle
Fengliaoxing Yaojiu	*Caulis Erycibes, Radix Angelicae Dahuricae, Cortex Acanthopanacis Radicis, Herba Ephedrae, Herba Artemisiae Annuae, Radix Angelicae Sinensis, Rhizoma Ligustici Chuanxiong, Fructus Foeniculi, Ramulus Cinnamomi, Radix Clematidis, Radix Stephaniae Tetrandrae, Fructus Gardeniae, Rhizoma seu Radix Notopterygii, Radix Angelicae Pubescentis, liquor*	Dispelling wind and removing obstruction in meridians, expelling cold and relieving pain	Arthralgia-syndrome due to wind, cold and dampness manifested as numbness of limbs, sore and painful tendons and bones, weakness of the waist and knees, relapse of old trauma	10 –15 ml each time orally and twice daily	250 ml or 500 ml per bottle

（七）祛风舒筋活络类

方　名	组　成	功　用	主　治	用法与用量	规　格
豨桐丸	豨莶草，臭梧桐叶。	祛风通络，平肝定眩。	风湿痹证，肢体麻木疼痛，活动不利，或肝风上扰，头晕目眩，手足麻木，腰膝酸软。	口服：每次10粒，每日2次。	每瓶装120丸。
天麻丸	天麻，羌活，独活，萆薢，杜仲，牛膝，附子，地黄，玄参，当归。	祛风除湿，舒筋通络，活血止痛。	风湿痹痛，肢体拘挛，手足麻木，腰膝酸痛。	口服：水蜜丸每次6g，大蜜丸每次1丸，每日2～3次。	大蜜丸每丸重9g。
木瓜丸	木瓜，当归，川芎，白芷，威灵仙，狗脊，牛膝，鸡血藤，海风藤，人参，川乌，草乌。	散风祛寒，活络止痛。	风寒湿痹，四肢麻木，遍身疼痛，腰膝无力，行步艰难。	口服：每次50粒，每日2次。	每10粒重1.8g。
舒筋活络丸	五加皮，胆星，川芎，豨莶草，桂枝，地骨皮，独活，牛膝，当归，木瓜，威灵仙，羌活。	祛风除湿，舒筋活络。	风湿痹证，关节疼痛，筋脉拘急，手足麻木，腰膝酸软无力。	口服：每次1丸，每日2次。	每丸重6g。
尪痹冲剂	生地黄，熟地黄，附子，骨碎补，淫羊藿，独活，桂枝，防风，蜈蚣，知母，皂角刺，羊胫骨，白芍药，红花，威灵仙，伸筋草，补骨脂等。	补益肝肾，强筋壮骨，通络止痛。	肝肾不足，邪气痹阻筋骨，关节肿大疼痛变形，屈伸不利，甚则关节强直，腰膝酸软，畏寒喜温。	口服：每次1袋，重者加倍，每日2～3次。	每袋装10g。
人参再造丸	白花蛇，藿香，母丁香，细辛，玄参，香附，地龙，熟地黄，檀香，参三七，乳香，青皮，肉豆蔻，防风，何首乌，川芎，片姜黄，黄芪，甘草，桑寄生，茯苓，赤芍药，黄连，大黄，葛根，麻黄，全蝎，附子，荜茇，龟版，沉香，生姜，僵蚕，琥珀，白术，天麻，肉桂，当归，白芷，草豆蔻，没药，威灵仙，乌药，羌活，红参，神曲，橘红，血竭，天竺黄，朱砂，牛黄，冰片，麝香，水牛角。	益气养血，祛风化痰，活血通络。	肝肾气血不足，痰瘀痹阻经脉，半身不遂，口眼歪斜，四肢拘急麻木，关节疼痛。中老年肝肾气血不足，痰湿较重者服之可预防中风。	口服：每次1丸，每日2次。	每丸重7.5g。

续表

方　名	组　　成	功　用	主　治	用法与用量	规　格
华佗再造丸	当归,川芎,白芍药,红花,红参,五味子,马钱子,天南星,冰片等。	活血化瘀,祛痰通络,行气止痛。	中风半身不遂,口眼歪斜,手足麻木,拘挛不利;胸痹,胸痛心悸;风寒湿痹关节疼痛,肢体麻木,屈伸不利。	口服:每次 8 g,每日 2～3 次。	每瓶 8 g 或 80 g。
参茸木瓜药酒	麻黄,桑寄生,人参,狗脊,独活,制川乌,羌活,桃仁,甘草,秦艽,鹿茸,当归,续断,木瓜,苍术,五加皮,制草乌,威灵仙,乌梢蛇,青风藤,赤芍药,防风,老鹳草,地龙,桂枝,牛膝,红花,海风藤,川芎,白芷,细辛,白糖,白酒。	祛风散寒,舒筋活血,通络止痛。	肢体、关节、腰脊麻木或疼痛,关节屈伸不利,畏寒喜温。	口服:每次 10～15 ml,每日 3 次。	每瓶 450 ml。
蕲蛇药酒	蕲蛇,羌活,红花,防风,天麻,秦艽,五加皮,当归,白糖,白酒。	祛风散寒,除湿通络。	风寒湿痹,关节疼痛,活动不便。	口服:每次 30 ml,每日 2 次。	每瓶 500 ml。
史国公药酒	甘草,羌活,川芎,当归,独活,续断,蚕沙,木瓜,牛膝,防风,玉竹,桑寄生,白术,红花,鹿角胶,鳖甲胶,神曲,白酒。	祛风除湿,养血活络。	风寒湿痹,四肢麻木,骨节疼痛。	口服:每次温服 15～20 ml,每日 2～3 次。	每瓶 250 ml 或 500 ml。
冯了性药酒	丁公藤,白芷,五加皮,麻黄,青蒿子,当归,川芎,小茴香,桂枝,威灵仙,防己,栀子,羌活,独活,白酒。	祛风通络,散寒止痛。	风寒湿痹,四肢麻木,筋骨酸痛,腰膝乏力,老伤复发。	口服:每次 10～15 ml,每日 2 次。	每瓶 250 ml 或 500 ml。

Chart Eight　Medicines for Promoting Digestion，Regulating Stomach and Reinforcing Spleen

Name of the Recipe	Ingredients	Functions	Indications	Directions & Dosage	Specifications
Da Shanzha Wan	*Fructus Crataegi, Massa Fermentata Medicinalis, Fructus Hordei Germinatus*	Whetting appetite and promoting digestion	Poor appetite, indigestion, abdominal fullness	1 - 2 pill each time orally and once or twice or 3 times daily	9 g per pill

(**Following table**)

Name of the Recipe	Ingredients	Functions	Indications	Directions & Dosage	Specifications
Xiangsha Yangwei Wan	*Radix Platycodi, Rhizoma Pinelliae, Poria, Fructus Gardeniae, Fructus Aurantii Immaturus, Cortex Magnoliae Officinalis, Rhizoma Atractylodis, Fructus Crataegi, Fructus Amomi, Radix Aucklandiae, Rhizoma Cyperi, Pericarpium Citri Reticulatae, Rhizoma Ligustici Chuanxiong, Fructus Hordei Germinatus, Rhizoma Atractylodis Macrocephalae, Massa Fermentata Medicinalis, Herba Agastachis, Radix Glycyrrhizae*	Reinforcing the spleen and promoting digestion, regulating the stomach and relieving vomiting	Weakness of the spleen and stomach manifested as abdominal fullness, no appetite, vomiting of sour saliva, adverse flow of qi and discomfort	1 bag each time orally and twice daily	10 g per bag
Kaixiong Shunqi Wan	*Fructus Crataegi, Massa Fermentata Medicinalis, Fructus Hordei Germinatus, Semen Arecae, Fructus Aurantii Imaturus, Radix Aucklandiae, Radix Linderae, Semen Raphani, Cortex Magnoliae Officinalis, Radix et Rhizoma Rhei, Pericarpium Citri Reticulatae Viride, Radix Glycyrrhizae*	Promoting digestion, regulating the flow of qi and relieving fullness	Stagnated food and obstructed flow of qi manifested as abdominal fullness or pain, nausea and vomiting, belching and no appetite, loose stool or constipation	6 g each time orally and twice or 3 times daily	3 g per 50 pills
Qipi Wan	*Radix Ginseng, Rhizoma Atractylodis Macrocephalae, Poria, Radix Glycyrrhizae, Pericarpium Citri Reticulatae, Rhizoma Dioscoreae, Semen Nelumbinis, Fructus Crataegi, Massa Dermentata Medicinalis, Fructus Hordei Germinatus, Rhizoma Alismatis*	Reinforcing the spleen and stomach, promoting digestion and reliving diarrhea	Indigestion due to weakness of the spleen manifested as chest distress and distending pain, no appetite, nausea and vomiting, belching and regurgitation, loose stool with sour and foul smell or diarrhea with borborygmus, sallow complexion, lassitude	1 pill each time orally and twice or 3 times daily	3 g per pill

Name of the Recipe	Ingredients	Functions	Indications	Directions & Dosage	Specifications
Xiangsha Zhizhu Wan	*Rhizoma Atractylodis Macrocephalae, Fructus Aurantii Immaturus, Radix Aucklandiae, Fructus Amomi, Folium Nelumbinis*	Reinforcing the spleen and promoting digestion, regulating the flow of qi and relieving fullness	Indigestion due to weakness of the spleen and obstructed flow of qi manifested as abdominal fullness or pain, poor appetite and indigestion, loose stool or diarrhea	6 – 9 g each time orally and twice or 3 times daily	3 g per 50 pills
Zisheng Wan	*Radix Codonopsis Pilosulae, Rhizoma Dioscoreae, Semen Nelumbinis, Semen Coicis, Rhizoma Atractylodis Macrocephalae, Semen Euryales, Poria, Semen Dolichoris, Herba Agastachis, Fructus Amomi Rotundus, Massa Fermentata Medicinalis, Fructus Hordei Germinatus, Fructus Crataegi, Rhizoma Coptidis, Radix Platycodi*	Reinforcing the spleen and promoting digestion, inducing diuresis and arresting diarrhea	Stagnated food complicated with dampness-heat due to weakness of the spleen manifested as chest and abdominal fullness, no appetite, nausea and vomiting, dry mouth with sticky sensation, loose stool, mental fatigue and lassitude, greasy yellow fur.	3 g each time orally and 3 times daily	1 g per 20 pills
Kaiwei Jianpi Wan	*Rhizoma Atractylodis Macrocephalae, Fructus Crataegi, Massa Fermentata Medicinalis, Pericarpium Citri Reticulatae, Semen Coicis, Fructus Hordei Germinatus, Poria, Radix Codonopsis Pilosulae, Rhizoma Dioscoreae, Cortex Magnoliae Officinalis, Radix Aucklandiae, Radix Paeoniae Alba, Fructus Amomi, Semen Nelumbinis, Polyporus Umbellatus, Radix Glycyrrhizae*	Reinforcing the spleen, promoting digestion and whetting appetite	Indigestion due to weakness of the spleen and stomach manifested as no appetite, nausea, vomiting, lassitude, loose stool or diarrhea	6 g each time orally and twice daily	18 g per pack
Shanzha Huazhi Wan	*Fructus Crataegi, Semen Raphani, Semen Pharbitidis, Fructus Hordei Germinatus, Massa Fermentata Medicinalis*	Promoting digestion and removing stagnancy	Stagnated food in the stomach due to intemperance in diet	1 pill each time orally and twice or 3 times daily	9 g per pill

(Following table)

Name of the Recipe	Ingredients	Functions	Indications	Directions & Dosage	Specifications
Baochi San	*Massa Fermentata Medicinalis*, *Pulvis Crotonis Tiglium*, *Rhizoma Arisaematis*, *Cinnabaris*	Promoting digestion, removing phlegm and relieving convulsion	Indigestion due to cold in babies manifested as no appetite for milk or food, abdominal fullness, constipation, excessive phlegm, palpitation due to fright, restlessness	0.09 g each time orally for babies aging 6 months to 12 months; and 0.18 g each time orally for children aging 2 to 4 years	0.09 g per bottle
Feier Chongji	*Rhizoma Atractylodis Macrocephalae*, *Poria*, *Rhizoma Dioscoreae*, *Semen Coicis*, *Semen Dolichoris Album*, *Semen Euryales*, *Semen Nelumbinis*, *Fructus Hordei Germinatus*, *Fructus Crataegi*, *Radix Glehniae*	Reinforcing the spleen and promoting digestion, eliminating dampness and relieving diarrhea	Weakness of the spleen and stomach in children manifested as indigestion, abdominal fullness, poor appetite, diarrhea, sallow complexion, emaciated figure	3 - 6 g each time orally and 3 times daily	12 g per packet
Xiaoshi Jian'er Chongji	*Fructus Oryzae Germinatus*, *Fructus Hordei Germinatus*, *Rhizoma Atractylodis Macrocephalae*, *Rhizoam Dioscoreae*, *Radix Adenophorae*, *Aspongopus*, *cane sugar*	Reinforcing the spleen and regulating the stomach, promoting digestion and relieving diarrhea	Weakness of the spleen and stomach in children manifested as diarrhea, poor appetite, slim figure, profuse perspiration and mental fatigue	5 g each time orally for children under 3 years; and 10 g for those over 3 years; 3 times daily and taken after infused in hot boiled water	0.5 g available composition contained in every 1 g of the granule

(八) 消食和胃健脾类

方　名	组　成	功　用	主　治	用法与用量	规　格
大山楂丸	山楂,神曲,麦芽。	开胃消食。	食欲不振,消化不良,脘腹胀满。	口服:每次1~2丸,每日1~3次。	每丸重9g。
香砂养胃丸	桔梗,半夏,茯苓,栀子,枳实,厚朴,苍术,山楂,砂仁,木香,香附,陈皮,川芎,麦芽,白术,神曲,藿香,甘草。	健脾消食,和胃止呕。	脾胃虚弱,胃脘满闷,不思饮食,呕吐酸水,气逆不舒。	口服:每次1袋,每日2次。	每袋重10g。
开胸顺气丸	山楂,神曲,麦芽,槟榔,枳实,木香,乌药,莱菔子,厚朴,大黄,青皮,甘草。	消食导滞,理气除满。	食积气滞,脘腹胀满或疼痛,恶心呕吐,嗳气厌食,大便或溏泄或干结。	口服:每次6g,每日2~3次。	每50粒重3g。

方　名	组　成	功　用	主　治	用法与用量	规　格
启脾丸	人参,白术,茯苓,甘草,橘皮,山药,莲子,山楂,神曲,麦芽,泽泻。	健脾和胃,消食止泻。	脾虚食积,胸脘痞闷胀痛,不思饮食,恶心呕吐,嗳腐吞酸,便溏酸臭或泄泻肠鸣,面色萎黄,倦怠乏力。	口服:每次1丸,每日2～3次。	每丸重3 g。
香砂枳术丸	白术,枳实,木香,砂仁,荷叶。	健脾消食,理气除满。	脾虚食积,气机失畅,脘腹痞满或疼痛,食少不化,便溏或泄泻。	口服:每次6～9 g,每日2～3次。	每50粒重3 g。
资生丸	党参,山药,莲子,薏苡仁,白术,芡实,茯苓,扁豆,藿香,白蔻仁,神曲,麦芽,山楂,黄连,桔梗。	健脾消食,化湿止泻。	脾虚食积,兼夹湿热,胸脘胀满,不思饮食,恶心呕吐,口干而粘,大便溏泄,神疲乏力,舌苔黄腻。	口服:每次3 g,每日3次。	每20丸重1 g。
开胃健脾丸	白术,山楂,神曲,橘皮,薏苡仁,麦芽,茯苓,党参,山药,厚朴,木香,白芍药,砂仁,莲子,猪苓,甘草。	健脾开胃,增进饮食。	脾胃虚弱,饮食不化,不思饮食,恶心呕吐,倦怠乏力,便溏或泄泻。	口服:每次6 g,每日2次。	每袋重18 g。
山楂化滞丸	焦山楂,莱菔子,牵牛子,麦芽,神曲。	消食化滞。	饮食不节,食滞胃脘。	口服:每次1丸,每日2～3次。	每丸重9 g。
保赤散	神曲,巴豆霜,天南星,朱砂。	消食导滞,化痰定惊。	小儿冷积,停乳停食,腹部胀满,大便秘结,痰多,惊悸不安。	口服:小儿6个月～1岁,每次0.09 g;2～4岁,每次0.18 g。	每瓶重0.09 g。
肥儿冲剂	白术,茯苓,山药,薏苡仁,白扁豆,芡实,莲子,麦芽,山楂,北沙参。	健脾消食,化湿止泻。	小儿脾胃虚弱,食积不化,脘腹痞满,食少泄泻,面色萎黄,形体消瘦。	口服:每次3～6 g,每日3次。	每包重12 g。
消食健儿冲剂	谷芽,麦芽,白术,山药,南沙参,九香虫,蔗糖。	健脾和胃,消食止泻。	小儿脾胃虚弱,泄泻食少,形体消瘦,汗多神疲。	口服:3岁以下,每次5 g,3岁以上,每次10 g,每日3次,热开水冲服。	每克含药量0.5 g。

II. Index of the Prescriptions

二、方名索引

Postscript

The Compilation of *A Newly Compiled Practical English-Chinese Library of TCM* was started in 2000 and published in 2002. In order to demonstrate the academic theory and clinical practice of TCM and to meet the requirements of compilation, the compilers and translators have made great efforts to revise and polish the Chinese manuscript and English translation so as to make it systematic, accurate, scientific, standard and easy to understand. Shanghai University of TCM is in charge of the translation. Many scholars and universities have participated in the compilation and translation of the Library, i.e. Professor Shao Xundao from Xi'an Medical University (former Dean of English Department and Training Center of the Health Ministry), Professor Ou Ming from Guangzhou University of TCM (celebrated translator and chief professor), Henan College of TCM, Guangzhou University of TCM, Nanjing University of TCM, Shaanxi College of TCM, Liaoning College of TCM and Shandong University of TCM.

The compilation of this Library is also supported by the State Administrative Bureau and experts from other universities and colleges of TCM. The experts on the Compilation Committee and Approval Committee have directed the compilation and translation. Professor She

后　记

《(英汉对照)新编实用中医文库》(以下简称《文库》)从2000 年中文稿的动笔,到2002 年全书的付梓,完成了世纪的跨越。为了使本套《文库》尽可能展示传统中医学术理论和临床实践的精华,达到全面、系统、准确、科学、规范、通俗的编写要求,全体编译人员耗费了大量的心血,付出了艰辛的劳动。特别是上海中医药大学承担了英语翻译的主持工作,得到了著名医学英语翻译家、原西安医科大学英语系主任和卫生部外语培训中心主任邵循道教授,著名中医英语翻译家、广州中医药大学欧明首席教授的热心指导,河南中医学院、广州中医药大学、南京中医药大学、陕西中医学院、辽宁中医学院、山东中医药大学等中医院校英语专家的全力参与,确保了本套《文库》具有较高的英译水平。

在《文库》的编撰过程中,我们始终得到国家主管部门领导和各中医院校专家们的关心和帮助。编纂委员会的国内外学者及审定委员会的

Jing, Head of the State Administrative Bureau and Vice-Minister of the Health Ministry, has showed much concern for the Library. Professor Zhu Bangxian, head of the Publishing House of Shanghai University of TCM, Zhou Dunhua, former head of the Publishing House of Shanghai University of TCM, and Pan Zhaoxi, former editor-in-chief of the Publishing House of Shanghai University of TCM, have given full support to the compilation and translation of the Library.

With the coming of the new century, we have presented this Library to the readers all over the world, sincerely hoping to receive suggestions and criticism from the readers so as to make it perfect in the following revision.

Zuo Yanfu

Pingju Village, Nanjing

Spring 2002

专家对编写工作提出了指导性的意见和建议。尤其是卫生部副部长、国家中医药管理局局长佘靖教授对本书的编写给予了极大的关注,多次垂询编撰过程,并及时进行指导。上海中医药大学出版社社长兼总编辑朱邦贤教授,以及原社长周敦华先生、原总编辑潘朝曦先生及全体编辑对本书的编辑出版工作给予了全面的支持,使《文库》得以顺利面世。在此,一并致以诚挚的谢意。

在新世纪之初,我们将这套《文库》奉献给国内外中医界及广大中医爱好者,恳切希望有识之士对《文库》存在的不足之处给予批评、指教,以便在修订时更臻完善。

左言富

于金陵萍聚村

2002 年初春

A Newly Compiled Practical English-Chinese Library of Traditional Chinese Medicine

（英汉对照）新编实用中医文库

Basic Theory of Traditional Chinese Medicine	中医基础理论
Diagnostics of Traditional Chinese Medicine	中医诊断学
Science of Chinese Materia Medica	中药学
Science of Prescriptions	方剂学
Internal Medicine of Traditional Chinese Medicine	中医内科学
Surgery of Traditional Chinese Medicine	中医外科学
Gynecology of Traditional Chinese Medicine	中医妇科学
Pediatrics of Traditional Chinese Medicine	中医儿科学
Traumatology and Orthopedics of Traditional Chinese Medicine	中医骨伤科学
Ophthalmology of Traditional Chinese Medicine	中医眼科学
Otorhinolaryngology of Traditional Chinese Medicine	中医耳鼻喉科学
Chinese Acupuncture and Moxibustion	中国针灸
Chinese Tuina (Massage)	中国推拿
Life Cultivation and Rehabilitation of Traditional Chinese Medicine	中医养生康复学